Milestones in Drug Therapy
MDT

Proton Pump Inhibitors

Edited by L. Olbe

Birkhäuser Verlag
Basel · Boston · Berlin

Editor

Dr. Lars Olbe
Centre for Gastroenterological Research
University of Göteborg
S-41345 Göteborg
Sweden

Library of Congress Cataloging-in-Publication Data
A CIP catalogue record for this book is available from the library of Congress, Washington D.C., USA

Deutsche Bibliothek Cataloging-in-Publication Data
Proton pump inhibitors / ed. by L. Olbe. - Basel ; Boston ; Berlin :
Birkhäuser, 1999
(Milestones in drug therapy)
ISBN 3-7643-5897-1 (Basel ...)
ISBN 0-8176-5897-1 (Boston)

Printed on acid-free paper produced from chlorine-free pulp. TCF ∞
Printed in Germany
ISBN 3-7643-5897-1
ISBN 0-8176-5897-1

9 8 7 6 5 4 3 2 1

Contents

Preface VII

List of contributors. IX

The discovery and development of the proton pump inhibitor

S. E. Sjöstrand, L. Olbe and E. Fellenius
The discovery and development of the proton pump inhibitor 3

Mechanism of action

G. Sachs and B. Wallmark
The gastric H,K ATPase 23

B. Wallmark and G. Sachs
Inhibition of the gastric proton pump 47

The pharmacology of proton pump inhibitors

J.-Q. Huang and R. H. Hunt
Inhibition of gastric acid secretion 63

E. Carlsson and N. Havu
Consequences of gastric acid inihibition in animals 79

W. Creutzfeldt
Consequences of gastric acid inhibition in man 91

G. Sachs, D. Scott, D. Wecks and K. Melchers
The acid tolerance of *Helicobacter pylori* 117

A. L. Blum and J. Martínek
Interactions of proton pump inhibitors and *Helicobacter pylori in vivo* 131

K.-U. Petersen
Comparison of different proton pump inhibitors 143

Pharmaceutical considerations

Å. G. Pilbrant
Pharmaceutical considerations 161

Clinical experience with proton pump inhibitors

P. Malfertheiner
Helicobacter pylori infection and peptic ulcer disease 173

C.J. Hawkey
Non-steroidal anti-inflammatory drug-associated ulcers 193

R.T. Jensen
Zollinger-Ellison syndrome 205

L. Lundell and J. Dent
Gastro-oesophageal reflux disease 223

Socio-economic impact of acid-related diseases

H. Glise and B. Hallerbäck
Socio-economic impact of acid-related diseases 239

Subject index 249

Preface

Inhibition of the proton pump in the parietal cells has been established as the main therapeutic principle in the treatment of acid-related diseases, such as peptic ulcer and gastro-oesophageal reflux. The proton pump inhibitors are tailored for their purpose. They accumulate in the target cell, are activated by acid and bind strongly to the specific target – the proton pump. The clinical superiority of the proton pump inhibitors is due not only to their high efficacy but also to the long duration of the acid inhibition in comparison with other antisecretory drugs.

At present when drug discovery mostly relies on identification and characterization of potential targets by genome research, molecular biology, combinatorial chemistry and automated screening, it seems worthwhile to present the development of the first proton pump inhibitor – omeprazole – starting from a chemical structure with an observed antisecretory effect but also severe toxic effects that had to be eliminated. As always, basic and applied research operate hand in hand to optimize the delicate balance between efficacy and safety of a new drug. This goal often involves time and many different specialists.

The significant progress in the treatment of acid-related diseases by proton pump inhibition and the widespread use of these inhibitors are good reasons for reviewing their impact and current position. The monograph is written by eminently qualified specialists who cover a wide range of aspects of acid suppression, including the acid secretory machinery of the parietal cell, the mechanism of inhibition of the proton pump, and the pharmacology of proton pump inhibitors as well as a comparison of presently available proton pump inhibitors. There has been some concern about the safety of long-term suppression of gastric acid secretion, and consequently this issue is discussed. The proton pump inhibitors are transformed during storage and quickly degraded in an acid environment, which created a challenge for their pharmaceutical formulation. The problem and its solution are described. At present the optimal treatment of *Helicobacter pylori*-induced peptic ulcer disease is a combination of a proton pump inhibitor and two antibiotics. The mechanism and clinical results of this treatment are presented. The clinical experience with proton pump inhibitors in the treatment of other important acid-related diseases – peptic ulcer disease induced by antiinflammatory drugs, gastrin-producing tumours and gastro-oesophageal reflux disease – are separately discussed. Quality of life and the socio-economic effects of treatment with proton pump inhibitors are also considered.

Proton pump inhibition is probably not the final therapeutic solution for several of the acid-related diseases, but it undoubtedly represents a valuable and widely accepted therapeutic principle.

Lars Olbe
Göteborg

October, 1998

List of contributors

André Blum, Division de Gastro-Enterologie, Chuv, CH-Lausanne, Switzerland
Enar Carlsson, ASTRA Hässle, Preclinical Research, S-43183 Mölndal, Sweden; e-mail: enar.carlsson@hassle.se.astra.com
Werner Creutzfeldt, Department of Medicine, Georg-August-University, Robert-Koch-Strasse 40, D-37075 Göttingen, Germany
John Dent, Department of Gastrointestinal Medicine, Royal Adelaide Hospital, Adelaide, South Australia, e-mail: jdent@medicine.adelaide.edu.bu
Erik Fellenius, The Swedish Environmental Protection Agency, S-10648 Stockholm, Sweden
Hans Glise, ASTRA Hässle, Göteborg and Department of Surgery University Hospital, S-58185 Linköping, Sweden
Bengt Hallerbäck, Department of Surgery, NAL S-46185 Trollhätten, Sweden
Niilo Havu, ASTRA, Safety Assessment, S-15136 Södertälje, Sweden, e-mail: niilo.havu@astra.se.astra.com
Christopher Hawkey, Department of Medicine, Division of Gastroenterology, University Hospital, Queen's Medical Centre, Nottingham NG7 2UH, UK
Jia-Qing Huang, Division of Gastroenterology, Department of Medicine, McMaster University Medical Center, Hamilton, Ontario, Canada, e-mail: huangj@fhs.csu.McMaster.CA
Richard H. Hunt, Division of Gastroenterology, Department of Medicine, McMaster University Medical Center, 1200 Main Street West, Hamilton, Ontario, L8N 3Z5, Canada, e-mail: huntr@fhs.csu.McMaster.CA
Robert Jensen, NIH/NIDDK/DDB, Bldg. 10, Rm. 9C-103, 10 CENTER DR MSC 1804, Bethesda, MD 20892-18044, USA
Lars Lundell, Department of Surgery, Sahlgren's University Hospital, S-41345 Göteborg Sweden, e-mail: lars.lundell@surgery.gu.se
Peter Malfertheiner, Klinik für Gastroenterologie, Zentrum für Innere Medizin, Otto von Guericke-Universität, D-39120 Magdeburg, Germany
Jan Martínek, Division de Gastro-Enterologie, Chuv, CH-Lausanne, Switzerland
Klaus Melchers, Byk Gulden, Byk Gulden Str. 2, D-78467 Konstanz, Germany
Lars Olbe, Gastroenterology Laboratory, Department of Surgery, University of Göteborg, S-41345 Göteborg, Sweden
Karl-Uwe Petersen, Oberdorfstr. 22, D-52072 Aachen, Germany, e-mail: KarlUwe.Petersen@post.rwth-aachen.de

Åke Pilbrant, Pharmaceutical R & D, ASTRA Hässle AB, S-43183 Mölndal, Sweden, e-mail: ake.pilbrant@hassle.se.astra.com
Georg Sachs, Department of Medicine and Physiology UCLA and Wadsworth VA Hospital, Los Angeles, USA, e-mail: gsachs@ucla.edu
David Scott, Department of Medicine and Physiology UCLA and Wadsworth VA Hospital, Los Angeles, USA
Sven Erik Sjöstrand, ASTRA AB, R & D, S-15185 Södertälje, Sweden, e-mail: sven-erik.sjostrand@astra.se.astra.com
Björn Wallmark, ASTRA Hässle AB, S-43183 Mölndal, Sweden, e-mail: bjorn.wallmark@hassle.se.astra.com
David Wecks, Department of Medicine and Physiology UCLA and Wadsworth VA Hospital, Los Angeles, USA

The discovery and development of the proton pump inhibitor

Proton Pump Inhibitors
ed. by L. Olbe

The discovery and development of the proton pump inhibitor

Sven Erik Sjöstrand[1], Lars Olbe[2] and Erik Fellenius[3]

[1] *ASTRA AB, R & D, S-15185 Södertälje, Sweden*
[2] *Gastroent. lab. Dept. of Surgery, University of Göteborg, Sweden*
[3] *The Swedish Environmental Protection Agency, S-106 48 Stockholm, Sweden*

Introduction

In 1967 research director Ivan Östholm initiated an innovative research project in the gastrointestinal field at Astra Hässle. The aim was to develop an antisecretory drug to be used in peptic ulcer disease. Lars Olbe was appointed as an external consultant. The first idea was to block the release of the gastric acid stimulating hormone gastrin. This is released from the antrum of the stomach during meals and is a physiologically important stimulus of gastric acid secretion. It was known from animal experiments that local anesthesia of the antrum blocked the release of gastrin. The aim was to synthesize a local anesthetic drug that could be orally administrated and active in the antrum. All available local anesthetics were, however, protonated in an acidic environment and therefore inactive. The goal was therefore to change the chemical structure of lidocain – the established local anesthetic of Astra – into a nonbasic compound. The gastric fistula rat (the pylorus-ligated Shay rat) was used as a screening model. A large number of new chemical compounds were synthesized. It was found that the anesthetic property of selected compounds induced toxic effects in safety studies. The chemical development finally ended with antisecretory compounds, including carbamates, which were devoid of local anesthetic properties. The carbamates were found to be very effective as inhibitors of gastric acid secretion in the rat model [1–3] but rather ineffective in the dog. The most effective and nontoxic carbamate compound – H 81/75 – (Fig. 1)

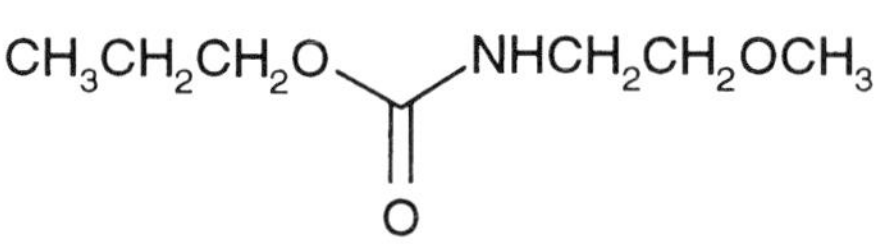

H 81/75

Figure 1. Molecular structure of H 81/75.

had no local anesthetic properties. It was finally tested in human volunteers in 1971–1972. It was found to be completely ineffective in human.

Restart of the project – the proton pump inhibitor project

The disappointing negative results of the carbamate series clearly showed that we had to change the screening procedures. It was decided that new compounds should first be tested for acute toxicity in rats and also in the dog. If considered atoxic, the screening for inhibitory effects on gastric acid secretion should be performed in conscious dogs provided with a gastric cannula. Acid secretion during the screening procedure was stimulated by pentagastrin or histamine. These stimuli were administered subcutaneously or intravenously and maintained a stable acid secretion for hours. The compounds to be tested should preferably be administered orally, but that caused problems in our screening model because of the open gastric cannula. Parenteral administration would have excluded water-insoluble compounds. Instead, we chosed to provide the gastric fistula dogs also with a duodenal fistula. A 10-cm-long section of the jejunum was sutured antiperistaltically between the skin and the duodenum in order to prevent leakage. During the screening procedure a plastic catheter was introduced through the skin fistula and the jejunal segment, after which the test compound could be injected into the duodenum.

When a clearly active compound was found in the screening procedure, its inhibitory characteristics were further tested in more sophisticated animal models. Active compounds were tested in dogs provided with isolated gastric pouches and conscious gastric cannula rats. Gastric acid secretion was also stimulated with meals as well as physiological or pharmacological vagal activation.

The research director had to reduce the staff at the gastrointestinal pharmacological department and could only allow limited time for continuation of the project without a breakthrough. At that time the project manager was the veterinary pharmacologist Sven Erik Sjöstrand, and the team involved the zoophysiologist Gunhild Sundell and the brilliant medicinal chemist Ulf Junggren, who regrettably did not live to see the successful end result, a surgeon as an external consultant, Lars Olbe and five laboratory technicians.

Instead of reviving the local anesthetic lead, a literature search was undertaken to look for new approaches. An abstract was found from a Hungarian pharmacological meeting in which a potent antisecretory compound called CMN 131 from the French pharmaceutical company Servier [4, 5] had been used. CMN 131 was reported to induce inhibition of stimulated gastric acid secretion in rats as well as anesthetized dogs. The research on this drug never continued, because of severe toxicological problems. It seemed quite obvious that the double-bonded sulphur (Fig. 2) should be

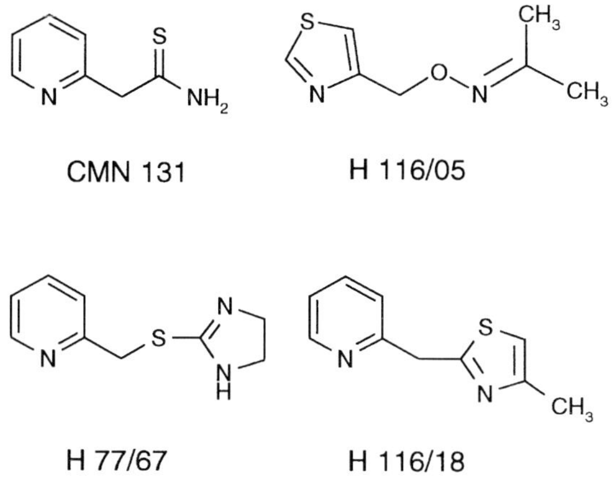

Figure 2. Molecular structures of CMN 131, H 116/05, H 77/67 and H 116/18.

responsible for the toxicity. It was decided to use CMN 131 as an initial lead compound. Further literature searching and our own experimental data disclosed that thioamides – like CMN 131 – as well as thioureas – like metiamide, the second histamine H_2-receptor antagonist – were active acid inhibitory compounds but expected to be carcinogenic. The chemical synthesis program followed two main lines emanating from the pyridine ring coupled to thioamides or thioureas. The first line was the synthesis of sulphur-containing heterocycles like H 116/05 and H 116/18 (Fig. 2). The second line was to synthesize thioethers with an imidazoline ring, like H 77/67 (Fig. 2), and further development by variation at the imidazoline ring position, for example to benzimidazole. Several heterocycles were tested, but these mostly led to dead ends.

The small series of thioamides and thioureas made indicated that the pyridine ring or similar systems like the quinolines were an essential feature for the activity. The impression emerged that slightly basic compounds would be preferable to make. The first attempts to "mask" the sulphur atom of the thioamides by incorporating it into a ring system were H 116/05 and H 116/18 (Fig. 2). The latter was synthesized using CMN 131 as a starting material. They still retained a high degree of inhibitory activity in the Shay rat model. A few other heterocyclic compounds tested in 1972 showed a certain degree of activity. Taken together, H 116/18 and H 116/05 triggered some interest in sulphur heterocycles towards the end of the year. However, when H 116/18 was tested in the conscious dog model, it was practically inactive.

On the other hand, when CMN 131 and the first compound in the second line of the chemical synthesis program, H 77/67, were tested in the conscious dog model, both were clearly active in inhibiting gastric acid secretion. The benzimidazole analogue of H 77/67, H 124/26 (Fig. 3), was syn-

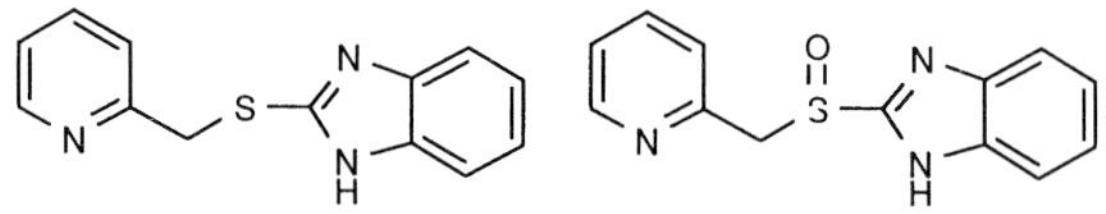

Figure 3. Molecular structures of H 124/26 and H 83/69.

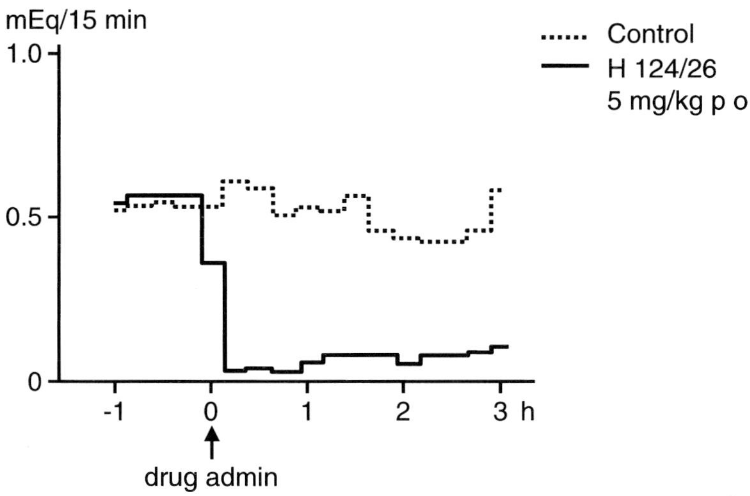

Figure 4. Gastric antisecretory effect of H 124/26 in a dog with a vagally denervated (Heidenhain) gastric pouch during stimulation with pentagastrin.

thesized in June 1973 and tested in October of the same year. It was the most powerful inhibitor of gastric acid secretion so far tested (Fig. 4). The project was now allowed to continue, but could only expand in the chemical synthesis and biological test programs by collaboration with Abbott Laboratories in Chicago and with their financial support. Obviously, H 124/26 became the new lead compound.

The first substituted benzimidazole H 124/26 and its metabolite H 83/69

In the initial chemical synthesis program the lead compound was treated as a molecular template consisting of two heterocyclic ring systems connected by a chain, that is three elements. Each element was systematically varied in the synthesis program during 1974. The original three elements of H 124/26 turned out to be optimal [6] (Fig. 5).

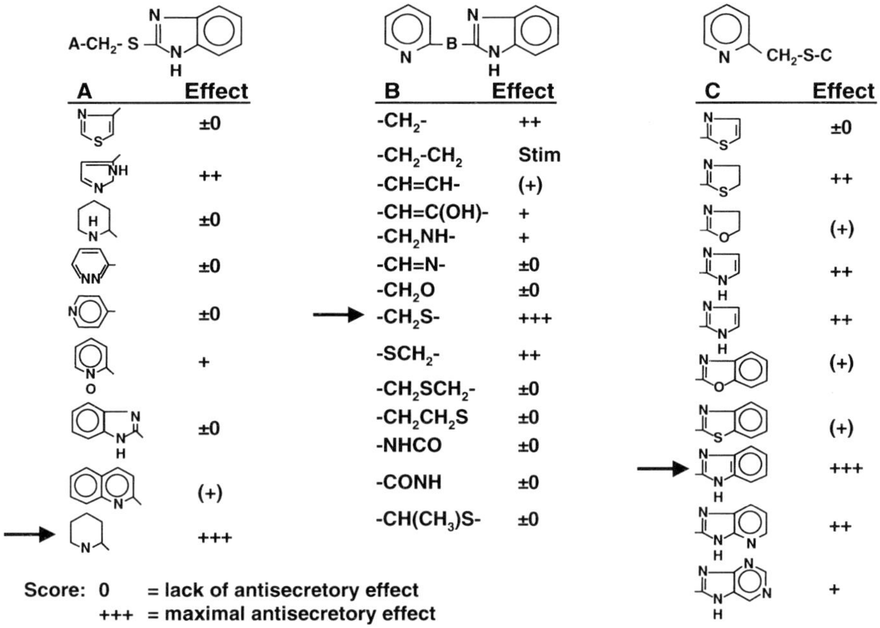

Figure 5. Gastric antisecretory effects in the dog by chemical variations of the three fundamental fragments (A, B, C) of H 83/69.

In 1974, however, it was realized that H 124/26 was included in a Hungarian patent for compounds aiming at treatment of, among others, tuberculosis. Again the project was on the verge of being stopped. Negotiations with the Hungarian authorities were difficult and ineffective. Meanwhile, the pharmacological screening program went ahead, and the potential metabolites of H 124/26, the sulphoxide and the sulphide, were tested. The sulphide, H 83/70, was found to be inactive as an inhibitor of gastric acid secretion. However, the sulphoxide, H 83/69, was found to be a very potent secretion inhibitor. Pharmacokinetic studies at Abbott Laboratories in Chicago indicated a rapid formation of two main metabolites of H 124/26. Analysis at Astra Hässle showed that those were identical to H 83/69 and H 83/70. H 83/69 was found to be even more potent as a gastric acid secretion inhibitor than the parent compound [7]. This compound was given the generic name timoprazole. Furthermore, it became apparent that the chemical structure of H 83/69 was not included in the Hungarian patent. The project was allowed to continue with the new lead compound H 83/69.

Development of pharmacological *in vitro* techniques

In the early 1970s the molecular structures and properties of the first two histamine-H_2-receptor antagonists – burimamide and metiamide – were published. Test methods, like the isolated guinea pig atrium, were available to establish interference with the histamine-H_2-receptor. It could be shown by various pharmacological methods that H 83/69 was neither a histamine H_2-receptor antagonist nor an anticholinergic drug. Furthermore, there was no evidence supporting any antigastrin activity of the compound. We needed new *in vitro* techniques to be able to study the inhibitory mechanism of H 83/69 close to the parietal cell level. A technique had been described using frog stomach mounted as a membrane in a two-compartment chamber – the Ussing chamber. This technique was modified in that the isolated mucosa was applied as a membrane on the end of a plastic funnel. This preparation was then immersed in a conventional organ bath. By addition of acid secretory stimuli or inhibitors to the nutrient side of the mounted gastric mucosa, acid was secreted or inhibited on the secretory side. However, we were more interested in using isolated gastric mucosa from a mammal. Isolated acid-secreting gastric mucosa from different species were tested. Most of them were poor responders to added secretory stimuli, probably due to a thick and impermeable submucosal layer. But isolated mucosa from guinea pig was very thin and upon stimulation resulted in a prominent secretory response for several hours.

Dose-response relationships for histamine were established. In the presence of a histamine-receptor antagonist the dose response for histamine was shifted to the right in a parallel manner, indicating conventional competitive receptor agonist-antagonist interaction [8]. H 83/69 was also found to inhibit histamine-stimulated acid secretion, although not in a competitive manner. In order to study drug action beyond the receptors on the basal side of the cell, the secretory process must be initiated from the interior of the cell. It was known that the intracellular content of cAMP increased in response to receptor activation, which led us to imitate this event by adding cAMP to the nutrient medium. However, no response was found, which was interpreted as an inability of exogenous cAMP to penetrate membranes. It was then replaced by dibutyryl-substituted cAMP, and we recorded a dose-dependent gastric acid secretory response [9] (Fig. 6). Intracellularly cAMP-stimulated acid secretion was not inhibited by administration of a histamine receptor antagonist, as expected, but H 83/69 induced a dose-dependent inhibition [10]. This was the first experimental evidence for a site of inhibitory action beyond the panel of stimulatory receptors. Interestingly, we found that our initial lead compound, CMN 131, had no inhibitory effect on dibutyryl-cAMP-stimulated acid secretion, nor was it a histamine H_2-receptor antagonist. The site of inhibitory action in the intracellular chain of events leading to acid secretion was still unknown.

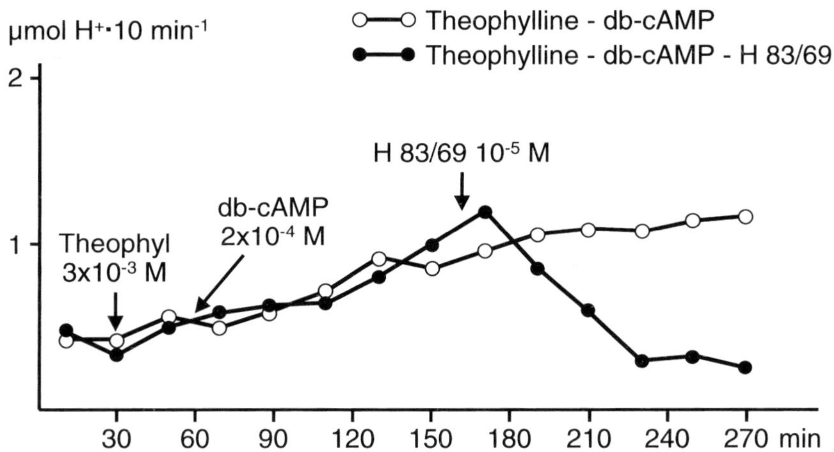

Figure 6. Effects of H 83/69 on db-cAMP-induced gastric acid secretion from isolated guinea pig gastric mucosa.

Side effects of H 83/69

In the toxicological studies of H 83/69 two observations caused concern. The pathology examination of animals treated with H 83/69 revealed atrophy of the thymus gland, which might indicate interference with immunodefence mechanisms. The other pathological observation was an enlargement of the whole thyroid gland. Further studies showed potent inhibition of iodine uptake. These side effects were seen in practically all experiments and resulted in a new proposal to cancel the project. Again, we were allowed a short period of time to try to eliminate the side effects and retain the antisecretory effect. This could only be done with financial support from other external sources (NUTEK, The Swedish National Board for Industrial and Technical Development), since the collaboration with Abbott Laboratories came to an end.

Thio-urea substances, like thiouracil, are commonly used as therapeutics to block the hormonal activity of the thyroid gland by inhibiting the iodine uptake. A publication was located that detailed how to substitute thiourea compounds for optimal effect on iodine uptake. The publication also showed a few substituted mercapto-benzimidazoles which had no effect at all on iodine uptake. These substituents were introduced into the corresponding ring of H 83/69. Specific studies in the rat were included as a new screening technique with the intention of selecting compounds devoid of inhibition of iodine uptake. The techniques were developed at our department of drug safety assessment. In many of the subsequent compounds the side effects on the thyroid and thymus were thus minimized without interfering with the antisecretory properties. Once again the project was allowed to continue. Later on it could be shown that separation of inhibi-

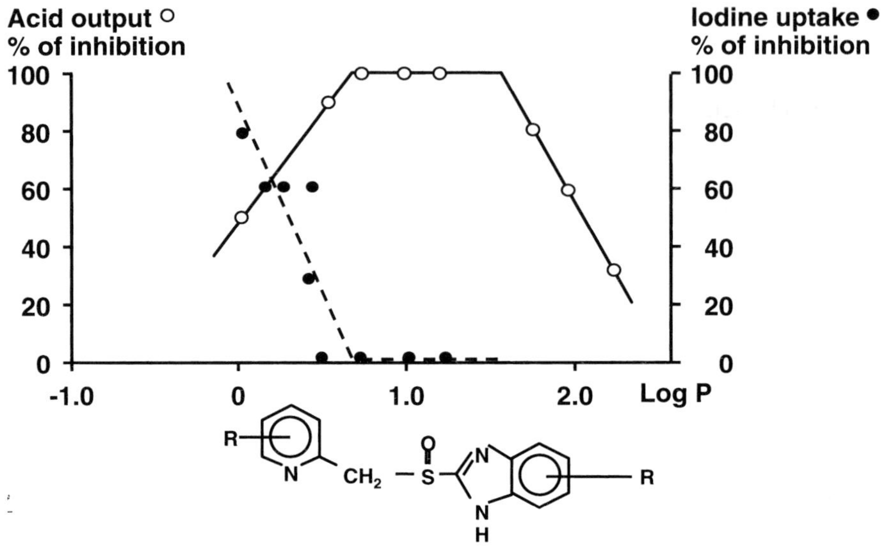

Figure 7. The effect of various substituted benzimidazoles on inhibition of acid secretion and iodine uptake in relation to their lipophilicity.

tion of iodine uptake and inhibition of acid secretion were obtained in a specific range of lipophilicity of the substituted benzimidazole (Fig. 7).

Development of biochemical techniques

With the knowledge of a site of inhibitory action beyond the cAMP step in isolated gastric mucosa, we needed to extend our project into the field of biochemical pharmacological techniques. Our intention was to perform pharmacological studies on the secretory process in different *in vitro* preparations such as isolated glandular preparation and in isolated fragments of parietal cell secretory membrane. The acid transport protein H^+/K^+-ATPase had just been discovered in the secretory membranes of the parietal cell [11–14].

Erik Fellenius in the biochemistry department of Astra Hässle was contacted and enthusiastically joined the project team as head of the biochemical staff. This also involved Björn Wallmark and two laboratory technicians. The initial aims were to test whether *in vitro* techniques could increase the screening capacity, whether these studies could improve our understanding of the mechanism of the inhibitory action and whether *in vitro* techniques could be used on human gastric mucosa. If these aims could be fulfilled, it would save time, improve the patent applications and also possibly give us information about drug effects on human tissue at an early stage, that is before taking the compounds to human pharmacological trials.

Isolated gastric glands from the rabbit

At Astra Hässle we started the biochemical program by adopting a technique published by Thomas Berglindh [15]. Gastric acid secretion was indirectly determined in isolated rabbit gastric glands. In this preparation the acid secretory response can be monitored semiquantitatively by measuring oxygen uptake or the uptake of a radiolabelled weak base, ^{14}C-aminopyrine (^{14}CAP), which accumulates in the gland in proportion to pH differences between the intraglandular acid compartments and the surrounding medium [15, 16]. The isolated glands had been shown to respond to a number of different secretagogues and inhibitors [15–17]. Secretagogues such as dibutyryl cAMP (db-cAMP) and K^+ stimulated acid secretion intracellularly, probably at a site close to the acid secretory membranes [18–20]. In contrast, histamine and acetylcholine have a site of action in the basal membrane at specific receptors [15, 16, 18, 21]. Stimulation at the receptor level initiates the physiological process of gastric acid secretion. By using receptor agonists and intracellularly active db-cAMP and K^+ for stimulating acid secretion in isolated gastric glands, a useful experimental model is available to study the pharmacological properties of potential acid secretion antagonists. The marked inhibition of K^+ and db-cAMP induced ^{14}CAP accumulation produced by the substituted benzimidazoles strongly supported the view that these compounds interfered with acid secretion at or close to the final site of acid secretion [22, 23] (Fig. 8). Receptor antagonists like cimetidine and atropine had no effect on K^+ and db-cAMP-stimulated secretion, as expected. In later extended studies we could rule out the possibility of an SCN^--like effect of the substituted benzimidazole [24]. SCN^- has been postulated to dissipate the proton gradient rather than inhibit acid secretion [25]. The aminopyrine uptake technique in isolated gastric glands from the rabbit was included in the screening system.

Isolated gastric vesicles containing the H^+/K^+-ATPase

In 1977 a scientific meeting was arranged in Uppsala on gastric ion transport. We presented our new technique and our results using isolated guinea pig gastric mucosa [9]. George Sachs and John Forte presented data about the properties of the acid pump, the H^+/K^+-ATPase [11–14], which was claimed to be the terminal step in the acid secretory process of the parietal cell. When acid secretory membranes are isolated from the parietal cells, they round up and form closed vesicles containing the H^+/K^+-ATPase. K^+ and H^+ transport and enzyme activity, for instance phosphate release, can be measured. Sachs also showed immunohistological data from various organs using antibodies against a crude preparation from the secretory membranes of the parietal cells, where the H^+/K^+-ATPase was supposed to be localized. He found strong immunoreactivity in the parietal

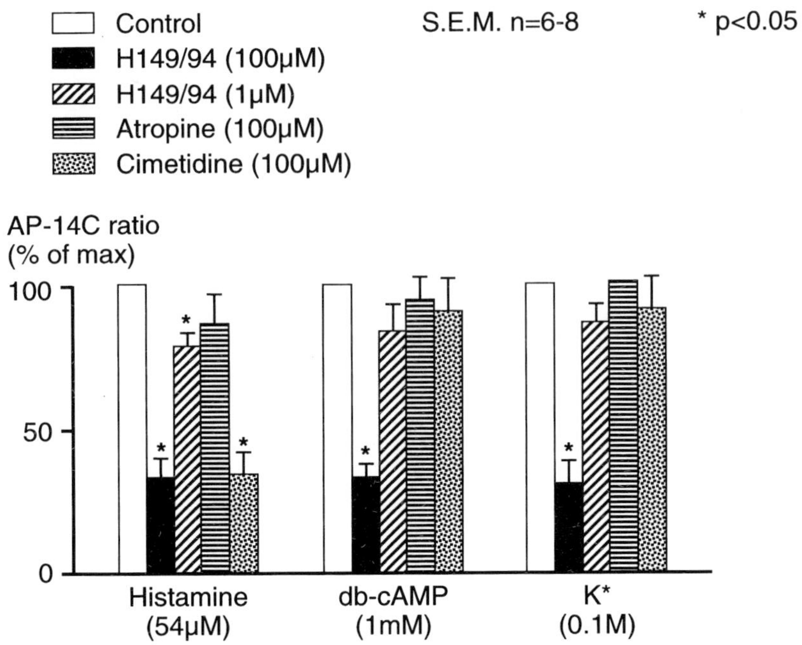

Figure 8. Gastric acid inhibitory effects on H 149/94, cimetidine and atropine on histamine-, db-cAMP- and K^+-induced ^{14}C-aminopyrine accumulation in the isolated rabbit glands. Adopted from ref. 27.

cell region of the stomach but also some activity in the thyroid gland. At this time we knew the inhibitory effects of H 83/69 on gastric acid secretion and its side effects on the thyroid and thymus. We told Sachs that if he had also studied the thymus immunohistologically, he would probably have found some reactivity. He looked clearly astonished and asked how we could know, because he had found immunoreactivity in the thymus but had not presented those data. We informed him about the properties of H 83/69. We also asked him whether he could envisage H 83/69 as an inhibitor of the H^+/K^+-ATPase. He shook his head, smiled and told us not to be too optimistic. We also asked him about collaboration, but he said that he was very much engaged with the new histamine-H_2-receptor antagonists.

One of our substituted benzimidazoles was, however, tested on isolated vesicles containing the acid pump enzyme in George Sachs's laboratory. To our disappointment, no effect was observed. Meanwhile, Björn Wallmark joined the project with the aim of studying the effects of substituted benzimidazole compounds on the acid pump mechanism. He introduced the technique with isolated gastric vesicles at the Astra Hässle biochemical laboratory and confirmed Sachs's negative results. We then decided to do more basic research on the H^+/K^+-ATPase, including characterization of

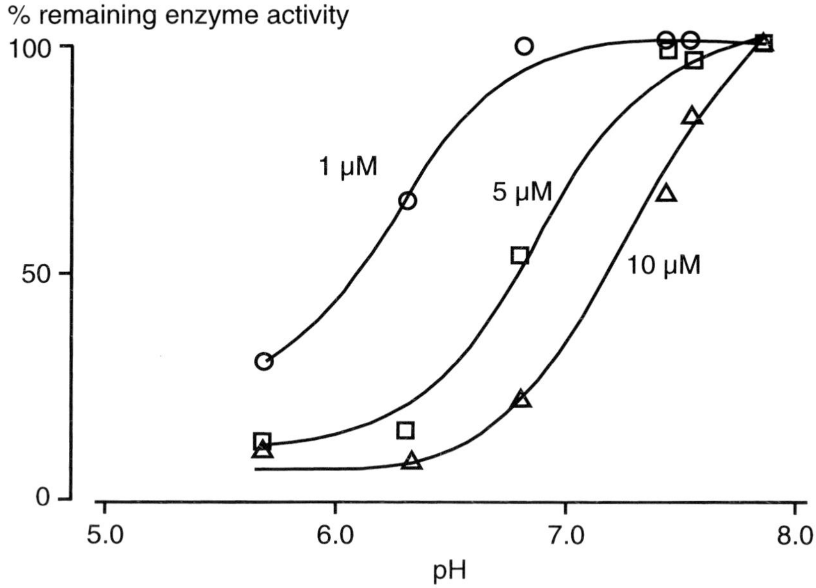

Figure 9. pH dependency for inhibition of H^+/K^+-ATPase by H 168/68 (omeprazole) in isolated gastric vesicles from rabbit. Adopted from ref. 24.

the enzyme-phosphate (E-P) complex. A collaboration with Sven Mårdh at the University of Uppsala was initiated. He was experienced in techniques using this type of complex with a related enzyme – the Na^+/K^+-ATPase. In one experiment his group included a substituted benzimidazole and found a slight but significant reduction of the E-P intermediate. Further testing of phosphate release by H^+/K^+-ATPase was undertaken with variations in incubation conditions, including preincubation with benzimidazoles. The results then showed distinct inhibition of H^+/K^+-ATPase. A real breakthrough was the finding that preincubation of isolated vesicles with substituted benzimidazoles resulted in inhibitory activity only when conditions were acidic. This was further verified in experiments where the compound solvent was acidified (Fig. 9). These data were the first indication that the substituted benzimidazoles probably had to be transformed in order to be active inhibitors. The first step in the transformation could be protonation of the compound. This was followed by a series of experiments using different test systems to study the interaction of substituted benzimidazoles with the H^+/K^+-ATPase, comprising acridine orange absorbance, phosphate release and *p*-nitrophenol release from *p*-nitrophenylphosphate [22, 26, 27]. Binding studies with the substituted benzimidazoles showed specific binding to H^+/K^+-ATPase [26]. All the results of the inhibitory effects of the substituted benzimidazoles in isolated gastric glands and isolated parietal vesicles containing H^+/K^+-ATPase supported the concept that the compounds interfered with the acid pump. The results were also confirmed in Sachs's laboratory, and he was then in favour of the concept. A long-lasting collaboration started between Sachs and the scientists at Astra Hässle.

Isolated human gastric glands and vesicles

Earlier experience in evaluating inhibitors of gastric acid secretion had indicated species differences in response to various chemical substances. Information about antisecretory effects on human tissue at an early stage would be an advantage. However, a direct transfer of the isolated gland technique to human tissue could be a problem. In rabbits, the gastric vascular system was perfused with digestive enzymes *in situ* prior to removing the secretory part for experimental studies [15]. An *in vitro* preparation technique was developed on human gastric mucosa that required new *in vitro* conditions [17]. Gastric mucosa was obtained from resected stomachs of patients with peptic ulcer. An advantage of resected specimens was that a rather large piece could be obtained. A disadvantage was that we could never exclude any influence by the surgical procedure, premedication or pathological condition in the area. However, this was overcome by the

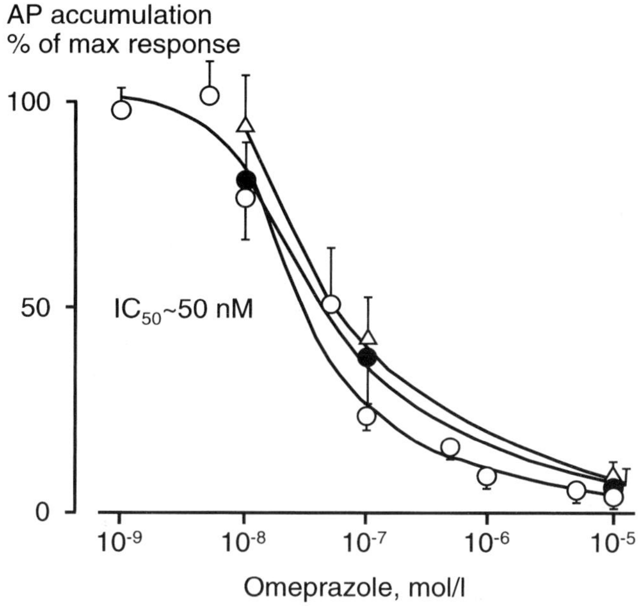

Figure 10. Inhibitory action of H 168/68 on histamine (○)-, db-cAMP (●)-, and K^+ (△)-stimulated human gastric glands. Adopted from ref. 31.

development of a micromethod which allowed isolation of gastric glands from gastric biopsies [28]. This technique represented a major step forward, because it increased the screening capacity and made it possible to include biopsy material from stomachs of healthy subjects. Furthermore, the isolated gastric gland preparation from human tissue could be used to study hormonal control of and pharmacological effects on human gastric acid secretion *in vitro* [29, 30]. Later on, preparations from human gastric biopsies also included isolation of H^+/K^+-ATPase [31]. The strong inhibition of the acid pump by the substituted benzimidazoles in animal preparations could now be confirmed in experiments with different *in vitro* techniques using human tissues [22, 23, 27, 31, 32] (Fig. 10).

The relative potency of the various substituted benzimidazoles was identical *in vivo* (dog) and *in vitro* (isolated guinea pig gastric mucosa, gastric glands and isolated vesicles) [27]. Kinetic studies of the inhibition in isolated human glands confirmed the noncompetitive type of inhibition found in isolated guinea pig gastric mucosal preparation.

Morphology studies

Information was needed about any morphological changes in the pareital cell during inhibition of gastric acid secretion after administration of substituted benzimidazoles. A collaboration was established with Herbert Helander at the University of Umeå, who had substantial experience in parietal cell morphology. Gastric acid secretion in the rat was stimulated with and without simultaneous administration of various antisecretory drugs. After sacrifice, specimens from the fundic mucosa were studied using electron microscopy. Stimulation of acid secretion induced an increase of the secretory surface area. After administration of an anticholinergic drug or a histamine H_2-receptor antagonist there was no increase of the secretory surface area. After administration of a substituted benzimidazole, on the other hand, the secretory membrane became significantly larger despite powerful inhibition of acid secretion. The results indicated that morphological changes of the parietal cell during stimulation of acid secretion were activated via the stimulatory receptors and unaffected by acid pump inhibitors [33].

Autoradiographic studies in mice using radiolabelled substituted benzimidazoles revealed rapid clearance of the intravenously injected compound to excretory organs. Retention in the stomach wall was observed which lasted for at least 16 h after a single injection with a selective uptake of the compound in parietal cells. Further electron microscopic autoradiographic investigations showed specific retention of radioactivity only in the secretory membranes of the parietal cell [34].

Search for a candidate drug

H 83/88 (Fig. 11) was the first compound devoid of any effects on the thyroid and thymus and as potent as H 83/69 in inhibiting gastric acid secretion. Extended toxicological studies showed no serious effects in the rat but necrotizing vasculitis in a few organs, including the small intestine, in some dogs, probably a hypersensitivity phenomenon. Once again the project was on the point of being stopped, but we were allowed a short period of time to solve the problem. We found a few occasions of necrotizing vasculitis in a previous toxicological study of a beta blocker compound. This finding raised the possibility that the antigen responsible for the immunological reaction was something other than the test compounds. Dogs used in the toxicological studies were heavily medicated against intestinal parasites just before the studies. The antiparasitic drugs or fragments of dead parasites might have been immunogenic factors in sensitive dogs. Two approaches were used to solve the problem. A study with H 83/88 was initiated in nonparasitic dogs that were available in the United States. And another new candidate was chosen for continuation of the project. H 149/94, picoprazole (Fig. 11), was the most potent antisecretory substituted benzimidazole found so far, and like all compounds from that time and onwards was

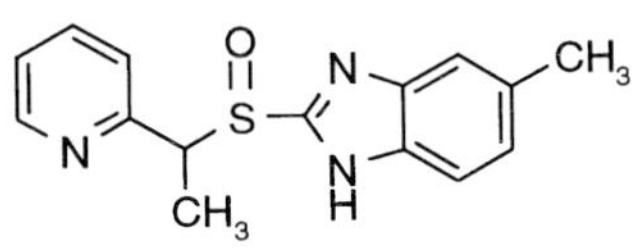

H 83/88

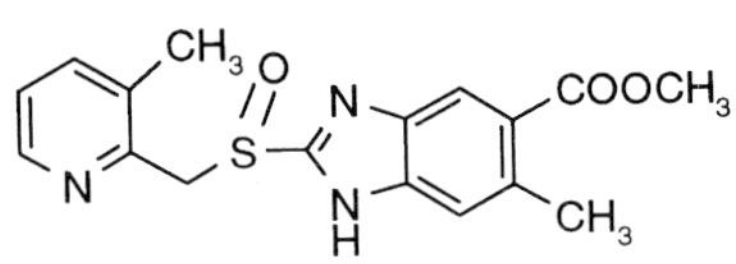

H 149/94

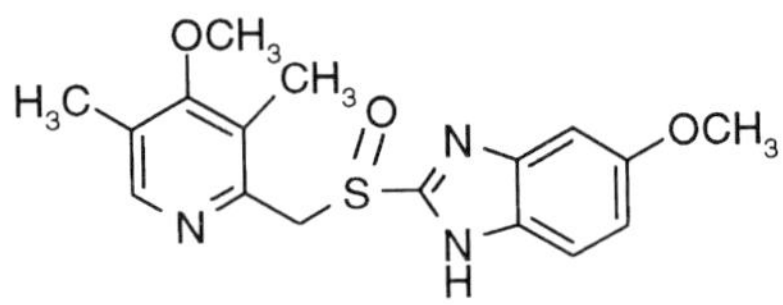

H 168/68

Figure 11. Molecular structures of H 83/88, H 149/94 (picoprazole) and H 168/68 (omeprazole).

without any effect on the thyroid and thymus. In 1978 the extended toxicological study on H 149/94 again showed necrotizing vasculitis in the small intestine of some dogs. The obvious conclusion of the toxicological experts was to terminate the project. However, one member of the scientific board called attention to the fact that one of the three dogs in the nonmedicated control group also showed vasculitis. The termination of the project was postponed, since this finding obviously suggested that the necrotizing vasculitis might be a non-drug-related phenomenon. The immunologist in the department of toxicology, Vera Stejskal, showed that drug-treated dogs with vasculitis had not developed antibodies against the test compounds but against epitopes on intestinal worms. Furthermore, all dogs that developed vasculitis emanated from one male dog, strongly suggesting that the necrotizing vasculitis was a hypersensitive reaction to fragments of intestinal worms as a result of the antiparasitic treatment in genetically predisposed dogs. Besides, the studies on parasite-free dogs in the United States did not show any vasculitis. In the light of these findings a new toxicological study was performed with H 149/94 after eliminating all genetically abnormal dogs. This second toxicological study was completely clean. H 149/94 was then tested in human volunteers and showed a very potent antisecretory action of very long duration [32], indicating the potential of high clinical efficacy. High clinical efficacy was further supported by treatment of a gastrinoma (Zollinger-Ellison syndrome) patient with H 149/94. This patient had severe ulcer bleeding and symptoms despite treatment with extremely high doses of cimetidine. Treatment with H 149/94 reduced the high basal acid secretion to normal values and quickly abolished the ulcer bleeding and symptoms (S. Rune, personal communication).

Weak bases like aminopyrine accumulate in the acidic compartment of the parietal cell. Our compounds behaved in a similar manner [23], confirmed in the autoradiographic studies described previously [34]. The chemists now changed the substituents on the heterocyclic rings to obtain a compound being a weak base with an optimal pK_a value (Fig. 12), thereby maximizing accumulation at the site of action. This compound, H 168/68 (Fig. 11), was synthesized in 1979 and given the generic name omeprazole. It was found to be the most powerful inhibitor of stimulated gastric acid secretion in experimental animals *in vivo* [35] and *in vitro* [24, 31] and also in human tissue *in vitro* [31]. No effect on iodine uptake, no induction of thymus atrophy, no necrotizing vasculitis and no other signs of toxicity were recorded from the early safety studies. It was very potent inhibitor of the proton pump *in vitro*, as well as in preparations from human stomach tissue. Pharmacological studies showed long-lasting inhibition of acid secretion, suggesting strong binding to the target site. An IND application on omeprazole was filed and it was taken to human trials. The first clinical results with omeprazole were presented at the satellite symposium "Substituted Benzimidazoles – A New Approach to Control of Gastric Acid Secretion" at the World Congress of Gastroenterology in Stockholm in

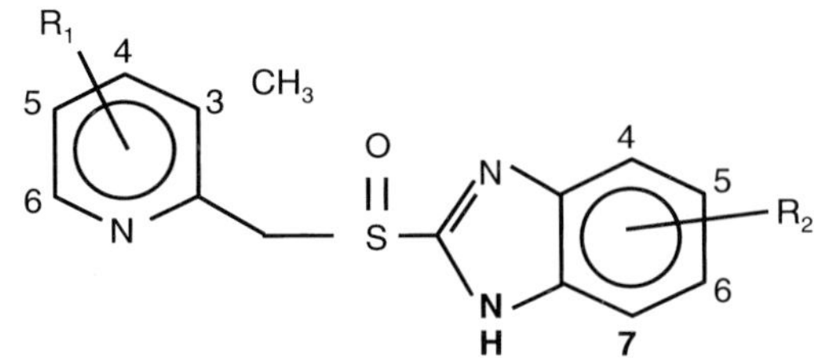

R1	R2	Calculated ΔpKa (pyridine)	Inhibition of acid secretion Dog, intraduodenally -log ED_{50}
H	5-OCH_3	0	-
4-CH_3	5-OCH_3	+0.76	5.2
3,5-$CH_3)_2$	5-OCH_3	+0.94	5.6
4,5-$CH_3)_2$	5-OCH_3	+1.23	5.3
5-CH_3, 4-OCH_3	5-OCH_3	+1.82	5.9
3,5-$(CH_3)_2$-4-OCH_3	5-OCH_3(omeprazole)	+2.29	6.6

Figure 12. The effect of variations of substituents on the pyridine ring of H 83/69 on acid-base properties (pK_a) and their influence on the inhibitory acton on gastric acid secretion in the dog. Data represent an extract from the chemical synthesis program.

1982. Treatment of 26 duodenal ulcer patients with 40 mg of omeprazole daily for 4 weeks resulted in ulcer healing in 25 out of the 26 patients [36]. After solving many problems during the research leading to omeprazole, it seemed to represent a successful new principle in the treatment of acid-related diseases. New problems were, however, waiting around the corner.

Acknowledgements
The authors thank Peder Berntsson, Ph.D., medicinal chemist at Astra Hässle, for contributing information about the chemical program in the development of proton pump inhibitors.

References

1 Berntsson P, Brändström A, Palmer L, Sjöstrand SE, Sundell G (1977) Gastric acid secretion inhibitors II. Carbamates and aromatic alcohols and phenols. *Acta Pharm Suecia* 14: 229–236
2 Sundell G, Borg K-O, Garberg L, Sjöstrand SE (1974) Effects of H 81/75 on gastric acid secretion in vagally innervated and denervated acute fistula rat preparations. *Acta Pharm Tox* 35: 83
3 Sundell G, Borg K-O, Garberg L, Palmer L, Sjöstrand SE (1973) Evaluation of a new gastric secretion inhibitor, H 81/75, in the rat. *Acta Phys Scand Suppl* 396: 131
4 Borsy J, Andrási F, Faraks L (1973) Experimental studies with 2-pyridyl-thioacetamide, a new antisecretory and antiulcer drug. In: J Borsy, G Móxsik (eds): *Gastrin and its antagonists*. Akadémiaik iadó. First Congress of the Hungarian Pharmacological Society, Budapest, 67–78
5 Malen CE, Danree BH, Pascaud XBL (1971) New thiocarboxamides derivatives with specific gastric antisecretory properties. *J Med Chem* 14: 244–246

6 Lindberg P, Brändström A, Wallmark B, Mattsson H, Rikner L, Hoffmann K-J (1990) Omeprazole, the first proton pump inhibitor. *Med Res Rev* 10: 1–54

7 Sundell G, Sjöstrand SE, Olbe L (1977) Gastric antisecretory effects of H 83/69, a benzimidazolyl-pyridyl-methyl-sulfoxide. *Acta Pharm Tox Suppl* 4: 77

8 Sjöstrand SE, Ryberg B, Olbe L (1977) Analysis of the actions of cimetidine and metiamide on gastric acid secretion in the guinea pig gastric mucosa. *Arch Pharmacol* 296: 139–142

9 Sjöstrand SE, Ryberg B, Olbe L (1978) Stimulation and inhibition of acid secretion by the isolated guinea pig gastric mucosa. *Acta Phys Scand Suppl Spec*: 181–185

10 Olbe L, Sjöstrand SE, Fellenius E (1979) Present situation and future prospects of medical treatment. In: JF Rehfeld, E Amdrup (eds): *Gastrins and the vagus*. Academic, New York, 245–250

11 Forte JG, Lee HC (1977) Gastric adenosine triphosphatases: a review of their possible role in HCl secretion. *Gastroenterology* 73: 921–927

12 Sachs G, Chang H, Rabon E, Shackman R, Sarau HM, Saccomani G (1977) Metabolic and membrane aspects of gastric H^+ transport. *Gastroenterology* 71: 931–940

13 Lee J, Simpson G, Scholes P (1974) An ATPase from dog gastric mucosa: changes of outer pH in suspensions of membrane vesicles accompanying ATP hydrolysis. *Biochem Biophys Res Com* 60: 825–832

14 Ray TK, Forte JG (1976) Studies on the phosphorylated intermediates of a K^+-stimulted ATPase from rabbit gastric mucosa. *Biochim Biophys Acta* 443: 451–467

15 Berglindh T, Öbrink KJ (1976) A method for preparing isolated glands from the rabbit gastric mucosa. *Acta Phys Scand* 96: 150–159

16 Berglindh T (1977) Effects of common inhibitors of gastric acid secretion on secretagogue-induced respiration and aminopyrine accumulation in isolated gastric glands. *Biochim Biophys Acta* 464: 217–233

17 Fellenius E, Elander B, Wallmark B, Haglund U, Olbe L, Helander HF (1979) Studies on acid secretory mechanisms and drug action in isolated gastric glands from man. In: G Rosselin, P Fromageot, S Bonfils (eds): *Hormone receptors in digestion and nutrition*. Elsevier, Amsterdam, 355–360

18 Chew CS, Hersey SJ, Sachs G, Berglindh T (1980) Histamine responsiveness of isolated gastric glands. *Am J Physiol* 238: G312–320

19 Berglindh T, Helander H, Sachs G (1979) Secretion at the parietal cell level – a look at rabbit gastric glands. *Scand J Gastroenterol* 55: 7–15

20 Berglindh T, Dibona DR, Ito S, Sachs G (1980) Probes of parietal cell function. *Am J Physiol* 238: G165–167

21 Soll AH (1980) Secretagogue stimulation of [^{14}C]aminopyrine accumulation by isolated canine parietal cells. *Am J Physiol* 238: G366–375

22 Fellenius E, Berglindh T, Sachs G, Olbe L, Elander B, Sjöstrand SE, Wallmark B (1981) Substituted benzimidazoles inhibit gastric acid secretion by blocking (H^+ + K^+)ATPase. *Nature* 290: 159–161

23 Fellenius E, Elander B, Wallmark B, Helander HF, Berglindh T (1982) Inhibition of acid secretion in isolated gastric glands by substituted benzimidazoles. *Am J Physiol* 243: G505–510

24 Wallmark B, Jaresten B-M, Larsson H, Ryberg B, Brandström A, Fellenius E (1983) Differentiation among inhibitory actions of omeprazole, cimetidine and SCN^- on gastric acid secretion. *Am J Physiol* 245: G64–G71

25 Gutnecht J, Walter A (1982) SCN^- and HSCN transport through lipid bilayer membranes a model for SCN^- inhibition of gastric acid secretion. *Biochim Biophys Acta* 685: 233–240

26 Wallmark B, Sachs G, Mårdh S, Fellenius E (1983) Inhibition of gastric (H^+ + K^+)ATPase by the substituted benzimidazole, picoprazole. *Biochim Biophys Acta* 728: 31–38

27 Fellenius E, Berglindh T, Brändström A, Elander B, Helander HF, Olbe L, Sachs G, Sjöstrand SE, Wallmark B (1980) The inhibitory action of substituted benzimidazoles on isolated oxyntic glands and H^+/K^+-ATPase. In: I Schultz, G Sachs, J Forte, KJ Ullrich (eds): *Hydrogen Ion Transport in Epithelia*. Elsevier, Amsterdam, 193–202

28 Fellenius E, Elander B, Wallmark B, Haglund H, Helander HF, Olbe L (1983) A micromethod for the study of secretory function in isolated human oxyntic glands from gastroscopic biopsies. *Clin Sci* 64: 423–431

29 Leth R, Elander B, Haglund U, Olbe L, Fellenius E (1987) Histamine H_2-receptor of human and rabbit parietal cells. *Am J Physiol* 253: G497–501

30 Haglund U, Elander B, Fellenius E, Leth R, Rehnberg O, Olbe L (1982) The effects of secretagogues of isolated human gastric glands. *Scand J Gastroenterol* 17: 455–460
31 Elander B, Fellenius E, Leth R, Olbe L, Wallmark B (1986) Inhibitory action of omeprazole on acid formation in gastric glands and on H^+,K^+-ATPase isolated from human gastric mucosa. *Scand J Gastroenterol* 21: 268–272
32 Olbe L, Haglund U, Leth R, Lind T, Cederberg C, Ekenved G, Elander B, Fellenius E, Lundborg P, Wallmark B (1982) Effects of substituted benzimidazole (H 149/94) on gastric acid secretion in humans. *Gastroenterology* 83: 193–198
33 Helander HF, Sundell G (1984) Ultrastructure of inhibited parietal cells in the rat. *Gastroenterology* 87: 1064–1071
34 Helander HF, Ramsay CH, Regårdh CG (1985) Localisation of omeprazole and metabolites in the mouse. *Scand J Gastroenterol* 108: 95–104
35 Larsson H, Carlsson E, Junggren U, Olbe L, Sjöstrand SE, Skånberg I, Sundell G (1983) Inhibition of acid secretion by omeprazole in the dog and rat. *Gastroenterology* 85: 900–907
36 Bonnevie O, Nielsen AM, Matzen P, Wandall J, Bendtsen F, Rune S, Bekker C, Bytzer P, Rask Madsen J, Bergsåker-Aspöy J et al (1984) Gastric acid secretion and duodenal ulcer healing during treatment with omeprazole. *Scand J Gastroenterol* 19: 882–884

Mechanism of action

Proton Pump Inhibitors
ed. by L. Olbe

The gastric H,K ATPase

George Sachs and Björn Wallmark

Department of Medicine and Physiology UCLA and Wadsworth VA Hospital, Los Angeles, USA and ASTRA-Hässle, Göteborg, Sweden

Introduction

On 11 December 1823, at the Royal Society, William Prout presented his landmark paper "*On the Nature of Acid and Saline Matters Usually Existing in the Stomach of Animals*". This presentation was unique in two ways. First, Prout had specifically identified hydrochloric acid in the gastric juice of many species (man, dog, rabbit, horse, calf and hare), and second, he was able to quantify the free and total hydrochloric acid and chloride present. The acid was measured by neutralization with potash solution of known strength and the chloride by titration with silver nitrate. He also proposed that chloride may be secreted from blood to lumen by electrical means and that, when gastric acid was secreted, the blood would become alkaline (now recognized as the postprandial alkaline tide). More than 100 years were to elapse before his subsequent proposal was confirmed.

Once acid was recognized, it became the source of all evils, and medicine and biology dedicated themselves to eradication of this clear liquid. First we were fascinated by its mechanism of stimulation and for three quarters of a century managed to produce compounds clearly effectively dealing with nighttime acidity. Daytime acidity remained a problem, so our fascination switched to the mechanism of secretion itself, recognising the difficulty of making drugs that did not have leads equivalent to molecules such as gastric, acetylcholine or histamine that stimulated acid secretion. Now with the establishment of *Helicobacter pylori* as causal or contributory to gastric ulcer/duodenal ulcer (GU/DU) and malt lymphoma, it seems that eradication of this organism must supplant other methods of therapy of peptic ulcer disease. Or combine with them. Yet there are those that claim that eradication without sensitivity to the proteins produced by *H. pylori* might well be removing a commensal from our midriff, producing rather than removing problems.

Theories of the mechanism of acid secretion

Work on acid secretion by isolated frog mucosae in the 1960s had started to point towards an ATP rather than the electrogenic, redox-based mecha-

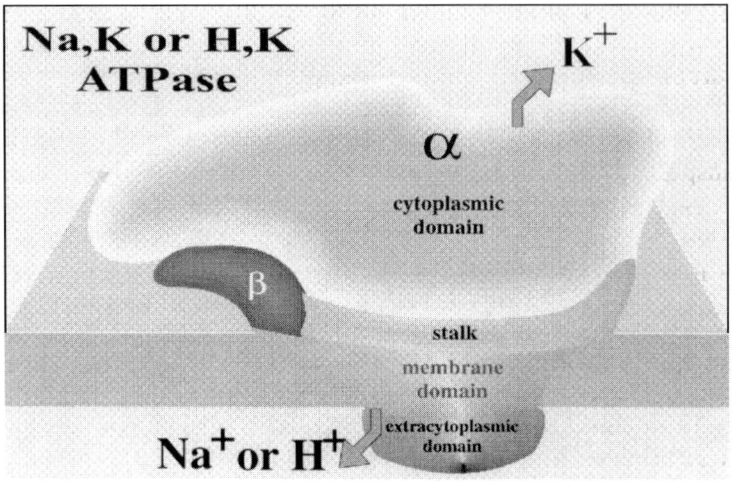

Figure 1. A general model of the sodium and gastric acid pumps identifying their domains and their two subunits. The cytoplasmic domain binds ATP, becomes phosphorylated and releases ADP and Pi. The stalk transduces the conformational change due to phosphorylation/dephosphorylation to the membrane domain which contains the ion transport pathway, binding Na or H with high affinity (ion "in") in one conformational state, and with low affinity in a second conformational state (ion "out") [7].

nism that had been in vogue since the 1930s. In the early 1970s, a K^+-stimulated ATPase was found in frog stomach [1]. A K^+-dependent acid transport was found in isolated gastric vesicles [2]. Then it was shown that the mechanism of this ATPase was similar to that of the Na pump but was an electroneutral ATP-driven H^+ for K^+ exchange [3]. Permeabilized gastric parietal cells in rabbit gastric glands were able to secrete acid when ATP was added to the bathing solution in the presence of high concentrations of K^+ [4]. Inhibition of acid secretion by the pyridyl methylsulfinyl benzimidazole class of drugs was shown to be due to inhibition of the ATPase [5]. Omeprazole inhibition of ATPase activity correlated with the rate of acid secretion [6]. These are the major observations that led to the definition of H,K ATPase as the final step in acid secretion, the gastric proton pump.

The acid pump is a drug target. A general model for this type of pump is shown in Figure 1. It is an α-β heterodimer as shown in the illustration and this property is shared by the Na,K and colonic K ATPases.

The H,K ATPase

General

The enzyme class to which the gastric H,K ATPase belongs is called the P-type ATPase class of ion motive ATPases. These P-type ATPases are phosphorylated and dephosphorylated during their enzyme/transport cycle. Enzymes of this family, with similar functions, transport or counter-transport of small cations or transition metals across membranes, often use similar amino acid sequences in regions that perform the same function, such as the binding of ATP or the sequence that is phosphorylated during the transport cycle. These are signature sequences that enable recognition of these ATPases in bacteria and eukaryotes from sequence alone [8]. Often the arrangement of their transmembrane segments is retained to give a similar placement of relatively hydrophobic regions, producing recognizable transmembrane footprints with either 8 or 10 transmembrane or membrane-inserted segments [9, 10].

There appear to be two subfamilies within the family of P-type ATPases. One family transports small cations such as Na, K, H, Ca and Mg, the other transition metals such as Cu, Cd, Zn or Co. The latter group has 8, the former 10 transmembrane segments [11].

Transport reaction pathway

Gastric H,K ATPase exchanges H for K at equal stoichiometry. Even though the outward and inward parts of the transport cycle are electrogenic, the net effect of pump transport is electroneutral and is not able to generate a transmembrane potential [12]. It is composed of two subunits. The α (catalytic) subunit contains the phosphorylation consensus sequence and ATP-binding domain. The β subunit has seven N-linked glycosylated consensus sequences, and this subunit is required for stability of the gastric pump and perhaps also for membrane recycling. The α subunit is about 75% homologous to the α subunit of the Na pump, and the β subunit is about 40% homologous to the $\beta 2$ subunit of the Na pump. The colonic K ATPase has a similar homology to the gastric and Na pumps and although called the colonic H,K ATPase, probably transports K but not H [12–15].

The general reaction that the α subunit of this pump catalyzes is shown in Figure 2 [16].

In order to achieve uphill transport of an ion against its electrochemical gradient at a significant rate, there has to be a decrease in binding site affinity on the whence side and orientation of this site towards the thence side. A conceptual model for this, which has experimental foundation, is that the transported ion enters the membrane domain from one side and binds to a site with relatively high affinity before the membrane domain closes to occlude the ion. A second conformational change then opens the membrane domain to allow the ion being removed from the cytoplasm to escape from the other side of the membrane from a lower-affinity site. Binding of the countertransported ion induces the converse changes in affinity and conformation, the ion binding with relatively high affinity to the outside face, occluding and releasing from the low-affinity state to the cytoplasm.

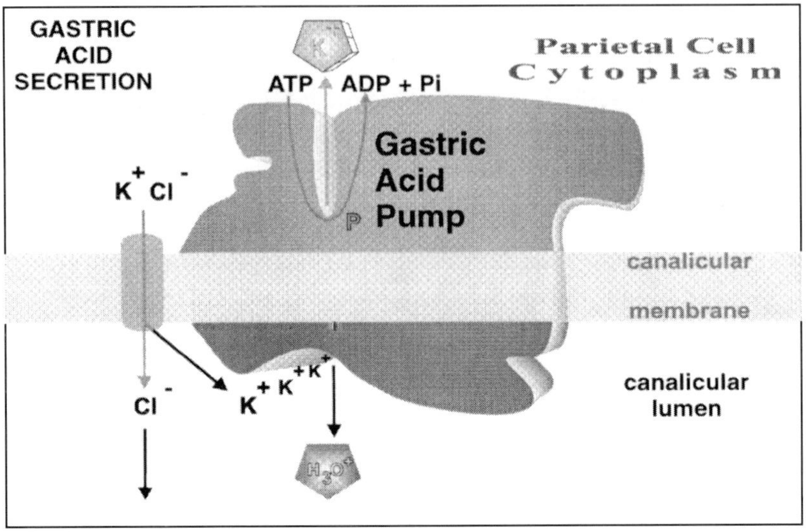

Figure 2. This illustrates the general mechanism of acid secretion catalyzed by H,K ATPase. It secretes acid only when present in the canalicular membrane. There is activation of a K^+/Cl^- pathway that enables efflux of KCl and H_2O from the cytoplasm of the parietal cell. The K secreted into the lumen of the secretory canaliculus of the parietal cell is transported inward in exchange for H_3O^+ by the cycle of phosphorylation/dephosphorylation on the catalytic subunit of the H,K ATPase, leaving HCl in the canalicular lumen.

The scheme of the chemical reaction shown in Figure 3 is illustrated for H,K ATPase but is similar to that of Na and Ca ATPases [17–19]. This shows that the enzyme exists in three major conformations, with ion-binding sites facing inward, the "in" conformation (E_1); ion-binding sites facing outward, the "out" conformation (E_2); and ion sites occluded in the membrane, the E_{occ} conformation. The transition between these conformations is driven by ATP binding, trans-phosphorylation and dephosphorylation. We are far from an adequately detailed understanding of the structure of these conformers to allow the building of a molecular model of transport by these pumps. Much experimental effort has gone into using different methods to outline the means whereby these pumps countertransport ions.

Kinetics

The rate of formation of the phosphoenzyme and the K^+-dependent rate of breakdown are sufficiently fast to allow the phosphoenzyme to be an intermediate in the overall ATPase reaction. The initial step is the reversible binding of ATP to the enzyme in the absence of added K^+ ion, followed by an Mg^{2+} (and proton)-dependent transfer of the terminal phosphate of ATP to the catalytic subunit (E_1-P · H^+). The Mg^{2+} remains occluded until dephosphorylation. The addition of K^+ to the enzyme-bound acyl phosphate

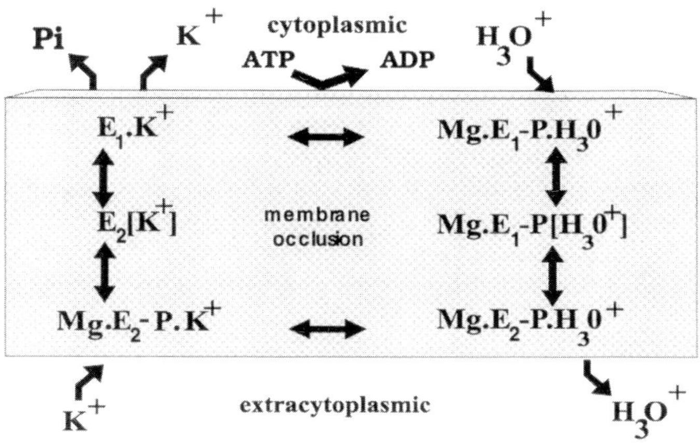

Figure 3. The enzymic reaction cycle for the gastric H,K ATPase. Similar cycles have been postulated for the other mammalian small cation P-type ATPases. With binding of hydronium and MgATP to the enzyme in the ion site "in" conformer, the phosphorylated form MgE_1-P · H_3O^+ is generated. This spontaneously moves into the occluded conformer and thence to the ion site "out" form, E_2. The hydronium ion binding has reduced affinity when the enzyme is in the E_2 state, but K is bound with relatively high affinity to this phosphorylated E_2 form. The enzyme is dephosphorylated as the occluded E_2. K^+ conformer is generated which then decays spontaneously to the E_1 · K^+ form, and K^+ release is stimulated by rebinding of Mg · ATP.

results in a two-step dephosphorylation. The faster initial step is dependent on the concentration of K^+. The second phase of EP breakdown is accelerated in the presence of K^+, but at K^+ concentration exceeding 500 μM, the rate becomes independent of K^+ concentration. This shows that two forms of EP exist. The first form, E_1P, is K^+-insensitive and converts spontaneously in the rate-limiting step to E_2P, the K^+-sensitive form. ATP binding to the H,K ATPase occurs in both the E_1 and the E_2 states, but with a lower affinity in the E_2 state (2000 times lower compared with E_1).

The selectivity of the "in" conformation of the cation binding site is for small cations such as H_3O^+ as opposed to the bulkier K^+. The converse is true for the "out" conformation of the cation-binding site. H^+ or K^+ interact competitively on the cytoplasmic surface of the pump, suggesting that they bind to similar regions of the enzyme that change in spatial characteristics in the two conformations. The effects of H^+ and K^+ on formation and breakdown of the phosphoenzyme were determined using transient kinetic analysis. Increasing hydrogen ion concentrations on the ATP-binding face of the vesicles accelerated phosphorylation, whereas increasing potassium ion concentrations inhibited phosphorylation. Increasing hydrogen ion concentration reduced K^+ inhibition of the phosphorylation rate. Decreasing hydrogen ion concentration accelerated dephosphorylation in the absence of K^+, and K^+ on the luminal surface accelerated dephosphorylation. Increasing K^+ concentrations at constant ATP decreased the rate of phosphorylation, and increasing ATP concentrations at constant K^+ concentration accelerated ATPase activity and increased the steady-state phosphoenzyme level. Therefore, inhibition by cations is due to cation stabilization of a dephospho form at a cytosolically accessible cation-binding site. Occlusion was demonstrated directly by showing ^{86}Rb binding to the enzyme at low temperature that was released by the addition of ATP [20–22].

As for the Na pump, various cations such as Rb^+, Cs^+, NH_4^+ and Tl^+ can act as K^+ surrogates. As will be seen later, design of K^+ competitive inhibitors of the H,K ATPase can take advantage of the surrogate properties of NH_4^+.

Stoichiometry

The gastric H,K ATPase is electroneutral, in contrast to the Na,K ATPase. The H^+ for K^+ stoichiometry of the H,K ATPase was reported to be one or two per ATP hydrolyzed. The H^+/ATP ratio was independent of external KCl and ATP concentrations. When care was taken to measure initial rates in tight vesicles, the ratio found was 1ATP:2H:2K. Lower stoichiometries imply leaky or damaged vesicles. Since at full pH gradient the stoichiometry must fall to 1ATP:1H:1K, this pump displays a variable stoichiometry. This may be explained by the presence of two groups, such as carboxylic acids, of different pK_a such that 2H or 2K can release or bind at low acid concentrations, but only 1H or 1K can bind at highly acidic pH [23].

Activation of the gastric H,K ATPase

Stimulation of acid secretion by the parietal cell is due mainly to gastrin- or pituary adenylate cyclase activating peptide (PACAP)-stimulated release of histamine from the enterochromaffin-like (ECL) cell of the fundic epithelium and activation of the H_2 receptor. Direct stimulation by acetylcholine occurs at an M3 receptor on the parietal cell. The parietal cell also has a cholecystokinin B (CCK-B) receptor which appears to require permissive activation of the H_2 receptor for elevation of parietal cell calcium. The H_2 receptor is coupled to mainly Gs with elevation of cAMP but also to Gq, resulting in a small stimulation of intracellular calcium levels. The final event is activation of the H,K ATPase, which is in a resting, non-secreting state in cytoplasmic membranes [24–26].

The complex pathways of stimulation using at least three endocrine cells for stimulation and inhibition of acid secretion are illustrated in Figure 4 [28].

In contrast to the regulation of many other enzymes, there is no evidence for any chemical factors which directly influence the activity of the H,K ATPase other than the availability of the necessary substrates Mg ATP, H^+ and K^+. Since within the parietal cell the availability of protons and Mg ATP are not likely to be rate-limiting given the large number of mitochondria, it follows that the major, if not the only, factor which controls proton transport is the availability of K^+ at the extracytosolic surface of the H,K

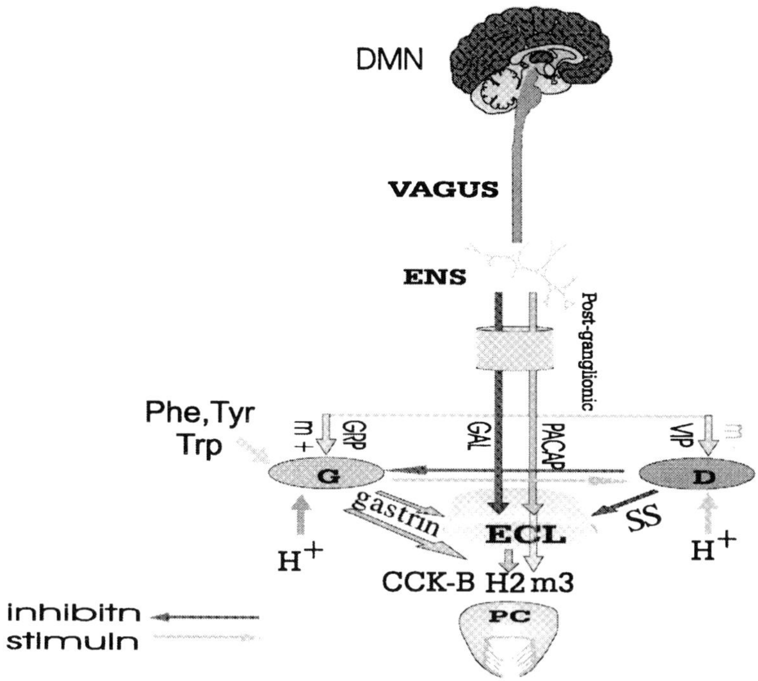

Figure 4. Stimulatory pathways of the mammalian parietal cell. The ECL cell is the central endocrine cell releasing histamine for activation of the parietal cell. Its function is regulated centrally by PACAP and galanin and peripherally by gastrin and somatostatin released from G and D cells, respectively.

ATPase. Substantial evidence has accumulated to indicate that this is indeed the case and that activation of the proton pump results from association of the H,K ATPase with a K^+ permeability in the membrane of the secretory canaliculus [27]. A simplified model for the activation process is depicted in Figure 5.

The nature and origin of the K^+ permeability which is associated with the H,K ATPase in the canaliculus remain undefined. It has been proposed that the canalicular membrane contains parallel conductances for K^+ and Cl^- or alternatively that there is a KCl cotransporter. Further, the proteins that interact with the enzyme in the cytoplasmic membranes that enable stimulus-dependent conversion to the canalicular form remain elusive, although ezrin and actin are clearly associated with the enzyme in its stimulated form.

Recruitment of the pump into the canalicular membrane is thought to involve a fusion process of the cytoplasmic tubules into the microvilli which is followed by a process of eversion so that the cytoplasmic surface of the pump is on the inner surface of the microvillus. Retrieval of the pump involves inversion and presumably separation of the tubule membrane from the apical membrane, as shown in Figure 6.

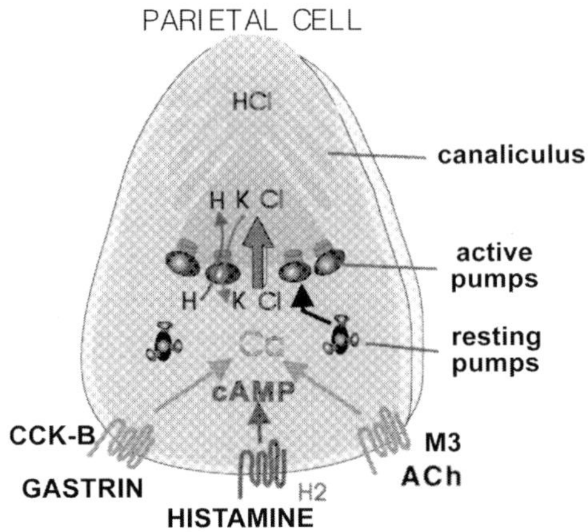

Figure 5. A model of the receptors present on the basolateral surface of the parietal cell and their intracellular effects, which lead to movement of the H,K ATPase from the cytoplasmic tubule to the microvillus of the secretory canaliculus. The cholinergic receptor is of the M3 subtype and increases intracellular calcium. The gastrin receptor is the CCK-B receptor and also generates calcium signaling, although it appears that elevation of cAMP is required for this signaling cascade. The histamine 2 (H_2) receptor is coupled mainly to adenylate cyclase and is the major regulatory receptor for acid secretion. The substrates for the A kinase are not known.

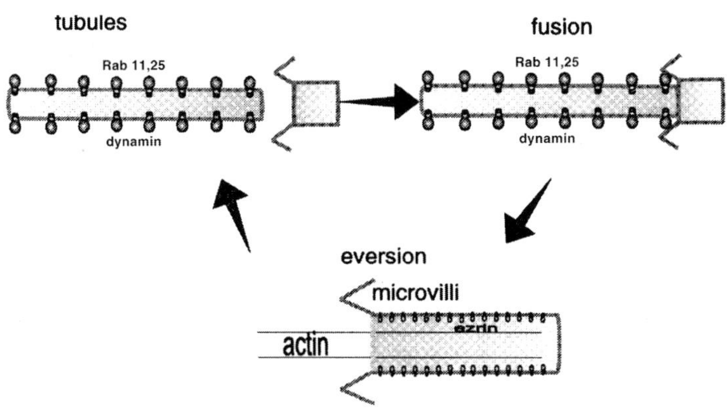

Figure 6. A model of the cycling of the H,K ATPase between the cytoplasmic tubule and the microvillus of the secretory canaliculus of the parietal cell.

Synthesis and turnover of the H,K ATPase

Biosynthesis of the two subunits of the ATPase takes place in the endoplasmic reticulum of the parietal cell. It appears that there is a need for coassembly of the two pump subunits for stabilization of the α subunit and for targeting of the dimer to the post-Golgi membrane compartment and the plasma membrane. The rate of synthesis of the H,K ATPase is directly relevant to the duration of action of proton pump inhibitors (PPIs).

The half-life of the α subunit has usually been inferred rather than directly measured. Thus, treatment of rats with cycloheximide resulted in a loss of ATPase activity with a half-life of 72 h [29]. Recovery from inhibition with the covalent inhibitor, omeprazole, showed a half-life of 30 h in the same series of experiments. Other workers have claimed a half-life of recovery from proton pump inhibition of as short as 15 h [30].

Direct measurement of the half-life of the catalytic subunit of the H,K ATPase in the rat gave a value of 54 h. Treatment with omeprazole did not change this value, whereas treatment with the H_2 receptor antagonist, ranitidine, gave a value of 125 h, a statistically significant increase [31].

2D structure of the gastric H,K ATPase

The catalytic subunit is similar in general structure to that of other mammalian small cation P-type ATPases. Composed of 1034 or 1035 amino acids, it has a large cytoplasmic domain, a connecting stalk or energy transduction domain, a transmembrane domain and a small extracytoplasmic domain. The β subunit has an N-terminal cytoplasmic sequence of about 60 amino acids, a transmembrane domain of about 30 amino acids and a C-terminal domain containing about 200 amino acids with seven N-linked glycosylation sites. Although the function of the pumps that have been sequenced is usually known, it is not possible by inspection of the sequence to predict which ion is transported by which sequence. In the 1980s, when complementary DNA cDNA and hence amino acid sequences became available, there was hope that linear sequencing would provide mechanistic clues as to protein function. Amino acid sequencing has enabled enormous advances in the fields of phenotyping cells, analyzing families of proteins, defining interacting proteins and signature sequences but has not fully enabled functional or mechanistic analysis. Biochemical, molecular and structural features are necessary in addition to be able to call the function of a protein sequence.

The catalytic subunit

The primary sequences of the α subunits deduced from cDNA have been reported for several species such as pig, rat, rabbit and human. The hog gastric H,K ATPase α subunit sequence deduced from its cDNA consists of 1034 amino acids and has a MW of 114,285. The sequence based on the known N-terminal amino acid sequence is one less than the cDNA-derived sequence and begins with glycine. The degree of conservation among the α subunits is extremely high (over 97% identity). The human gastric H,K ATPase gene has 22 exons and encodes a protein of 1035 residues including the initiator methionine residue (MWt = 114,047). These H,K ATPase

α subunits show high homology (~ 60% identity) with the Na,K ATPase catalytic α subunit. The distal colon K ATPase α subunit has also been sequenced and shares 75% homology with both the H,K and Na,K ATPases.

The gastric α subunit has conserved sequences, along with the other P-type ATPases, for the ATP-binding site, the phosphorylation site, the pyridoxal 5′-phosphate-binding site and the fluorescein isothiocyanate (FITC)-binding site. These sites are thought to be within the ATP-binding domain in the large cytoplasmic loop between membrane-spanning segments 4 and 5 and have detected different regions of the enzyme surface.

In the case of the hog gastric H,K ATPase, pyridoxal 5′-phosphate is bound at lys^{497} of the α subunit in the absence but not the presence of ATP, suggesting that lys^{497} is present in the ATP-binding site or in its vicinity [32]. The phosphorylation site was observed to be at asp^{386}. FITC covalently labels the Na,K and the gastric H,K ATPases in the absence of ATP. The binding site of FITC was at lys^{518}. However, several additional lysines, such as those at positions 497 and 783, were shown to react with FITC during inactivation of the Na,K ATPase and to be protected from reaction with FITC when ATP was present in the incubation. Based on these data, similar lysines of the H,K ATPase could be near or in the ATP-binding site, which is formed by several nonadjacent stretches of the cytoplasmic amino acid sequence [33]. The region between 386 and at least 518 clearly encloses the ATP-binding regions of the enzyme and may even extend to position 783.

The membrane domain contains the ion transport region of the enzyme, and hence is structurally fascinating for those with a penchant for ion transport mechanisms and drugs able to block such transport.

The hydropathy plot of H,K ATPase is shown in Figure 7 and is similar in the P-tye ATPases that transport the small cations H, Na, K, Ca and Mg. This plot defines the potential transmembrane or membrane-inserted segments, and the methods that have been used to define these segments of the acid pump are also illustrated in this figure.

Within this 10-membrane segment model, regions of the membrane domain are concerned with transporting H_3O^+ outward and K^+ inward. A variety of sites have been mutated in this pump but more extensively in the sr Ca pump and the Na,K ATPase. Measurements have been made of enzyme activity, cation binding and transport in these mutants. In the membrane domain, mutations especially of carboxylic and hydrophilic amino acids in the region of TM4, 5, 6 and 8 affect ion binding and transport [37, 38]. It is therefore considered that these transmembrane sequences enclose the ion pathway across the membrane. The carboxylic and other hydrophilic side chains of the amino acids provide binding sites for the cations, but the carbonyl of the peptide bond is probably also involved. When the amino acid sequences of the Na,K, H,K and sarcoplasmic reticulum (SR) Ca ATPases are compared, there is conservation of several of these carboxylic or hydrophilic amino acids in certain transmembrane segments. The carboxylic acids in TM4, 5, 6 and 8 are conserved as well as the

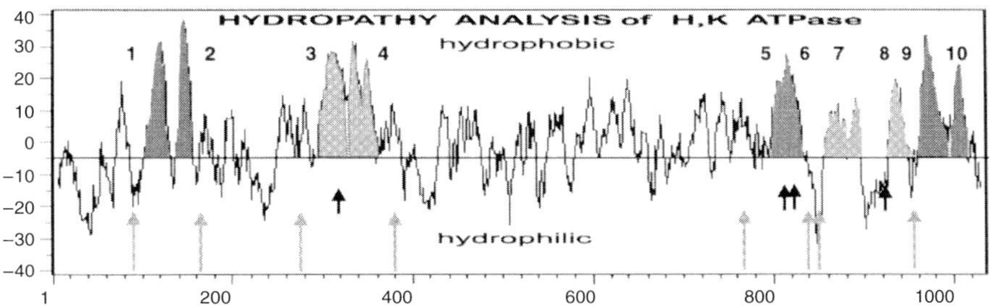

Figure 7. Determination of membrane topology. Methods used to determine the number and position of transmembrane segments shaded and numbered in the hydropathy plot. The lower set of arrows denotes sites determined to be tryptic cleavage sites by amino acid sequencing of the digested, separated fragments; the darker, shorter arrows indicate cysteins derivatized by one or another of the PPIs. TM9 and 10 were detected by *in vitro* transcription/translation. The membrane domain of the enzyme contains the ion transport pathways where there must be a hydrophilic pathway that the ions traverse as the cytoplasmic domain changes conformation as a function of phosphorylation and dephosphorylation. It can be seen that there are five regions of hydrophobicity, suggesting the possible presence of 10 membrane segments. These have been established experimentally by determining the residual membrane domains after removal of the cytoplasmic sectors by tryptic digestion of cytoplasmic side-out vesicles, by *in vitro* translation scanning and by sites of labeling with extracytoplasmic inhibitors of the enzyme such as omeprazole, lansoprazole and pantoprazole and a photoaffinity derivative of SCH 28080 [34–36]. 1. Tryptic cleavage sites in cytoplasmic side out vesicles. 2. Labelling with extracytoplasmic thiol reagents. 3. *In vitro* translation/investion of hydrophobic sequences.

motifs surrounding these amino acids, suggesting a commonality of function such as ion binding. The amino acid sequences thought to be within the membrane domain and on the outside face of the pump are illustrated in Figure 8.

The relationship between the cytoplasmic domain and the transmembrane domain changes as a function of transport conformation. This statement is based on findings with fluorescent probes that change their quantum yield as a function of the hydrophobicity of their environment. When the H,K ATPase is in the ion-binding site "in" conformation, the distance between the inner boundary of the cytoplasmic domain and the inner boundary of the membrane domain is small. With the ion-binding site in the "out" conformation, this distance increases as measured by the K-dependent quenching of fluorescence of FITC bound to lys 516 of the amino acid sequence [39]. Conversely, the distance between the outer edge of the membrane domain and the inner surface is larger with the ion site "in" conformation and smaller with the ion site "out" conformation. The enzyme therefore contracts its cytoplasmic domain as the ion is transported outward, and associated with this is a degree of extrusion of the membrane domain. As the countertransported ion binds to the outside surface, the outside binding site moves towards the cytoplasm.

There is evidence that the more mobile part of the membrane domain is the fifth and sixth transmembrane segment pair and its connecting loop.

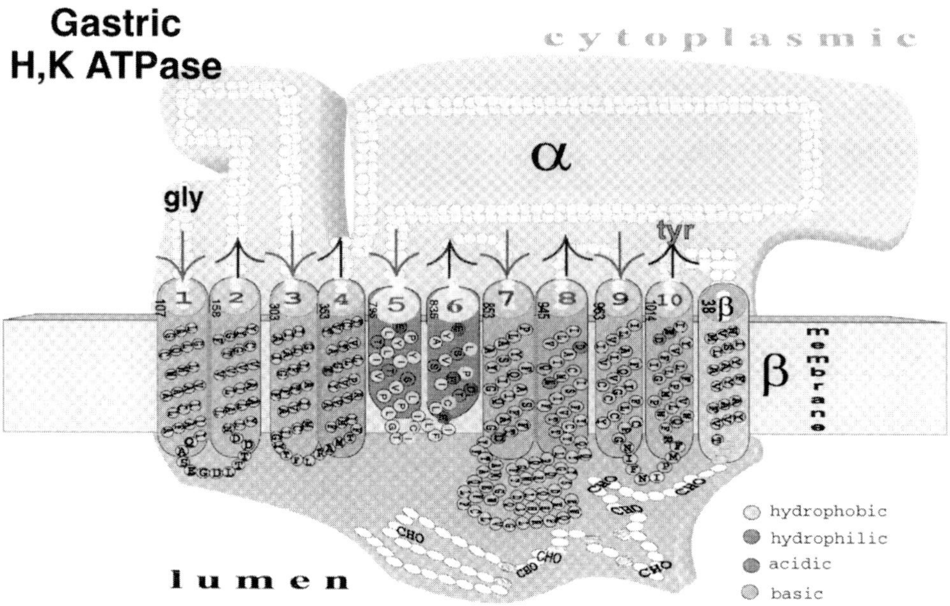

Figure 8. Schematic diagram of the arrangement of the membrane segments with their constituent amino acids of the α and β subunits of the gastric H,K ATPase. Highlighted are the transport segments in TM4, M5, M6 and TM8, the hydrophilic and charged amino acids in the membrane domain. The M5 and M6 segments are presented here as a membrane-inserted hairpin, and this structure may reflect mobility of this segment of the pump.

For example, tryptic cleavage of cytoplasmic side-out vesicles cuts the cytoplasmic chain prior to M5 at different places depending on either the length of digestion or the absence or presence of K^+. The first N-terminal cutting site is at position 776 and then at 784 and finally at 792 after longer digestion or in the presence of K, whereas the C-terminal cutting site does not change [40]. After digestion in the presence of K, if the membrane residue is washed in the absence of K, of the five transmembrane segment pairs, most of the M5/M6 is removed and then at higher pH TM7/loop/TM8 also [41]. *In vitro* translation of M5/M6 also shows that these relatively hydrophilic membrane segments probably do not insert during translation of the protein and may require subsequent protein surfaces of other transmembrane segments for membrane insertion. TM7 also does not act as a membrane insertion sequence in *in vitro* translation [42]. The cluster of M5/M6 and TM7/TM8 may provide the flexibility within the membrane domain that is necessary for transport competence. Mutation of the glutamyl residue at position 820 to other amino acids resulted in K-independent turnover of the enzyme, suggesting that K is required to be bound at this anionic site for the E_2 to E_1 transition to be rate-limiting [42] and that absence of an anionic site allows K-independent pump cycling.

The β subunit

The primary sequences of the β subunits have been reported for rabbit, hog, rat, mouse and human enzymes and contain about 290 amino acids. The hydropathy profile of the β subunit appears less ambiguous than the α subunit. There is one membrane-spanning region predicted by the hydropathy analysis, which is located at the region between positions 38 and 63 near the N terminus. Tryptic digestion of intact gastric H,K ATPase produces only one small cleavage of the N-terminal segment of the β subunit on SDS gels. Wheat germ agglutinin (WGA)-binding of the β subunit is retained. These data indicate that most of the β subunit is extracytoplasmic and glycosylated. When lyophilized hog vesicles are cleaved by trypsin followed by reduction, a small, nonglycosylated peptide fragment is seen on SDS gels with the N-terminal sequence, AQPHYS, which represents the C-terminal region beginning at position 236 in the pig sequence [43]. This small fragment is not found either after trypsinolysis of intact vesicles nor in the absence of reducing agents. A disulfide bridge must therefore connect this cleaved fragment to the β subunit containing the carbohydrates. The C-terminal end of the disulfide is at position 262. This leaves little room for an additional membrane-spanning α helix. Hence the β subunit has only one membrane-spanning segment.

Region of association of the α and β subunits

The β subunit of both the Na,K and H,K ATPases is necessary for targeting the complex from the endoplasmic reticulum to the plasma membrane. It also stabilizes a functional form of both the gastric H,K and Na,K ATPases. Rupture of the disulfide bonds interferes with catalytic function. In the case of the Na,K ATPase, the last 161 amino acids of the α subunit are essential for effective association with the β subunit [44].

Further the last four or five C-terminal hydrophobic amino acids of the Na^+ pump β subunit are essential for interaction with the α subunit, whereas the last few hydrophilic amino acids are not [45]. The H,K ATPase α subunit requires its β subunit for efficient cell surface expression. However, expression of the sodium pump α subunit along with the β subunit of either sodium or proton pump in *Xenopus* oocytes has shown that the β subunit of the gastric proton pump can act as a surrogate for the β subunit of the sodium pump for membrane targeting and $^{86}Rb^+$ uptake [46]. The coupling in mammalian systems was less impressive [47]. Nevertheless, this implies homology in the associative domains of the β subunits of the two pumps [46].

In experiments aimed at finding the region of the α subunit associated with the β subunit, tryptic fragments were adsorbed to a WGA-affinity column and free and associated peptides eluted successively. The β subunit was associated almost quantitatively with the M7/loop/M8 sector of the α subunit [48], and no other segment remained associated. Other experiments carried out in the presence of K^+ showed that a fragment of 19 to 21 kDa results, which begins with the M7 segment and continues to the C-terminal end of the enzyme, that is associated with the β subunit. A fragment representing the M5/loop/M6 sector is now also retained by the β subunit. Hence, provided there is no hydrolysis between M8 and M9, an additional interaction is present between the α and β subunits or between the M5, 6 and M9, 10 regions of the α subunit. When tryptic digestion is carried out on solubilized enzyme, WGA fractionation of fluorescein maleimide (FMI)-labeled tryptic fragments of detergent-solubilized H,K ATPase showed that a fragment Leu^{854} to Arg^{922} of the α subunit was bound to the β subunit, that is the region of the loop between TM7 and TM8.

Yeast two-hybrid analysis takes advantage of the split β-galactosidase nuclear transcription factor, so that a protein fragment expressed on the binding domain when it interacts with a protein fragment on the activating domain reconstitutes translation of the transcription factor with synthesis of β-galactosidase, a molecular method for detecting strong interaction between proteins or fragments of proteins. Analysis of α-β interaction by the yeast two-hybrid system of the two subunits of the H,K ATPase [49] showed that only the region containing a part of TM7, the loop and part of TM8 was capable of giving positive interaction signals with the ectodomain of the β subunit, in agreement with the data from digeston [48]. We deduced that there is strong interaction within the sequence Arg^{897} to Arg^{922} in the α subunit and the extracytoplasmic domain of the β subunit. Again, using yeast two-hybrid analysis, two different sequences in the β subunit – Gln^{64} to Val^{126} and Ala^{156} to Arg^{188} – were identified as containing association domains in the extracytoplasmic sequence of the β subunit. Figure 9 illustrates a model arising from these observations.

Role of the M5/M6 domain in cation transport

This region of the membrane domain of the enzyme may well be mobile and is thought to be intimately involved with the ion transport pathway. This is based on site-directed mutagenesis, extractability from trypsin-digested membranes and conformationally sensitive cutting sites at the N-terminal end of this region. It is also the effective covalent binding region for the active form of the PPI class of drug. These are thiophilic reagents and therefore can bind covalently to the –SH group of cysteines. There are two cysteines in the M5/M6 domain, at positions 813 and 822, and both seem to be involved in reaction with PPIs. Ion transport by H,K ATPase probably involves transport of H_3O^+ rather than H^+, since at high pH the bulky Na ion is transported by the enzyme. The maximal transport of

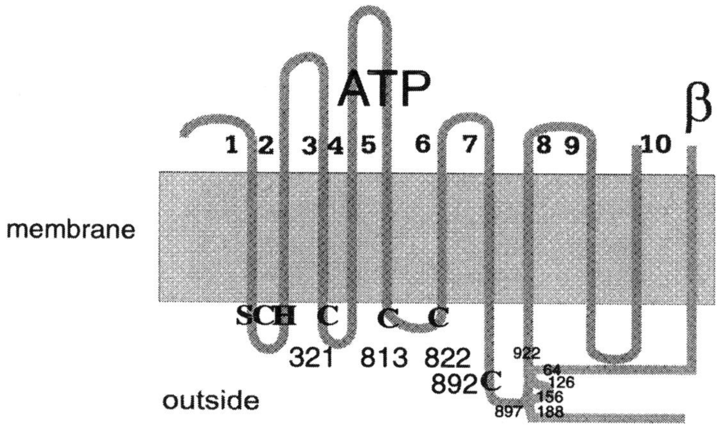

Figure 9. A schematic illustration of the regions of association between the α and β subunits of the H,K ATPase of gastric mucosa and the positions of the cysteines in the α sequence accessed by various proton pump inhibitors.

160 mM H_3O^+ is similar to the 160 mM Na^+ transported by the sodium pump and would account for the pH of 0.8 that can be achieved by the gastric acid pump [50].

Transmembrane insertion of the native M5 of either Na or H,K sequences does not occur in *in vitro* translation or in translation of truncated sequences of the ATPase in oocytes [42]. After digestion in the presence of K and removal of K, these segments are easily removed from the membrane domain both for the Na,K and H,K ATPases [51]. The M5/M6 region is also involved in inhibition of the Na pump by ouabain, distal to the TM1/2 site, where mutations confer ouabain resistance [52], or SCH28080 resistance in the H,K ATPase [53]. However, in the Na,K ATPase mutation of either proline in the sequence PLPL or the asparagine preceding this sequence permitted full membrane insertion but resulted in nonfunctional enzyme. This would suggest that the actual structure of M5/M6 is not a hairpin with two transmembrane segments but that the sequence PLPL results in a turn preventing full transmembrane insertion [54]. It is likely that M5 and M6 are membrane-inserted between other membrane peptide segments but not fully transmembraned to explain their ready extractability after trypsinolysis as compared with the other membrane segments, as suggested by the model of Figure 10. This structure is similar in concept to the structure proposed for the S4 segment of the shaker K channel, the movement of which is thought to gate this channel.

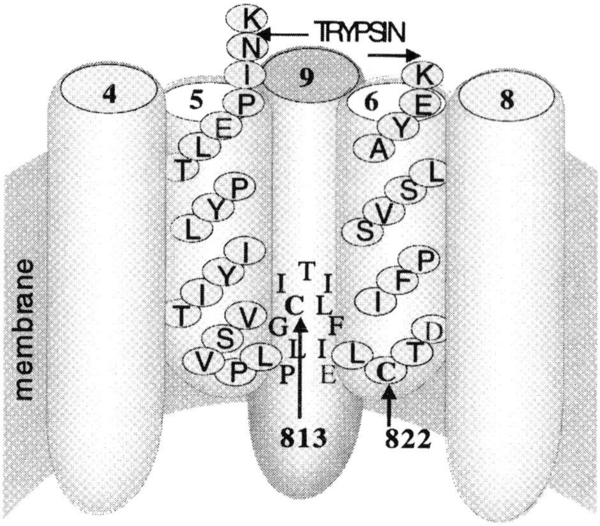

Figure 10. A tentative model of the M5 M6 region of H,K ATPase with only partial membrane insertion of these sequences enabling access of PPIs to both cys 813 and 822 and also placing the glutamate at position 820 at a boundary position prior to M6.

3D structure of P-type ATPases

The analysis of crystals of this type of pump is most advanced for the sr Ca ATPase and *Neurospora* H ATPase. Given that the transmembrane topology of these pumps is similar, it is likely that the analysis carried out on these pumps will apply in general to all P-type ATPases. Reconstruction of two-dimensional 2D crystals of Ca^{2+} ATPase showed that this P-type enzyme consisted of three distinct segments fitting into a box of 120 Å (height) × 50 Å (perpendicular to the dimer ribbons) × 85 Å (along the dimer ribbons). The enzyme has a highly asymmetric mass distribution across the lipid bilayer. The cytoplasmic region comprises ~70% of the total mass, whereas the luminal region takes up only ~5%. The cytoplasmic domain was shown to have a complex structure similar to the shape of the head and neck of a bird. The "head" is responsible for forming dimer ribbons and contains the ATP-binding domain. The "neck" represents the stalk domain about 25 Å long, consisting of two segments. Ten transmembrane segments could be discerned [55, 56]. This enzyme was in the E_2 conformation, whereas analysis of the *Neurospora* ATPase was of the enzyme in the E_1 conformation. If these two enzymes can be compared, it would appear that the cytoplasmic domain is extended in the E_1 form and contracted in the E_2 form.

The 2D crystal structure of H,K ATPase formed in an imidazole buffer containing HVO_4^- (vanadate, a Pi surrogate inhibitor) and Mg^{2+} ions was

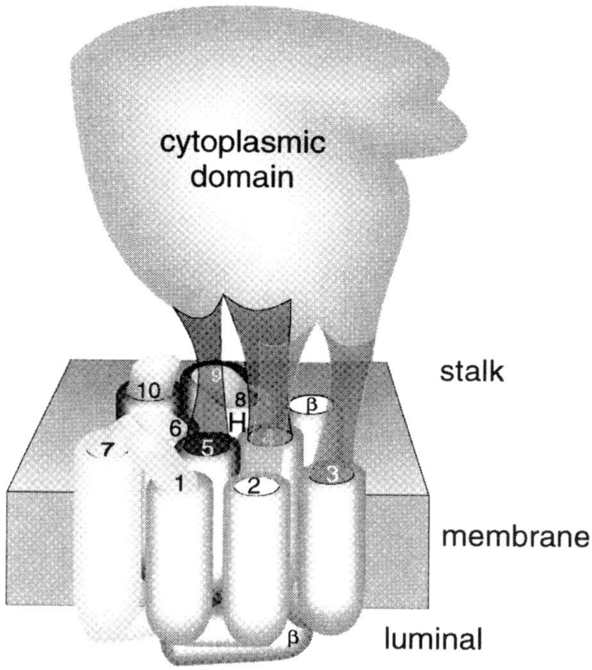

Figure 11. Schematic illustration of the domains of the gastric H,K ATPase, also showing a postulated arrangement for the 10 membrane segments of the α subunit and the single transmembrane domain of the β subunit. The positions as illustrated are derived from the crystals of the SR and *Neurospora* ATPases, analysis of α, β association, of M5/M6 with TM7-10, cross-linking of TM3-5 with M5/M6, nonconserved hydrophobic amino acids in TM1–3 and mutations in the TM4, M5/M6 and TM8 regions that affect ion transport.

resolved at about 25 Å. The average cell edge of the H,K ATPase was 115 Å, containing four asymmetric protein units of 50 Å × 30 Å, whereas the unit cell dimension of $Co(NH_3)_4$ATP-induced crystals of Na,K ATPase was 141 Å. This suggests a more compact packing of the H,K ATPase than the Ca ATPase or the Na,K ATPase.

Figure 11 shows the hypothetical arrangement of the protein of the H,K ATPase, providing a more refined model of the structure shown in Figure 1. The position of the membrane segments is derived from the structure of the crystals of the sr Ca and *Neurospora* H ATPases [55, 56] and from biochemical analysis of α, β association as well as α, α association.

A structure function model of the H,K ATPase

The above data show the presence of 10 membrane-spanning segments of the catalytic subunit of the H,K ATPase, and generally similar data have

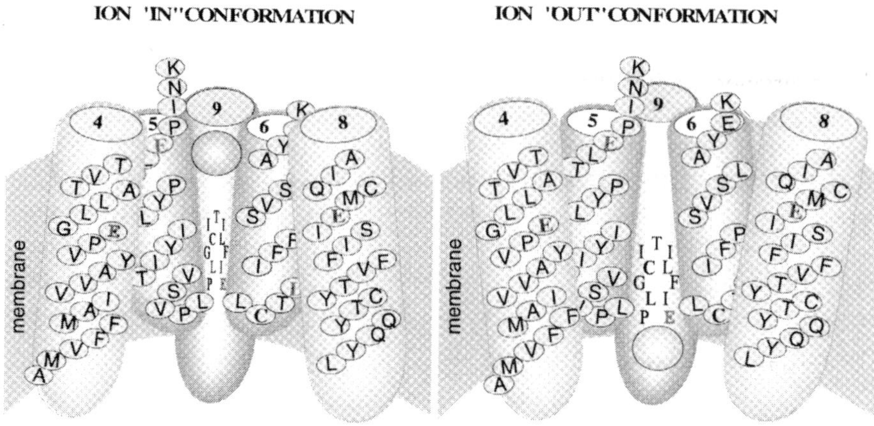

Figure 12. Magnification of the transport region of the H,K ATPase that includes TM4, M5, M6 and TM8. The binding of the ion (H_3O^+) in the "in" configuration allows ATP binding and protein phosphorylation. This changes the protein to the ion "out" conformation by altering the tilt of the four helices. From this form, H_3O^+ can be released, but binding of K is necessary to reverse the position of the ion-binding sites. The M5/M6 membrane sequences are membrane-inserted but not transmembrane segments, whereas TM4 and TM8 are transmembrane.

been found for the mammalian P-type family, consistent with those found for the Mg ATPase of *S. typhimurium* using a fusion protein approach [10]. The boundary amino acids of these transmembrane segments are defined by a combination of these techniques along with alignment with other P-type ATPases and molecular modeling. A model of the transport 4 transmembrane segment core structure is presented in Figure 12. The fourth, fifth, sixth and eight membrane segments of the α subunit are shown with TM9 at the back. Illustrated in this model is the putative transport pathway contained within these membrane segments. A series of site-directed mutagenesis studies in the Na,K and sr Ca ATPases have defined these regions (M4, 5, 6 and 8) as important for transport and occlusion [57, 58]. The ion "in" conformation is shown with ion binding in the region of these membrane segments close to the interface of the membrane domain and the stalk of Figure 11. A change of tilt in these segments places the ion-binding site at the outside face of this region of the pump.

H,K ATPase as a target for drugs

There are several isoforms of each of the mammalian ATPases, and even if largely homologous, there are sufficient differences in amino acid sequence to provide specificity of inhibitory agents. For example, the cardioglycosides such as digoxin have only one known target, the NaK ATPase, and thapsigargin the endoplasmic reticulum (ER), not the plasma membrane Ca ATPase. Bafilomycin targets only the V-type ATPases, and oligomycin largely F_1F_0 ATPase. There was thus good reason to expect that drugs targeted against the gastric H,K ATPase would have strict specificity if properly designed.

In 1968, SK & F initiated a program in Philadelphia for regulation of acid secretion by inhibiting the acid pump. A screen was set up using the K^+-stimulated pNPPase (a partial reaction of the H,K ATPase) as a target for a variety of compounds, and by 1971 some hits had been found by the group led by Virgil Wiebelhaus. However, the rapid progress in discovery of H_2-receptor antagonists led to the abandonment of the pump project in 1973.

In 1975, Astra Hässle in Göteborg, Sweden, synthesized pyridyl-2-methylsulfinyl-1*H*-benzimidazole and found that this was a potent inhibitor of acid secretion irrespective of the stimulatory pathway. This compound showed efficacy but also toxicity for the thyroid and the thymus. There was no understanding of either target or mechanism of reaction by 1977. In a meeting that year on acid secretion in Uppsala, Sweden, data were presented in the cross-reactivity of a polyclonal antibody against the gastric H,K ATPase, but whereas activity agains the thyroid was presented, no mention was made of thymus radial immunodiffusion recognition [59]. At the break, Eric Fellenius asked one of the authors of this and the succeeding chapter whether the antibody recognized anything in the thymus. The answer was that it did, and the question then arose whether the compound they were studying had as its target the gastric acid pump. This seemed an attractive hypothesis, since the compound was a weak base which would be expected to accumulate, like aminopyrine, in the active canaliculus of the parietal cell. Very recently it has been claimed that the α subunit of the H,K ATPase is expressed in the thymus, perhaps explaining these early observations [60]. A subsequent compound, picoprazole, was not thyrotoxic or thymotoxic to the same degree as this earlier, less neutral pH stable compound, timoprazole.

Some months later the compound was sent from Sweden and disappointingly was inactive against the pump when assayed at neutral pH. However, after finding out that the compound was acid labile, the correct experiments were done, and by 1978 activity was shown to be due to acid activation of the core structure. The key experiment was the demonstration that acid transport by H,K ATPase vesicles was inhibited only after a lag phase. Hence, inhibition was due to accumulation and acid activation to the active form [61]. It was also shown that these compounds bound covalently to the pump. Some time later, it was shown that the sulfenamide was the stable solution form after acid activation and considered responsible for inhibition of the acid pump [62]. The development of the PPI omeprazole was the result of mutual convictions and close interactions between preclinical research and development at Hässle and academic laboratories in the United States and Sweden.

Similar serendipity surrounded the discovery of the K-competitive class of compounds. In searching for effects of changes of intracellular Ca on acid secretion, it was recognized that a series of Ca-active drugs such as verapamil or *t*-butylamine had effects on acid secretion at concentrations at least 10-fold lower than those described on calcium. These effects turned out to be due to inhibition of the ATPase by K competition [63]. A drug being developed for secretory inhibition by Schering, an imidazo-1,2α pyridine, SCH28080, was then classified as a high-affinity K-competitive inhibitor of acid secretion, and further development of this class of anti-secretory agents continues [64].

The target amino acids in the gastric H,K ATPase

The three-dimensional structure of the pump is not known, and therefore cannot provide a template for design of specific inhibitory ligands. However, if an acid-activated compound generates a reactive inhibitor, it is possible to define the amino acids in proteins that are able to react under biological conditions. Whereas relatively harsh conditions are used for reaction with carboxylic acids, histidines, lysines, arginines and tyrosines, the most reactive amino acids under biological conditions are cysteines, by virtue of the higher reactivity of the –SH group. Given that an –SH reactive group has to be generated in the canalicular space, it is the cysteines accessible from the luminal space that are targets for thiol reactive (thiophilic) prodrugs. Cysteines of this nature are present between M3 and M4, M5 and M6, and M7 and M8, and all have been shown to react with one PPI or another. The cysteine at the end of M9 persists in nonreactivity to any reagent we have tried.

K^+-competitive ligands such as the imidazopyridines bind noncovalently, and their specific site of attachment is much harder to predict, since the region of the protein that binds K^+ or whose conformation prevents K^+ binding is not known. But when a photoaffinity derivative, such as an azido derivative of the methylated imidazopyridine, SCH 28080, is shown to have properties essentially identical to SCH 28080 and its binding site(s) is defined, this region of the ATPase is revealed [36] and turns out to be contained within the M1/M2 domain.

The inhibitory sites on ATPase are discussed in the next chapter.

Acknowledgements
Supported in part by NIH grant nos DK 46917, 41301 and 53462, and USVA SMI grant.

References

1 Forte JG, Ganser A, Beesley R, Forte TM (1975) Unique enzymes of purified microsomes from pig fundic mucosa. *Gastroenterology* 69: 175–189
2 Lee J, Simpson G, Scholes P (1974) An ATPase from dog gastric mucosa: changes of outer pH in suspensions of dog membrane vesicles accompanying ATP hydrolysis. *Biochem Biophys Res Commun* 60: 825–832
3 Sachs G, Chang HH, Rabon E, Schackman R, Lewin M, Saccomani G (1976) A nonelectrogenic H^+ pump in plasma membranes of hog stomach. *J Biol Chem* 251: 7690–7698
4 Berglind T, Dibona DR, Pace CS, Sachs GG (1980) ATP dependence of hydrogen ion secretion. *J Cell Biol* 85: 392–401
5 Fellenius E, Berglindh T, Sachs G, Olbe L, Elander B, Sjöstrand SE, Wallmark B (1981) Substituted benzimidazoles inhibit gastric acid secretion by blocking $(H^+ + K^+)$ATPase. *Nature* 290: 159–161
6 Wallmark B, Larsson H, Humble L (1985) The relationship between gastric acid secretion and gastric H^+, K^+-ATPase activity. *J Biol Chem* 260: 13681–13684
7 Glynn IM, Karlish SJ (1990) Occluded ions in active transport. *Ann Rev Biochem* 59: 171
8 Walderhaug, MO, Post RL, Saccomani G, Leonard RT, Briskin DP (1985) Structural relatedness of three ion-transport adenosine triphosphatases around their active sites of phosphorylation. *J Biol Chem* 260: 3852–3859
9 Melchers K, Weitzenegger T, Buhmann A, Steinhilber W, Sachs G, Schafer KP (1996) Cloning and membrane topology of a P type ATPase from *Helicobacter pylori*. *J Biol Chem* 271: 446–457
10 Smith DL, Tao T, Maguire ME (1993) Membrane topology of a P-type ATPase. The MgtB magnesium transport protein of *Salmonella typhimurium*. *J Biol Chem* 268: 22469–22479
11 Lutsenko S, Kaplan JH (1995) Organization of P-type ATPases: significance of structural diversity. *Biochemistry* 34: 15607–15613
12 Rabon EC, Reuben MA (1990) The mechanism and structure of the gastric H,K-ATPase. *Ann Rev Physiol* 52: 321–344
13 Shull GE (1990) cDNA cloning of the beta-subunit of the rat gastric H,K-ATPase. *J Biol Chem* 265: 12123–12126
14 Shull GE, Lingrel JB (1986) Molecular cloning of the rat stomach $(H^+ + K^+)$-ATPase. *J Biol Chem* 261: 16788–16791
15 Reuben MA, Lasater LS, Sachs G (1990) Characterization of a beta subunit of the gastric H+/K(+)-transporting ATPase. *Proc Natl Acad Sci USA* 87: 6767–6771
16 Post RL (1974) A reminiscence about sodium, potassium-ATPase. *Ann N Y Acad Sci* 242: 6–11
17 MacLennan DH, Brandl CJ, Coreczak B, Green NM (1985) Amino acid sequence of the Ca^{2+} Mg^{2+} dependent ATPase from rabbit muscle sarcoplasmic reticulum, deduced from its complementary DNA sequence. *Nature* 316: 696–700
18 Maeda M, Ishizaki J, Futai M (1988) cDNA cloning and sequence determination of pig gastric $(H^+ + K^+)$-ATPase. *Biochem Biophys Res Commun* 157: 203–209
19 Stewart B, Wallmark B, Sachs G (1981) The interaction of H+ and K+ with the partial reactions of gastric H,K-ATPase. *J Biol Chem* 256: 2682–2690
20 Rabon EC, Smillie K, Seru V, Rabon R (1993) Rubidium occlusion within tryptic peptides of the H,K-ATPase. *J Biol Chem* 268: 8012–8018
21 Lorentzon P, Sachs G, Wallmark B (1988) Inhibitory effects of cations on the gastric H^+,K^+-ATPase. A potential-sensitive step in the K^+ limb of the pump cycle. *J Biol Chem* 263: 10705–10710
22 Wallmark B, Stewart HB, Rabon E, Saccomani G, Sachs G (1980) The catalytic cycle of gastric $(H^+ + K^+)$-ATPase. *J Biol Chem* 255: 5313–5319
23 Rabon EC, McFall TL, Sachs G (1982) The gastric [H,K]ATPase: H^+/ATP stoichiometry. *J Biol Chem* 257: 6296–6299
24 Helander HF, Hirschowitz BI (1972) Quantitative ultrastructural studies on gastric parietal cells. *Gastroenterology* 63: 951–961
25 Gibert AJ, Hersey SJ (1982) Morphometric analysis of parietal cell membrane transformations in isolated gastric glands. *J Membr Biol* 67: 113–124
26 Forte TM, Machen TE, Forte JG (1977) Ultrastructural changes in oxyntic cells associated with secretory function. A membrane recycling hypothesis. *Gastroenterology* 73: 941

27 Wolosin JM, Forte JG (1984) Stimulation of oxyntic cell triggers K^+ and Cl^- conductances in apical H^+-K^+-ATPase membrane. *Am J Physiol* 246: C537–C545
28 Sachs G, Zeng N, Prinz C (1997) Physiology of isolated gastric endocrine cells. *Ann Rev Physiol* 59: 243–256
29 Im WB, Blakeman DP, Davis JP (1985) Irreversible inactivation of rat gastric (H^+-K^+)-ATPase *in vivo* by omeparzole. *Biochem Biophys Res Commun* 126: 78–82
30 Wallmark B, Larsson H, Humble L (1985) The relationship between gastric acid secretion and gastric H^+,K^+-ATPase activity. *J Biol Chem* 260: 13681–13684
31 Gedda K, Scott D, Besancon M et al (1995) Turnover of the gastric H^+,K^+-ATPase α subunit and its effect on inhibition of gastric acid secretion. *Gastroenterology* 109: 1134–1141
32 Maeda M, Tagaya M, Futai M (1988) Modification of gastric ($H^+ + K^+$)-ATPase with pyridoxal 5′-phosphate. *J Biol Chem* 263: 3652–3656
33 Xu K-Y (1989) Any of several lysines can react with 5′-isothiocyanatofluorescein to inactivate sodium and potassium ion activated adenosine triphosphatase. *Biochemistry* 28: 5764–5772
34 Besancon M, Shin JM, Mercier F, Munson K, Miller M, Hersey S, Sachs G (1993) Membrane topology and omeprazole labeling of the gastric H,K-adenosinetriphosphatase. *Biochemistry* 32: 2345–2355
35 Bamberg K, Sachs G (1994) Topological analysis of the HK ATPase using *in vitro* translation. *J Biol Chem* 269: 16909–16919
36 Munson KB, Gutierrez C, Balaji VN, Ramnarayan K, Sachs G (1991) Identification of an extracytoplasmic region of H^+,K^+-ATPase labeled by a K^+-competitive photoaffinity inhibitor. *J Biol Chem* 266: 18976–18988
37 Jewell EA, Lingrel JB (1993) Site-directed mutagenesis of the Na,K-ATPase. Consequences of the substitutions of negatively charged amino acids localized in the transmembrane domains. *Biochem* 32: 13523–13530
38 Swarts HG, Klaassen CH, de Boer M, Fransen JA, De Pont JJ (1996) Role of negatively charged residues in the fifth and sixth transmembrane domains of the catalytic subunit of gastric H+,K+-ATPase. *J Biol Chem* 271: 29764–29772
39 Rabon E, Sachs G, Bassilian S, Leach C, Keeling D (1991) A K^+-competitive fluorescent inhibitor of the H,K-ATPase. *J Biol Chem* 266: 12395–12401
40 Sachs G, Shin JM, Besancon M, Prinz C (1993) The continuing development of gastric acid pump inhibitors (lansoprazole). *Aliment Pharmacol Ther 7* (Suppl 1): 4–12
41 Besancon M, Simon A, Sachs G, Shin JM (1997) Sites of reaction of the gastric H,K-ATPase with extracytoplsmic thiol reagents. *J Biol Chem* 272: 22438–22446
42 Bamberg K, Sachs G (1994) Topological analysis of the HK ATPase using *in vitro* translation. *J Biol Chem* 269: 16909–16919
43 Hall K, Perez G, Mayer P, Gutierrez C, Munson K, Hersey, SJ, Kaplan JH, Sachs G (1990) Location of the carbohydrates present in the HK-ATPase vesicles isolated from hog gastric mucosa. *Biochemistry* 29: 701–706
44 Lemas MV, Hamrich M, Takeyasu K, Fambrough DM (1994) 26 Amino acids of an extracellular domain of the Na,K-ATPase alpha-subunit are sufficient for assembly with the Na,K-ATPase beta-subunit. *J Biol Chem* 269: 8255–8259
45 Beggah AT, Beguin P, Jaunin P, Peittshc MC, Geering K (1993) Hydrophobic C terminal amino acids in the β subunit are involved in assembly with the a subunit of Na,K ATPase. *Biochemistry* 32: 14117–14124
46 Horisberger JD, Jaunin P, Reuben MA, Lasater LS, Chow DC, Forte JG, Sachs G, Rossier BC, Geering K (1991) The H,K-ATPase beta-subunit can act as a surrogate for the beta-subunit of Na,K-pumps. *J Biol Chem* 266: 19131–19134
47 Gottardi CJ, Caplan MJ (1993) Molecular requirements for the cell-surface expression of multisubunit ion-transporting ATPases. *J Biol Chem* 268: 14342–14347
48 Shin JM, Sachs G (1996) Identification of a region of the H,K ATPase alpha subunit associated with the beta subunit. *J Biol Chem* 269: 8642–8646
49 Melle-Milovanovic D, Milovanovic M, Nagpal S, Sachs G, Shin JM (1998) Regions of association between the alpha and the beta subunit of the gastric H,K-ATPase. *J Biol Chem* 273: 11075–11081
50 Polvani C, Sachs G, Blostein R (1989) Sodium ions as substitutes for protons in the gastric H+K+-ATPase. *J Biol Chem* 264: 17854

51 Lutsenko S, Anderko R, Kaplan JH (1995) Membrane disposition of the M5-M6 hairpin of Na+,K(+)-ATPase alpha subunit is ligand dependent. *Proc Natl Acad Sci USA* 92(17): 7936–7940
52 Palasis M, Kuntzweiler TA, Arguello JM, Lingrel JB (1996) Ouabain interactions with the H5-H6 hairpin of the Na,K-ATPase reveal a possible inhibition mechanism via the cation binding domain. *J Biol Chem* 271: 14176–14182
53 Beguin P, Geering K (1997) Structural domain implication in ER degradation of alpha subunit of Na,K-ATPase. *Ann N Y Acad Sci* 834: 540–542
54 Lyu RM, Farley RA (1977) Amino acids Val115-Ile126 of rat gastric H(+)-K(+)-ATPase confer high affinity for SCH-28080 to (Na(+)-(K+)-ATPase. *Am J Physiol* 272: C1717–1725
55 Zhang P, Toyoshima C, Yonekra K, Green NM, Stokes DL (1998) Structure of the calcium pump from sarcoplasmic reticulum at 8A resolution. *Nature* 992: 835–839
56 Auer M, Scarbrough GA, Kuhlbrandt W (1998) Three dimensional map of the plasma membrane H^+ ATPase in the open conformation. *Nature* 392: 840–843
57 Feng J, Lingrel JB (1994) Analysis of amino acid residues in the H5-H6 transmembrane and extracellular domains of Na,K-ATPase alpha subunit identifies threonine 797 as a determinant of ouabain sensitivity. *Biochemistry* 33: 4218–4224
58 Clarke DM, Loo TW, MacLennan DM (1990) Functional consequences of alterations to polar amino acids located in the transmembrane domain of the Ca-ATPase of the sarcoplasmic reticulum. *J Biol Chem* 265: 6262–6267
59 Saccomani G, Crago S, Mihas A, Dailey DW, Sachs G (1978) Tissue and cell localization of hog gastrin plasma membrane by antibody techniques. *Acta Physiol Scand* Suppl: 1978: 293–305
60 Alderuccio F, Gleeson PA, Berzins SP, Martin M, Van Driel IR (1997) Toh BH Expression of the gastric H/K-ATPase alpha-subunit in the thymus may explain the dominant role of the beta-subunit in the pathogenesis of autoimmune gastritis. *Autoimmunity* 25: 167–175
61 Wallmark B, Sachs G, Mardh S, Fellenius E (1983) Inhibition of gastric hydrogen potassium ATPase by the substituted benzimidazole, picroprazole. *Biochim Biophys Acta* 728: 31–38
62 Brandstrom A, Lindberg P, Bergman N-A, Alminger T, Ankner K, Junggren U, Lamm B, Nordberg P, Erickson M, Grundevik I et al (1989) Chemical reactions of omeprazole and omeprazole analogues. I. A survey of the chemical transformations of omeprazole and its analogues. *Acta Chem Scand* 43: 536–611
63 Im WB, Blakeman DP, Mendlein J, Sachs G (1984) Inhibition of proton potassium ATPase and proton accumulation in hog gastric membranes by trifluoperaz, verapamil and 8 N,N-diethylaminooctyl-3,4-5-trimethoxybenzoate. *Biochim Biophys Acta* 770: 65–75
64 Wallmark B, Briving C, Fryklund J, Munson K, Jackson R, Mendlein J, Rabon E, Sachs G (1987) Inhibition of gastric H+,K+-ATPase and acid secretion by SCH 28080, a substituted pyridyl(1,2a)imidazole. *J Biol Chem* 262: 2077–2084

Proton Pump Inhibitors
ed. by L. Olbe

Inhibition of the gastric proton pump

Björn Wallmark[1] and George Sachs[2]

[1] *Astra Hässle AB, Preclinical R&D, S-431 83 Mölndal, Sweden*
[2] *UCLA, VA Wadsworth, Los Angeles, CA 90073, USA*

Introduction

For many years pharmacologists have utilized knowledge of the regulation of gastric acid secretion to discover and develop antisecretory agents. The first agents to emerge were the anticholinergic ones. These were associated with side effects, such as blurred vision, and also with a relatively modest level of efficacy. Success came with the discovery of histamine H_2-receptor antagonists, which were found to be both efficacious and selective. The introduction of these agents, in particular cimetidine, revolutionized the treatment of peptic ulcer disorders. Formerly, substantial efforts were also made to discover selective gastrin-receptor antagonists, since gastrin was known to play a central role in stimulating gastric acid secretion. Despite these efforts, no clinically useful agents of this type emerged. Only more recently have nonpeptide, selective CCK-B receptor subtype antagonists been synthesized and tested experimentally.

From many points of view, the gastric H^+,K^+-ATPase represents a unique molecular target for novel antisecretory agents:

- In contrast to its congeners, the ubiquitous Na,K^+-ATPase and Ca-ATPase, the H^+,K^+-ATPase is located in the apical (secretory) membrane of the parietal cell. Although other locations have been described in the kidneys and in the colon [1–3], the parietal cell has the highest density of H^+,K^+-ATPase and is consequently by far the most acidified location in the body during acid secretion. The secretory canaliculi of the parietal cell generate a primary acidity of about 160 mM HCl. This highly acidic environment can be used for selective targeting by inhibitors of the H^+,K^+-ATPase. Hence, drugs that are targeted for H^+,K^+-ATPase can be anticipated to be very selective in their action.
- The H^+,K^+-ATPase is the final common mediator of hydrochloric acid secretion. Thus, irrespective of the mechanism of activation of the parietal cell, cholinergic, histaminergic or gastrinergic, inhibition of H^+,K^+-ATPase will effectively prevent acid secretion from occurring.
- The H^+,K^+-ATPase is a unique enzyme and has biochemical properties that make it suitable for the selective targeting of antisecretory drugs.

These unique properties of the H^+,K^+-ATPase were instrumental in the discovery of selective drugs, as will be described below.

Classes of inhibitors of H^+,K^+-ATPase

Two very different approaches to inhibition of the H^+,K^+-ATPase exist today. By far the most well documented class of compounds is that of the substituted pyridinemethylsulphinylbenzimidazoles. These compounds covalently inhibit H^+,K^+-ATPase, which means that the pump is inhibited in an irreversible manner. Omeprazole, pantoprazole, lansoprazole, rabeprazole and others (see Fig. 1) belong to this class of agents.

The second class of agents comprises the reversible K-site antagonists of H^+,K^+-ATPase. These compounds have not reached regulatory approval and medical use. They differ from the covalent inhibitors in that they interact reversibly with H^+,K^+-ATPase. Therefore, the duration of their antisecretory effect is proportional to their elimination from plasma (Fig. 2).

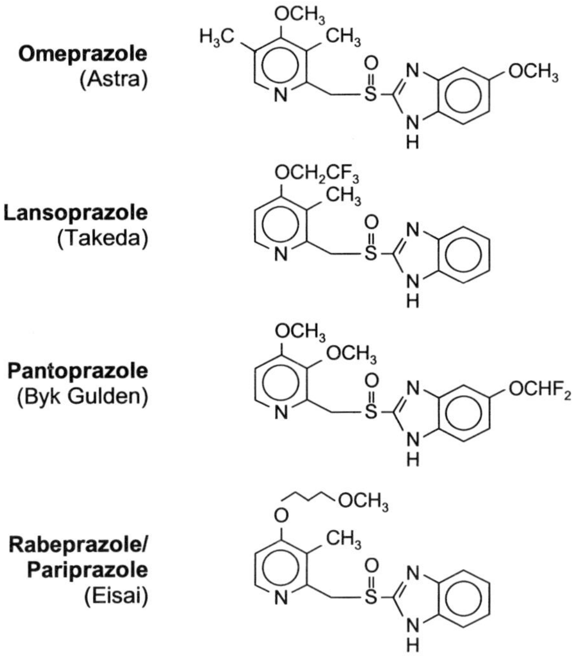

Figure 1. Structures of covalent inhibitors of H^+,K^+-ATPase inhibitors.

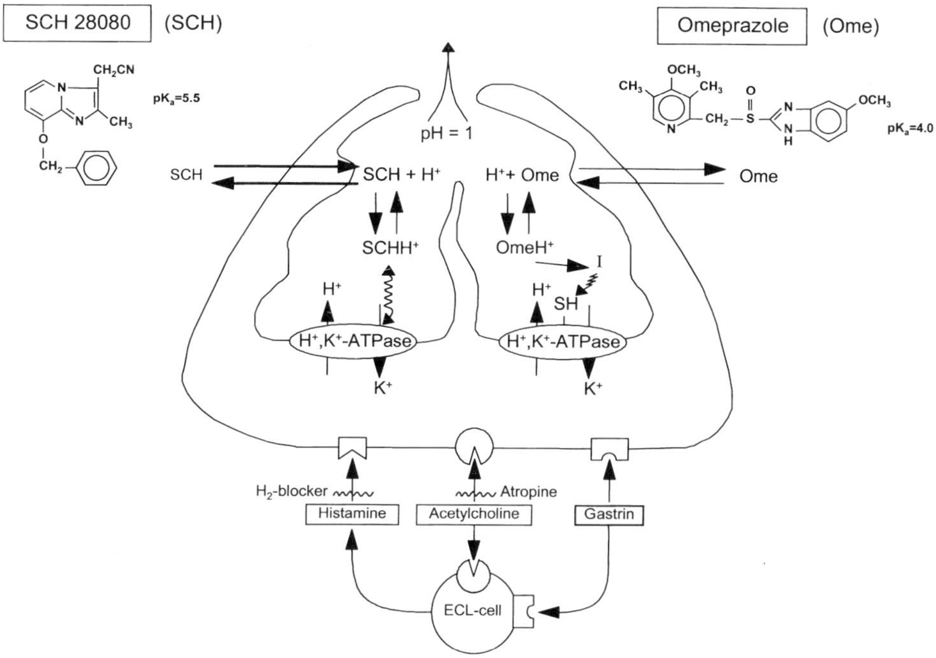

Figure 2. Mechanisms for secretagogue-induced acid secretion of the parietal cell and for inhibitory mechanisms of covalent omeprazole and reversible (SCH 28080) H^+,K^+-ATPase inhibitors.

Covalent H^+,K^+-ATPase inhibitors

Introduction

The discovery of the substituted pyridinemethylsulphinylbenzimidazoles as effective acid secretion inhibitors involved chemical substitution and screening in rats and dogs without prior knowledge of the molecular target. Substitutions on this core structure improved efficacy and reduced toxicity. For subsequent elucidation of the molecular mechanism of action, investigation of the *in vitro* pharmacological behavior (gastric glands and H^+,K^+-ATPase) and *in vitro* screening was of great importance, as outlined later in this chapter [4]. The following description of the molecular mechanisms of action will focus on omeprazole, since this compound is the most thoroughly documented and characterized.

The duration of the antisecretory effect was observed to be long, approximately 4 days in humans and dogs and 2 days in rats [5]. This should be compared with a terminal plasma half-life time of 1 h in these species. Thus, the active compound is retained at its site of action well after elimination of omeprazole or its metabolites from the blood compartment. We will now see how these pharmacological findings correlate with the molecular mechanism of action.

Mechanism of action of omeprazole

Omeprazole was found to inhibit both basal and stimulated acid secretion. In addition, the potency for inhibition of stimulated acid secretion was independent of the stimulus used [6, 7]. Furthermore, the level of antisecretory effect at any given time point after administration of omeprazole did not correlate to its plasma concentration. However, a strict correlation was found between the area under the plasma concentration curve (AUC) for omeprazole and the antisecretory effect. This indicates that the antisecretory effect is determined by the amount of omeprazole that reaches the target site rather than by the plasma concentration [6, 8].

A generalized model for the mechanism of action of H^+,K^+-ATPase inhibitors is found in Figure 2.

Evidence that the H^+,K^+-ATPase was the target enzyme for omeprazole came from autoradiographic studies in which the tubulovesicular and canalicular membranes of the parietal cell were selectively labeled from radiolabeled omeprazole. Other studies including monoclonal antibodies showed that these membrane structures harbor the H^+,K^+-ATPase [9–11]. Direct proof that omeprazole inhibited the H^+,K^+-ATPase under *in vivo* conditions came from studies in the rat in which a linear relationship was found between inhibition of the H^+,K^+-ATPase and acid secretion [12, 13]. Thus, both direct binding studies and measurements of H^+,K^+-ATPase activity provided strong evidence that omeprazole selectively inhibited acid secretion under *in vivo* conditions.

Omeprazole is a weak base, $pK_a = 4$ for the pyridine nitrogen, and this causes it to concentrate in the acidic locations of the parietal cell (Fig. 2). Given that the primary acidity generated by the parietal cell is 160 mM, the drug will be enriched at least 1000-fold in this acid compartment compared with compartments of physiological pH, such as plasma. In this manner, the very acidic compartment provides a trapping mechanism for omeprazole.

In vivo, it was found that reduction of acid secretion led to prevention of the inhibitory effect of omeprazole [13–15]. This confirmed *in vitro* experiments where it was found that neutralization of acid compartments in isolated gastric glands prevented acid-catalyzed conversion of omeprazole and its subsequent blockade of acid secretion [16]. In addition, in isolated gastric membranes containing the H^+,K^+-ATPase, neutralization of the acidic vesicle compartment prevented the inhibition normally observed after omeprazole [17, 18]. That omeprazole is targeted for the secretory canaliculus, rather than the cytoplasmic tubules, is illustrated in Figure 3 [19]. Under resting conditions, a low level of labeling was found both in cytoplasmic tubules and in the secretory canaliculus as a function of incubation time. This low level is probably due to the low basal rate of

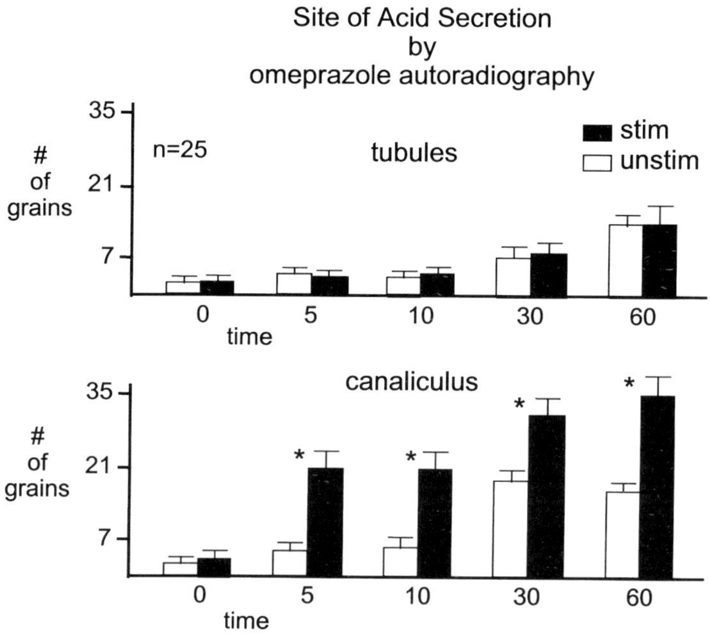

Figure 3. Radiolabeling from 3H-omeprazole in isolated resting and stimulated gastric glands.

secretion taking place under resting or nonstimulated conditions. During stimulation the situation is markedly different: with short incubation times labeling occurs predominantly in the secretory canaliculus; with longer incubation times the cytoplasmic vesicles are also labeled. This indicates internal recycling of the apical membrane pool.

All these experiments clearly indicate that acid-catalyzed conversion of omeprazole to an active inhibitor is a necessary prerequisite for inhibition of the H^+,K^+-ATPase.

The stoichiometry of binding has been investigated in a number of experimental settings. From *in vivo* labeling of the H^+,K^+-ATPase with ^{3}H-omeprazole, it was found that approximately 2 mol of radiolabel were bound per mole of active site. The active site concentration was estimated by phosphorylation from ^{32}P-ATP in the absence of potassium ions. Under those conditions, dephosphorylation is very slow, and the level of ^{32}P labeling can be used as a measure of the active-site concentration of the H^+,K^+-ATPase [15, 17, 18, 20].

The nature of the chemical reactions of omeprazole is outlined in Figure 4. This inhibitory mechanism has been deduced under different conditions and in different laboratories [21–25].

Under acid-catalyzed degradation of omeprazole, the inhibitory compound, the sulphenamide, has been isolated as an intermediate. The reaction leading to formation of the sulphenamide in acid involves nucleophilic

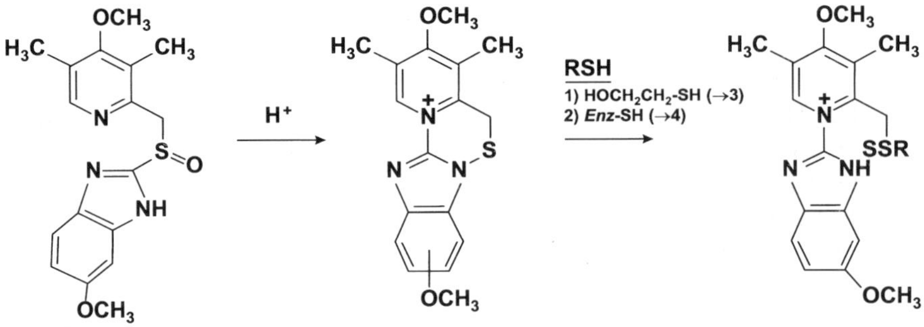

Figure 4. Acid catalyzed reactions of omeprazole and related compounds leading to inhibition of the H^+,K^+-ATPase.

attack by the unprotonated pyridine nitrogen atom on the benzimidazole 2 carbon atom. Substitutions that enhance the nucleophilicity (and also the pK_a) of the pyridine nitrogen will lead to faster formation of the tetracyclic sulphenamide.

The sulphenamide readily reacts with the purified H^+,K^+-ATPase and causes inhibition [16]. This inhibition can be both prevented and reversed by the addition of mercaptans, such as 2-mercaptoethanol or glutathione [15, 18]. The protection and reversibility of inhibition induced by exogenous mercaptanes indicated that the sulphenamide forms a disulphide linkage to a cysteine residue in the H^+,K^+-ATPase. Hence, the inhibitory bond is covalent. This explains not only why inhibited H^+,K^+-ATPase can be isolated under *in vivo* conditions but also why the anti-secretory effect persists well after the decline of plasma levels of omeprazole.

A very intriguing observation was that the sulphenamide was without inhibitory effect in more integrated biological preparations, such as isolated gastric glands [26]. There are several explanations for this. First, the sulphenamide is very labile at pH 7 and relatively stable at pH 1. Second, the compound is a permanent cation and will not penetrate biological membranes. Third, the sulphenamide will react with mercaptanes like glutathione in the cell cytoplasm. All these properties of the sulphenamide indicate that, in order for the compound to act *in vivo* as an inhibitor of H^+,K^+-ATPase, the following steps must take place:

- Omeprazole reaches the acidic compartments of the parietal cell after intestinal absorption into the bloodstream. Gastroprotection is essential for omeprazole to reach the duodenum for absorption.
- In the acidic compartments, omeprazole is concentrated and undergoes conversion to the active drug, the sulphenamide.
- The sulphenamide subsequently reacts with luminally accessible cysteine residues, forming a covalent inhibitory bond.

The location of the cysteines in the H^+,K^+-ATPase that react with the sulphenamide has been deduced in a series of experiments [27]. The H^+,K^+-ATPase contains 28 cysteine residues in its α subunit and 9 in the β subunit. The H^+,K^+-ATPase is a heterodimer of its α and β subunits, respectively. Under no experimental conditions has binding of the omeprazole-derived inhibitor been localized to the β subunit. This indicates that those cysteines are either oxidized or not sterically accessible for inhibition. It has been postulated, based on hydrophobicity analyses and other biochemical studies, that five cysteines in the α subunit would be accessible from the luminal phase of the membrane. These are cysteines 321, 813, 822, 892 and 981, located in the 3rd, 5th, 6th transmembrane segments, the hairpin loop between transmembrane segments 7 and 8 and at the end of transmembrane segment 9, respectively. In order to correlate binding of inhibitor to inhibition of the H^+,K^+-ATPase, acid-transporting membrane vesicles were used. It was found that labeling to cys 813 and cys 822 correlated with inhibition. Isolation and sequencing of the fragment containing the radioactive material defined binding to cys 813 in the TM5/6 domain (Fig. 5a).

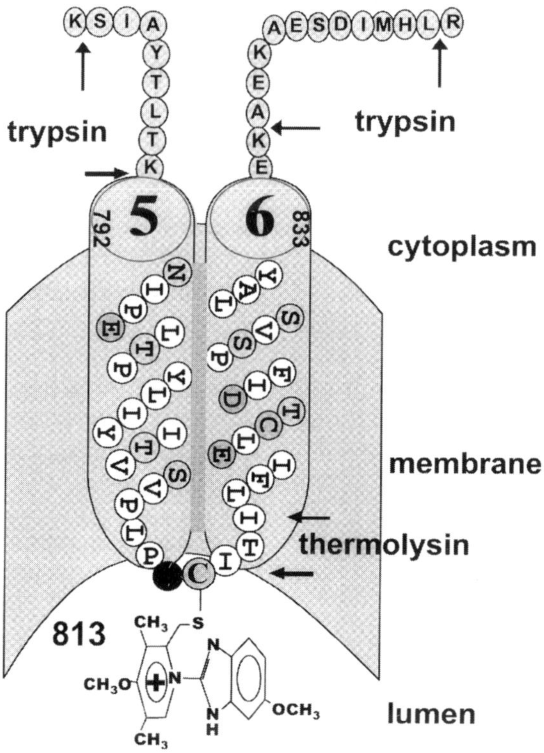

a

Figure 5a. Binding site of the omeprazole-derived sulphenamide in the TM5/TM6 luminal hairpin loop of the H^+,K^+-ATPase.

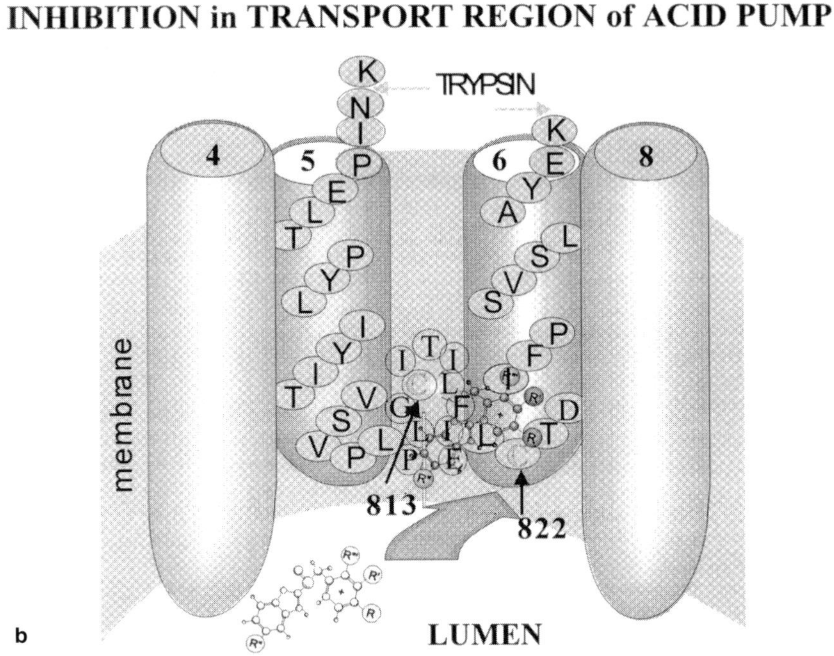

b

Figure 5b. Binding of sulphenamide derivatives to cysteins 813 and 822 in the luminal domain of the H^+,K^+-ATPase.

Figure 5 shows a model derived from the assumption that cys 813, the site of covalent binding of omeprazole, is the more exposed of the two cysteines in the M5/6 fragment. This model is similar to models proposed for this region in the Na, K and sacroplasmic reticular Ca ATPases. However, in a series of mutation experiments, cys 813 and cys 822 were converted to 813 thr and 822 gly, respectively, in an α-β fusion protein expressed in HEK 293 cells. These mutations did not affect the catalytic activity of the H^+,K^+-ATPase. In studies of 86Rb uptake with wild-type and mutated fusion proteins, acid-activated omeprazole failed to inhibit the 822 thr mutant but did inhibit the 813 gly mutant. The conclusions appear to contradict the results of chemical labeling. However, if both cysteines are accessible either to the protonated omeprazole or its sulfenamide derivative, the data can be reconciled. Pantoprazole had been shown to label both cysteines in the M5/6 region, showing that indeed these were both accessible [28]. Cys 822 is in a pocket between two carboxylic acids, which would be compatible with a binding site for a positively charged molecule such as K^+ or a protonated benzimidazole. If binding here is essential prior to covalent labeling, and the cys-gly mutation prevents benzimidazole binding, then removal of cys 822 would prevent omeprazole inhibition. Once docked at this site either cysteine could react, cys 813 being the preferred cysteine in the natural enzyme. Cys 822 or cys 321 might be the covalent site of modification of the cys 813 thr mutant. A model allowing access to both cysteines in M5/6 is shown in Figure 5b.

From the experiments described above, it can be concluded that the mechanism of action of omeprazole has been elucidated to a detailed molecular level. This forms the basis for our understanding of the unique selectivity of this class of agents.

Selectivity of action

It has been outlined elsewhere in this volume that the only major toxicological finding of omeprazole was enterochromaffin like (ECL) cell carcinoids in the rat. This finding relates to the reduction of gastric acid and the corresponding increase in gastrin levels, which in turn leads to the proliferation of gastric ECL cells. Hence, this is not an effect of the drug itself but a consequence of inhibition of gastric acid secretion. This has been shown in several studies where simply hypergastrinaemia exerted a similar effect on ECL cells. Isolated rat ECL cells respond to gastrin both by secretion of histamine and by growth. Omeprazole is without effect on these cells [29]. Omeprazole also exhibits a low side-effect profile in controlled clinical trials and in routine clinical use and has been shown to be well tolerated even at high doses.

In accordance with the above-described molecular mechanism of action of omeprazole, this favorable side-effect profile can be anticipated for the following reasons:

- The H^+,K^+-ATPase is uniquely located in the parietal cell and generates the most acidic compartment in the body.
- Omeprazole is concentrated in and converted by the acid in the parietal cell canaliculus to the active compound, the sulphenamide (the "prodrug" principle), which inhibits the H^+,K^+-ATPase. Other acidic compartments are not able to accumulate omeprazole, since their pH > 4.0.
- Once formed in the canaliculus, the sulphenamide cannot permeate into other compartments due to its positive charge and short half-life at higher pH.

Although the principles above appear to be logical design features for novel H^+,K^+-ATPase inhibitors and the patent literature describing compounds of this class is extensive, only four such compounds have found clinical utility today (Fig. 1). This implies that even though many compounds meet the basic design features of omeprazole, their intrinsic toxicity or pharmacokinetic properties are not satisfactory. The long period of research and development needed for omeprazole described elsewhere is indicative of the hurdles in this respect.

Duration of antisecretory effect

Omeprazole has a long duration of antisecretory effect. The duration is about 2 days in the rat and 4 days in the dog and humans [6, 8]. This implies that a certain level of inhibition of acid secretion will remain after the first dose upon administration of the second dose. Provided that a once-daily dose regimen is used, the antisecretory effect will therefore increase to a steady-state level during the first few days of use. However, irrespective of the length of treatment, the duration of antisecretory effect is the same [5]. This pharmacodynamic behavior of omeprazole allows convenient once-daily administration of omeprazole.

The mechanisms for the recovery of acid secretion following administration of omeprazole have been somewhat controversial. Since inhibition of acid secretion persists well after clearance of the drug, it would appear logical that *de novo* synthesis of H^+,K^+-ATPase is the major determinant of the antisecretory effect. This would imply that the rate of recovery is independent of the chemical substitution of the pyridine methylsuphinylbenzimidazole used. This has indeed been verified experimentally (Fig. 6a–c).

Rabeprazole has been claimed to exert a shorter duration of antisecretory effect compared with omeprazole. Clearly this is not the case, as may be seen in the *in vivo* experiments below. In order to correlate the turnover rate of H^+,K^+-ATPase to the duration of antisecretory effects, the half-life of the rat H^+,K^+-ATPase was determined and found to be 48 h. However, the half-life for recovery of H^+,K^+-ATPase activity in the same experimental setting was found to be 15 h [30]. This anomaly would imply that other

a

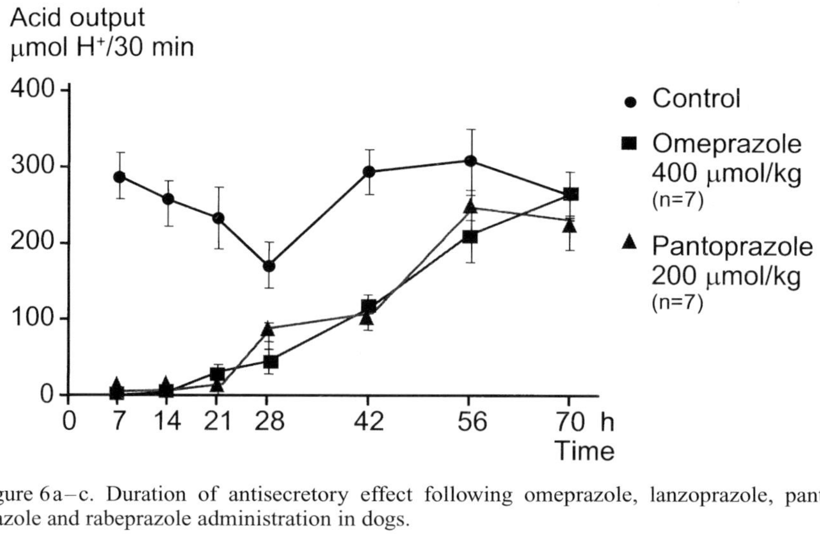

Figure 6a–c. Duration of antisecretory effect following omeprazole, lanzoprazole, pantoprazole and rabeprazole administration in dogs.

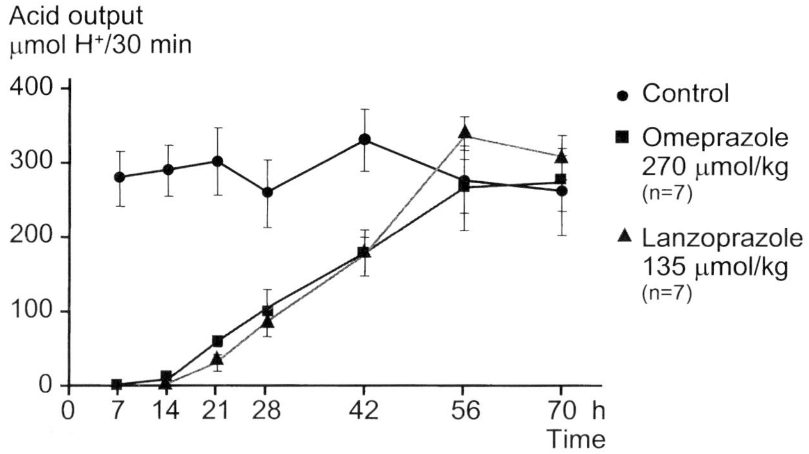

b

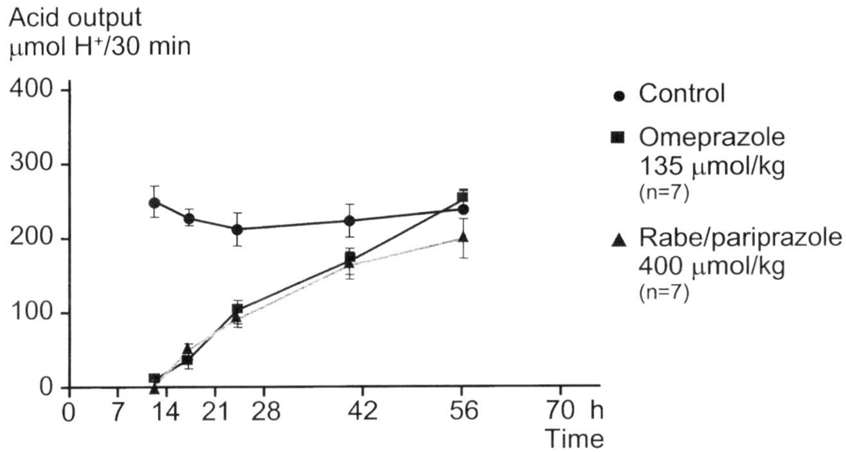

c

Figure 6b and c

mechanisms besides the turnover of H^+,K^+-ATPase would play an active role in the recovery of secretion. It has been speculated that breakage of the disulphide linkage between the sulphenamide and the extracytoplasmic cysteine(s) of the H^+,K^+-ATPase by endogenous mercaptanes like glutathione would be important in the recovery mechanism. Whatever the mechanisms for recovery, it is significant that the rate of recovery is very predictable irrespective of the length of treatment and the drug used.

Conclusions and future treatment perspectives

The introduction of safe long-acting covalent inhibitors of the H^+,K^+-ATPase has taken treatment of peptic ulcer disease forward, and the combination of omeprazole and antibiotics gives rapid symptom relief and high eradication rates of *Helicobacter pylori* infections, thereby providing a cure for the disease. In reflux disease, covalent H^+,K^+-ATPase blockers have provided a higher level of symptom relief and a higher level of healing in oesophagitis patients. The long duration of action allows convenient once-daily administration, and the specificity of omeprazole permits higher doses to be taken for long periods in severe cases without side effects.

With regard to the future treatment of peptic ulcer and reflux disease, several trends are apparent. In peptic ulcer disease, attempts are being made to discover new *Helicobacter pylori*-selective antimicrobial agents and therapeutic vaccines that are devoid of the resistance problems associated with today's agents. For reflux disease, new reversible H^+,K^+-ATPase inhibitors intended for use in symptomatic disease are being developed. These agents are targeted to protect patients at the time of their maximal exposure to acid reflux, such as after meals. Novel therapies aiming to correct lower oesophageal sphincter function are also under development. Hence, as for many other disease areas, more "tailor-made" remedies are likely to emerge and provide physicians and patients with better treatments.

References

1 Crawson MA, Shull GE (1992) Isolation and characterization of a cDNA encoding the putative distal colonic proton potassium ATPase: similarity of deduced animo acid sequence to proton potassium ATPase and sodium potassium ATPase and mRNA expression in distal colon and uterus. *J Biol Chem* 267: 13740–13748

2 Kraut JA, Starr F, Birmingham S, Sachs G, Reuben MA (1993) Expression of colonic and gastric hydrogen potassium ATPase mRNA in the rat kidney. *J Am Soc Nephrol* 4: 870

3 Wingo CS, Armitage FE (1993) Rubidium absorption and proton secretion by rabbit outer medullary collecting duct via H^+,K^+-ATPase. *Am J Physiol* 263: F849–857

4 Fellenius E, Berglindh T, Sachs G, Olbe L, Elander B, Sjöstrand SE, Wallmark B (1981) Substituted benzimidazoles inhibit gastric acid secretion by blocking (H^+,K^+) ATPase. *Nature* 290: 159–161

5 Carlsson E, Larsson H, Mattsson H, Ryberg B, Sundell G (1986) Pharmacology and toxicology of omeprazole with special reference to effects on the gastric mucosa. *Scand J Gastroenterol* 118 (Suppl): 31–38

6 Lind T, Cederberg C, Ekenved G, Haglund U, Olbe L (1983) Effect of omeprazole – a gastric proton pump inhibitor – on pentagastrin stimulated acid secretion in man. *Gut* 24: 270–276

7 Lind T, Cederberg C, Ekenved G, Olbe L (1986) Inhibition of basal and betazole- and sham feeding-induced acid secretion by omeprazole in man. *Scand J Gastroenterol* 21: 1004–1010

8 Larsson H, Carlsson E, Ljunggren U (1983) Inhibition of gastric acid secretion by omeprazole in the dog and rat. *Gastroenterology* 85: 900–907

9 Helander HF, Ramsey C-H, Regårdh C-G (1985) Localisation of omeprazole and metabolites in the mouse. *Scand J Gastroenterol* 20 (Suppl 108): 95–104

10 Fryklund J, Gedda K, Wallmark B (1988) Specific labeling of gastric H^+,K^+-ATPase by omeprazole. *Biochem Pharmacol* 37: 2543–2549

11 Smolka A, Helander HF, Sachs G (1983) Monoclonal antibodies against gastric H^+,K^+-ATPase. *Am J Physiol* 245: G589–596
12 Wallmark B, Larsson H, Humble L (1985) The relationship between gastric acid secretion and gastric H^+,K^+-ATPase activity. *J Biol Chem* 260: 13681–13684
13 Im WB, Blakeman DP, Davis JP (1985) Irreversible inactivation of rat gastric H^+,K^+-ATPase *in vivo* by omeprazole. *Biochem Biophys Res Commun* 126: 78–82
14 de Graaf J, Woursen-Colle M-L (1986) Influence of the stimulation state of the parietal cells in the inhibitory effect of omeprazole on gastric acid secretion in dogs. *Gastroenterology* 91: 333–337
15 Fryklund J, Helander HF, Elander B, Wallmark B (1988) Function and structure of parietal cells after H^+,K^+-ATPase blockade. *Am J Physiol* 254: G399–407
16 Wallmark B, Brändström A, Larsson H (1984) Evidence for acid-induced transformation of omeprazole into an active inhibitor of proton potassium ATPase within the parietal cell. *Biochim Biophys Acta* 778: 549–558
17 Keeling DJ, Fallowfield C, Underwood AH (1987) The specificity of omeprazole as an H^+,K^+-ATPase inhibitor depends upon the means of its activation. *Biochemical Pharmacology* 36: 399–344
18 Lorentzon P, Jackson R, Wallmark G, Sachs G (1987) Inhibition of H^+,K^+-ATPase by omeprazole in isolated gastric vesicles requires proton transport. *Biochim Biophys Acta* 897: 41–51
19 Scott DR, Helander HF, Hersey SJ, Sachs G (1993) The site of acid secretion in the mammalian parietal cell. *Biochim Biophys Acta* 1146: 73–80
20 Wallmark B, Stewart HB, Rabon E, Saccomani G, Sachs G (1980) The catalytic cycle of gastric H^+,K^+-ATPase. *J Biol Chem* 255: 5313–5319
21 Im WB, Sih JC, Blakeman DP, Mc Grath JP (1985) Omeprazole, a specific inhibitor of gastric H^+,K^+-ATPase is an H-activated oxidizing agent of sulphytyl groups. *J Biol Chem* 260: 4591–4571
22 Lindberg P, Nordberg P, Alminger T, Brändström A, Wallmark B (1986) The mechanism of action of the gastric acid secretion inhibitor omeprazole. *J Med Chem* 29: 1327–1329
23 Brändström A, Lindberg P, Bergman N-Å, Alminger T, Ankner K, Ljunggren U et al (1989) Chemical reactions of omeprazole analogues I–VI. (Six articles). *Aster Chemical Scandinavica* 43: 536–611
24 Figala V, Klemm K, Kohl B, Krüger U, Rainer G, Schaefer H et al (1986) Acid activation of H^+,K^+-ATPase inhibiting 2-[(2-pyridylmethyl)sulfinyl] benzimidazoles: isolation and characterization of the thiophilic "active principle" and its reactions. *J Chem Soc Chem Commun* 1: 125–127
25 Senn-Bilfinger J, Krüger U, Storm E, Figala V, Klemm K, Kohl B et al (1987) 1. H^+,K^+-ATPase inhibiting 2-[(2-pyridylmethyl)sulfinyl] benzimidazoles. 2. The reaction cascade induced by treatment with acids. Formation of 5H-pyrido-(1′,2′:4,5)(1,2,4,) thiadiazino (2,3-a) benzimidazol13-ium salts and their reaction with thiols. *J Org Chem* 52: 4573–4581
26 Lindberg P, Brändström A, Wallmark B, Mattsson H, Rikner L, Hoffmann K-J (1990) Omeprazole: the first proton pump inhibitor. *Med Res Rev* 10: 1–54
27 Lambrecht N, Corbett Z, Bayle D, Karlish SJD, Sachs G (1998) Identification of the site of inhibition by omeprazole of a $\alpha-\beta$ fusion protein of the H^+,K^+-ATPase using site-directed mutagnesis. *J Biol Chem* 273: 13719–13728
28 Sachs G, Shin JM, Besancon M, Prinz C (1993) The continuing development of gastric acid pump inhibitors. *Aliment Pharmacol Ther* 7 (Suppl 1): 4–12
29 Prinz C, Scott DR, Hurwitz D, Helander HF, Sachs G (1994) Gastrin effects on isolated rat enterochromaffinlike cells in primary culture. *Am J Physiol* 267: G663–G675
30 Gedda K, Scott D, Besancon M, Lorentzon P, Sachs G (1995) Turnover of the gastric H^+,K^+-adenosine triphosphatase α subunit and its effect on inhibition of rat gastric acid secretion. *Gastroenterology* 109: 1134–1141

The pharmacology of proton pump inhibitors

Proton Pump Inhibitors
ed. by L. Olbe

Inhibition of gastric acid secretion

Jia-Qing Huang and Richard H. Hunt

Division of Gastroenterology, Department of Medicine, McMaster University Medical Center, Hamilton, Ontario, Canada

Introduction

Gastric acid has been considered an important physiological factor in maintaining normal upper gastrointestinal functions since its presence in the stomach was first confirmed more than a century ago. Although its physiological role is not fully understood, classic studies have shown that gastric acid activates pepsin and initiates protein digestion, modulates gastrin release, facilitates calcium and iron absorption and also has protective action against a variety of bacterial infections. The regulation of gastric acid secretion is complex and involves extensive coordination between the gut and brain. Historical physiology studies have demonstrated that at least three types of receptors on the parietal cell are involved in the regulation of gastric acid secretion. Receptors are stimulated by acetylcholine through the neurocrine pathway (M3 receptors), by gastrin through a hormonal pathway (gastrin receptors) and by histamine through a paracrine pathway (histamine receptors) [1]. The relevance and importance of postreceptor interactions between these receptors have been discussed for many years; however, the H^+,K^+-ATPase or proton pump located in the secretory canaliculus of the parietal cell is recognized as the final pathway to acid secretion for these three receptors [2]. Abnormalities in acid secretion are associated with many diseases such as duodenal ulcer, Zollinger-Ellison syndrome and so on. Treatments to inhibit gastric acid secretion have been the mainstay of medical management for patients with peptic ulcer disease and gastroesophageal reflux disease and have proven to be very effective. Currently two major forms of antisecretory agents are used in clinical practice: the histamine H_2-receptor antagonists and the proton pump inhibitors (PPIs). However, proton pump inhibitors have been shown in numerous studies to be significantly better than H_2-receptor antagonists for inhibiting gastric acid secretion and superior in the treatment of acid-related diseases. The intention of this paper is to review mainly the effect of PPIs on gastric acid secretion, since the consequences of inhibition of gastric acid secretion and its relation with *Helicobacter pylori* infection are covered in other chapters.

Regulation of gastric acid secretion

Gastric acid is secreted from the parietal cells and pepsinogen from the chief cells in the gastric fundus in response to a variety of stimuli that originate in the central nervous system (CNS) and in the gastric and intestinal mucosa. Although many other peptides, prostanoids and cytokines may also play a role in regulating gastric acid secretion, histamine, acetylcholine and gastrin are considered the three principle stimuli to gastric acid secretion, whereas somatostatin serves as the most important inhibitor that modulates acid secretion. The many early descriptions of gastric acid secretion in physiological "phases" are no longer accurate, since our current understanding of the regulatory mechanisms suggest that both the brain and the gut actively and concurrently participate in all phases of the process of gastric acid secretion in response to meals. Therefore, the regulation of gastric acid secretion at all stages is a continuous, interactive and dynamic process [3].

Central Regulation

The CNS, primarily the dorsomotor nucleus of the vagus, the hypothalamus and the nucleus tractus solitarius, regulate activity of the parasympathetic outflow to the myenteric plexus in the gastric wall [3]. By modulating the activity of a variety of nuclei through chemical and peptide transmitters, the CNS regulates gastric acid secretion through a sophisticated network of afferent and efferent reflex circuits [4]. The sight, smell, taste or thought of food can stimulate gastric acid secretion to as much as 60% of the response seen with modified sham feeding [5]. Vagally stimulated gastrin release has also proved to play a role in the regulation of sham feeding-stimulated gastric acid secretion in animals [6].

Peripheral Regulation

The peripheral regulation of gastric acid secretion involves several mechanisms including neural, hormonal, paracrine and autocrine elements. The common goal of these regulatory mechanisms is to modulate gastric acid secretion by the parietal cell in response to different levels of stimuli such as acetylcholine, histamine and gastrin.

Muscarinic receptor
Acetylcholine is released from the postganglionic fibers of the enteric nervous system and regulates gastric acid secretion both by directly acting on the parietal cell and indirectly stimulating several endocrine cells, which in turn modulate the activity of the parietal cell [6]. Five subtypes of the

muscarinic receptor (M1–M5) have been cloned successfully [7, 8], but only the gene encoding the M3 receptor is expressed on the parietal cell [9, 10]. The action of the M3 receptor on the parietal cell depends upon the movement of intracellular Ca^{2+} in the parietal cell. Activation of the M3 receptor results in Ca^{2+} release from Ca^{2+} stores as well as Ca^{2+} entry into the cell, which may be activated by an alternative G protein coupled to the M3 receptor [11]. Atropine, a nonselective M receptor antagonist, given at high dose is able to inhibit acid secretion as effectively as H_2-receptor antagonists [12], whereas the possible mechanism by which the selective M1 receptor antagonist, pirenzipine, inhibits acid secretion is probably by interfering with either histamine release from the enterochromaffin like (ECL) cell or by preganglionic inhibition [13]. These results argue that both Ca^{2+} and cAMP (the second messenger for the H_2 receptor) are important factors in stimulating acid secretion.

Histamine receptor

Three known subtypes of histamine receptor have been identified in humans. The successful development of selective H_2RAs such as cimetidine, ranitidine, famotidine and nizatidine resulted in numerous clinical trials which confirmed the antisecretory effect and clinical value of H_2RAs in the management of acid-related diseases and also helped clarify some of the physiological pathways involved in the control of gastric acid secretion. H_2RAs markedly inhibit gastric acid secretion stimulated by histamine [14] and partially by cholinergic agents [15] or gastrin [16], suggesting that H_2RAs act directly on the parietal cell. Both vagal and gastrin stimulation of acid secretion is mediated in whole or in part by the release of histamine from the ECL cell. Two intracellular pathways are related to the activation of histamine-stimulated acid secretion: the cAMP and Ca^+ pathways [17–19].

Gastrin receptor

The presence of a gastrin receptor in the gastric mucosa was considered evidence for gastrin as the major mediator of acid secretion in the 1960s and 1970s [20], but this notion was soon disregarded following the discovery that the H_2RAs inhibited gastrin-stimulated acid secretion [16]. It appears that the major effect of gastrin on acid secretion is exerted through activation of the release of histamine from the ECL cell rather than by direct activation of the parietal cell, although an enriched population of gastrin-type binding sites exists on the parietal cell [21]. The gastrin receptor has also been successfully cloned from the parietal cells [22]. Activation of acid secretion is mediated by the gastrin receptor through a change in Ca^+ in individual parietal cells [23, 24], and activation of cAMP is dependent upon the change in cytosolic free Ca^+ [24]. However, since these experiments were performed without inhibition of the histamine receptor, a possible effect of H_2-receptor activity on the calcium response cannot be ruled out.

Gastric acid pump and H^+, K^+-ATPase

The discovery and increasing understanding of the importance of the H^+,K^+-ATPase in the late 1970s revolutionized our knowledge of the physiology of gastric acid secretion [25]. It is well accepted that the activation of H^+,K^+-ATPase is the final step in the stimulation of acid secretion and the specific PPIs, the substituted benzimidazoles, completely inhibit gastric acid secretion stimulated by cAMP and histamine [2].

Inhibition of gastric acid secretion

Many cells, pathways and receptors are involved in the regulation of acid secretion. Earlier antisecretory agents that regulate different receptors include those mediating muscarinic receptors (atropine and pirenzipine) and those targeting histamine receptors (cimetidine, ranitidine etc.). These drugs partially inhibit gastric acid secretion and are ineffective in overcoming acid secretion stimulated by a meal [26]. Four substituted benzimidazoles are now available for clinical use: omeprazole, lansoprazole, pantoprazole and rabeprazole [3, 27]. They all contain a pyridylmethylsulfinyl benzimidazole moiety but differ from each other due to substitutions on the pyridine or benzimidazole rings. They are all weak bases with a pK_a of about 4 and share a generally similar mechanism of action in the parietal cell. They are concentrated in the acidic compartment of the secretory canaliculus of the parietal cells and then undergo an acid-catalyzed transformation to a tetracyclic cationic sulfenamide. The sulfenamide reacts with specific cysteines, which results in inhibition of the H^+,K^+-ATPase proton pump [3, 27]. The binding is covalent with omeprazole, lansoprazole and pantoprazole, and inhibition of the activity of the acid pump is essentially irreversible; thus suppression of acid secretion is more complete than with other classes of antisecretory drugs. However, the substituted benzimidazoles bind only to those pumps that are actively secreting acid, sparing inactive pumps which are resting in the cytosol [27]. Inhibition of the secreting pumps results in an initially profound but transient elevation of intragastric pH. Recovery of acid secretion depends largely on the rate of *de novo* synthesis of new acid pumps and the breakdown of the covalent complex. When the drug concentration, after the first dose, has decreased to below threshold, any pumps which become inserted into the secretory canaliculus are able to secrete acid until the second dose. Newly active pumps are inhibited by the second dose, which also has a cumulative effect on the preexisting pumps, although this cumulative inhibition of acid secretion will eventually be balanced out by newly synthesized pumps. Therefore, intragastric acidity is rapidly restored after a single oral dose of PPIs. Twenty-four-hour gastric anacidity does not happen with single or even twice-daily oral administration of the PPIs. In order to achieve anacidity, continuous intravenous administration of PPIs may be needed. Full restoration of acid secretion generally occurs 72 h after the last dose of PPI [27]. Therefore, acid inhibition achieved by PPIs targeting the proton pump is more effective than that achieved by agents which target the parietal cell receptors.

Successful treatment of acid-related diseases is significantly correlated with suppression of 24-h gastric acid secretion [28–30]. Three key parameters which determine the effect of treatment with antisecretory drugs have been identified through a series of meta-analyses of pharmacodynamic gastric secretory studies and clinical therapeutic trials: the degree of suppression of acid secretion, the duration of acid suppression over the 24-h period and the length of therapy in weeks [28–30].

The effect of acid inhibition on peptic activity

The activation of pepsin is highly pH dependent. *In vitro* and *in vivo* peptic activity is virtually eliminated when pH is above 4 [31–33]. H_2RAs are not effective in suppressing peptic activity and pepsin secretion, as shown in many 24-h pH-monitoring studies [13, 34, 35]. This is because of their ineffectiveness in elevating and maintaining intragastric pH above 4. PPIs are strong acid-suppressing agents. The impact of PPIs on peptic activity can be by direct and indirect effects. PPIs decrease pepsin output and reduce the secretory volume, which directly inhibits peptic activity [36, 37], while effectively increasing intragastric pH to a level of pH > 4 indirectly eliminates almost all peptic activity [13]. This may explain partly the difference between PPIs and H_2RAs in healing peptic ulcer disease and erosive esophagitis, since for the majority of the 24 h when taking H_2RAs, the intragastric pH is still acidic enough to allow pepsin to have proteolytic activity, whereas the 24-h intragastric pH achieved with PPI essentially abolishes peptic activity.

Omeprazole

Omeprazole was the first of the PPIs shown to be superior to the H_2RAs in suppressing gastric acid secretion, and relieving symptoms and healing peptic ulcer disease [28–30, 38]. Results from two meta-analyses have shown a clear advantage for omeprazole over various dosing regimens of H_2RAs in the inhibition of 24-h intragastric acidity [28–30]. Omeprazole inhibits basal and maximum acid secretion stimulated by all known stimuli and in a dose-dependent manner, although there are marked variations in individual responses to omeprazole at lower doses of 5 to 10 mg [39, 40]. In an early report, Howden et al. studied the effects of single and repeated doses of omeprazole 10 mg on gastric acid secretion in six healthy volunteers [39]. Analyses of gastric acid secretion were performed on the first and seventh days of treatment, and results were compared with those obtained from a previous placebo study. After single doses of omeprazole, no significant changes in basal acid output (BAO) or pentagastrin-stimulated peak acid output (PAO) were seen compared with the results achieved with placebo. However, after 7 days of treatment, there was a significant reduction in BAO (93.1%) and in PAO (66.5%). Pharmacokinetic studies confirmed a significant increase in the bioavailability of omeprazole after repeated dosing, since the C_{max} increased significantly in all subjects from 92 μg/l on the first day to 193 μg/l on the seventh day as did the area under the plasma omeprazole concentration time curve (AUC) from 218 μg/l/h to 399 μg/l/h [39]. However, in another study, omeprazole at doses lower than 20 mg did not reduce pentagastrin-stimulated acid secretion in all patients even after 5 days of treatment [40].

Higher doses of omeprazole (20–80 mg daily) provide a much more predictable inhibition of 24-h intragastric acidity. For example, omeprazole 40 mg given in the morning or in the evening increased the median 24-h intragastric pH to 5.0 and 4.5 compared with 1.9 with placebo after 5 days of treatment in eight healthy volunteers in a cross-over study. This is equivalent to inhibition of hydrogen ion activity of >99% for both omeprazole regimens [41]. The increase in the antisecretory effect of omeprazole was due to increased absorption of the drug as measured by C_{max} and AUC [41]. This enhanced drug absorption may in part, be due to the pharmacological characteristics of omeprazole as an acid-labile compound such that its absorption increases as intragastric acidity decreases. Indeed, as reported in many other studies, the bioavailability of omeprazole increases with the duration of treatment. In healthy volunteers, the bioavailability of enteric-coated omeprazole 20 mg was 40% on the first day, increasing to 65% on the seventh day of dosing [42]. As opposed to H_2RAs, morning administration of omeprazole is better than evening dosing for suppressing 24-h intragastric acidity. Chiverton et al. found that, in patients with healed duodenal ulcer, omeprazole 20 mg given in the morning was considerably better than dosing in the evening for inhibiting gastric acid secretion [43]. The mean 24-h intragastric pH was 3.9 ± 1.8 for dosing in the morning, 2.9 ± 1.1 for the evening dose and 1.7 ± 0.1 for placebo ($p < 0.01$ between morning dose and placebo) [43].

In comparison with H_2RAs, omeprazole (>20 mg daily) has been shown, consistently and significantly, to be better than any recommended doses of H_2RAs in the suppression of gastric acid secretion [28–30]. In a 7-day randomized, double-blind, double-dummy study, the antisecretory effect of omeprazole 30 mg given in the morning was compared with ranitidine 150 mg bid in patients with duodenal ulcer [44]. On day 7 of the treatment, BAO and PAO were reduced by 98 and 80% in the omeprazole group, compared with 50 and 25% in the ranitidine group, respectively ($p = 0.015$ and < 0.001) [44]. This was also true when omeprazole was compared with other H_2RAs, such as cimetidine, famotidine and nizatidine [28–30, 38, 45].

The profound suppression of 24-h intragastric acidity has an important clinical relevance for the treatment of acid-related diseases [46, 47]. The healing of peptic ulcer and gastroesophageal reflux disease is correlated significantly with the degree and duration of suppression of gastric acid secretion over 24 h and the duration of antisecretory treatment [28–30, 48]. By plotting the frequency distribution of 24-h intragastric pH against the peptic activity curve, Hirschowitz et al. found that the majority of pH values achieved during treatment with cimetidine 1 g and ranitidine 300 mg daily were below 3, whereas omeprazole 30 mg daily consistently increased intragastric pH above 4, a pH at which peptic activity is essentially abolished [13]. This additional advantage of omeprazole over H_2RAs may be particularly relevant to healing both peptic ulcers and especially ulcerative esophagitis.

Recently, there have been studies suggesting that the antisecretory effect of a standard dose of omeprazole 20 mg is significantly greater in patients with *H. pylori* infection than in noninfected subjects or in those following eradication of the infection [49–54].

Lansoprazole

Lansoprazole, after oral administration, has a higher bioavailability and faster onset of antisecretory effect than omeprazole, although both agents have many similarities in structure and mechanisms of action [42, 55]. Results from pharmacokinetic and pharmacodynamic studies have shown that, after a single dose of lansoprazole, the absolute bioavailability was 81% for the 15-mg and 85–91% for the 30 mg doses, respectively [56, 57], and these remained steady after repeated dosing [56]. This has been confirmed in a recent study in healthy volunteers in whom once-daily lansoprazole 30 mg was given for 4 days, and the maximum antisecretory effect was obtained 6 h after the first dose and remained consistent with subsequent dosing [58].

In animal studies, lansoprazole 10 mg/kg inhibited histamine-, cAMP- and gastrin-stimulated gastric acid secretion in rats similarly to that achieved by omeprazole 30 mg/kg and to a greater extent than that achieved with ranitidine 100 mg/kg [59, 60]. The inhibitory potency was 2.4 and 16.1 times that of omeprazole and ranitidine, respectively [59, 60]. In healthy volunteers, lansoprazole inhibits basal and stimulated gastric acid secretion dose-dependently [61]. In an early study of the effect of different doses of lansoprazole (15, 30 and 60 mg given for 1 week) on BAO and gastrin-stimulated MAO, Müller et al. found a significant and dose-dependent decrease in BAO and MAO in all subjects (raw data for BAO were not given, Tab. 1) [62]. On day 2 and day 8, a significant decrease in MAO was

Table 1. Gastric acid secretion before, during and after dosing with three doses of lansoprazole

Lansoprazole	Day–7	Day 2	Day 8	Day 15
MAO (mmol H⁻/h)				
15 mg	23.3 ± 1.6	11.3 ± 1.9*	7.3 ± 1.9*	21.0 ± 2.1
30 mg	21.4 ± 2.3	4.1 ± 1.6*	2.2 ± 0.5*	20.1 ± 2.0
60 mg	23.8 ± 2.1	1.8 ± 0.5*	1.3 ± 0.4*	19.8 ± 2.5
Stimulated volume (ml/h)				
15 mg	227.6 ± 17.7	143.7 ± 22.2*	129.1 ± 19.1*	198.6 ± 27.2
30 mg	222.3 ± 22.7	179.2 ± 17.9*	71.8 ± 11.2*	219.5 ± 32.7
60 mg	271.0 ± 44.9	62.7 ± 15.4*	64.4 ± 11.6*	188.0 ± 27.2

* $p<0.05$ vs day–7. Raw data for BAO were not given. Data were extracted from ref. 62.

seen with all three doses of lansoprazole, and the reductions observed on day 8 were more pronounced compared with the pretreatment MAO (a fall of 94% for the 60-mg, 90% for the 30-mg and 69% for the 15-mg doses of lansoprazole, respectively). Together with the decrease in MAO, the volume of gastric secretion was also reduced significantly. All these changes returned to normal 1 week after discontinuation of treatment, suggesting the end of inhibition of acid secretion by lansoprazole [62]. In patients with healed duodenal ulcer and acid hypersecretion, lansoprazole also inhibited dose-dependently and significantly BAO and pentagastrin-stimulated PAO [63]. All three doses of lansoprazole (10, 20, and 30 mg administered as single doses in the evening) significantly inhibited PAO after the first dose on day 1 and repeated doses on day 7. However, it seems that lansoprazole at a dose of 10 mg did not sufficiently inhibit BAO even after repeated dosing for 7 days, whereas BAO was effectively suppressed by doses of 20 and 30 mg but only on day 7 [63]. This might have resulted from the different dosing schedule used in this study, since the rate of absorption and bioavailability of lansoprazole when administered in the morning were twice that seen with dosing in the evening [56]. Furthermore, when compared with placebo, lansoprazole given in the morning was significantly more effective in suppressing daytime acid secretion than dosing in the evening, as shown in a randomized double-blind study [64].

In comparison with H_2RAs or omeprazole 20 mg, lansoprazole 30 mg is significantly more effective in suppressing 24-h intragastric acidity in many comparative trials [65–69]. There is an apparent dose-dependent antisecretory effect for lansoprazole and omeprazole with a potency order of lansoprazole 30 mg ≡ omeprazole 40 mg > lansoprazole 15 mg ≡ omeprazole 20 mg [65, 66, 69]. The advantage of lansoprazole 30 mg over omeprazole 20 mg in suppressing 24-h gastric acid secretion is understandable, since after oral administration lansoprazole 30 mg has a better oral bioavailability (85–91%) [56, 57] than omeprazole 20 mg (35%) and it is also a higher dose [70]. This leads to a faster onset of action with lansoprazole than with omeprazole.

Several studies have compared the antisecretory effect of lansoprazole 60 mg with 30 mg, and two studies showed greater suppression of intragastric acidity with lansoprazole 60 mg over 30 mg [71, 72], while one study did not find any significant difference in the suppression of intragastric acidity between these two doses [73]. However, lansoprazole 60 mg was shown to be significantly better than lansoprazole 30 mg in reducing the volume of meal-stimulated gastric acid secretion and pepsin output [71], which may have additional benefits for patients with gastroesophageal reflux disease. In a comparative study of multiple doses of lansoprazole and omeprazole 20 mg bid, Timmer et al. showed that lansoprazole 30 mg bid had the best antisecretory profile in terms of the holding time that intragastric pH was above 5 [72], which has been considered an optimal intragastric pH for combination with antibiotics in the eradication of *H. pylori* infection [27].

Pantoprazole

Like omeprazole and lansoprazole, pantoprazole binds convalently to H^+,K^+-ATPase and irreversibly inhibits acid secretion by the proton pump. Although it shares many similarities in structure and mechanism of action with the former two PPIs, pantoprazole is chemically more stable than omeprazole or lansoprazole under near-neutral conditions [74]. This greater acid stability may improve tissue selectivity of the drug to the parietal cell, since it reduces the likelihood of the compound reacting with thiol group-containing proteins outside the parietal cell. After a single oral dose, pantoprazole 40 mg is absorbed rapidly with an average t_{max} of about 2.5 h although it is slightly longer than the t_{max} achieved with omeprazole (1–3 h) and lansoprazole (2 h) [75]. The absolute bioavailability of pantoprazole was reported to be 75–80% [42, 75], and this increases with repeated dosing. Pantoprazole also shows dose linearity and thus a predictable antisecretory effect [76].

Oral administration of pantoprazole (20–60 mg once daily) produces dose-dependent inhibition of 24-h intragastric acidity in healthy volunteers [74, 77], with minimal additional benefit at higher doses (80 and 120 mg) [77, 78]. One early cross-over study performed in 16 healthy volunteers compared the effect on intragastric pH of pantoprazole 20, 40 and 60 mg given in the morning for 5 days, and found that pantoprazole dose-dependently increased intragastric pH from pH 1.5 at baseline to pH 2.0 with 20 mg, and to pH 3.2 with 40 mg, and to pH 2.5 with the 60-mg dose, respectively. There was no significant difference between doses of 40 and 60 mg [77]. Another study compared the effects of pantoprazole 40 mg and 60 mg given for 5 days, with placebo on 24-h intragastric acidity [79]. On day 5, the median 24-h intragastric pH values were significantly different between placebo (pH 1.4) and pantoprazole 40 mg (pH 2.3) and pantoprazole 60 mg (3.5). The holding time for the intragastric pH above 3 was also significantly longer with pantoprazole 40 mg (33%) and 60 mg (58%), compared with placebo (14.9%). This was equivalent to a decrease in 24-h intragastric acidity of 87% with 40 mg and 99% with 60 mg of pantoprazole, respectively [79]. However, in a more recent study reported by Koop et al., pantoprazole 40, 80 and 120 mg were found to be equally effective at inhibiting gastric acid secretion [78]. In a review of the pantoprazole literature, Fitton and Wiseman found that the median 24-h intragastric pH achieved with repeated dosing of pantoprazole 40 mg was 2.3–4.3, suggesting a considerable variation in the antisecretory effect of pantoprazole after oral administration [74]. Like the former two PPIs, pantoprazole given in the morning is significantly better than dosing in the evening [80]. This difference, however, was due largely to a greater suppression of daytime gastric acid secretion obtained with the morning dose than with dosing in the evening [80].

In comparison with H_2RAs, pantoprazole 40 mg was significantly superior to ranitidine 300 mg once daily with inhibition of median 24-h intragastric pH (4.2 vs 2.7) and daytime pH (4.4 vs 2.0) in healthy volunteers, respectively [74]. In patients with grade II–III esophagitis, pantoprazole 40 mg was significantly better than ranitidine 150 mg bid, at increasing median intragastric pH and maintaining a longer holding time with intragastric pH above 4, although there was no significant difference in healing esophagitis probably due to the small number of patients [81]. When compared with the two former PPIs, pantoprazole 40 mg was as effective or better than omeprazole 20 mg, but no better than lansoprazole 30 mg on the first day of dosing due to its relatively slower onset of action [42, 82].

Rabeprazole

Rabeprazole is a new PPI that has been approved for clinical use in Japan and is undergoing late-phase clinical trials in Europe and North America. Although rabeprazole was designed to be more potent than omeprazole for suppressing gastric acid secretion, it appears to dissociate more quickly and completely from H^+,K^+-ATPase than omeprazole or lansoprazole, suggesting a partially reversible inhibition of the proton pump [83]. Currently, published information on rabeprazole is scarce and mainly comes from animal studies and a limited number of studies performed in humans which have been published in abstract form only [83].

In animal studies *in vitro*, rabeprazole was more potent than omeprazole at inhibiting the proton pump [84], but the duration of inhibition was considerably shorter than that seen with omeprazole [84] and lansoprazole due to the rapid dissociation from the proton pump [85]. In healthy volunteers, after single oral doses of rabeprazole 1–80 mg, the maximum plasma concentration and AUC values increased with increasing doses, but the t_{max} and plasma half-life ($t_{1/2}$) were not dose-dependent [86]. After a single dose of rabeprazole 20 mg, the C_{max} was 0.406 mg/l, t_{max} 3.1 h, AUC 0.809 mg/l, and the $t_{1/2}$ was 1.02 h in healthy volunteers [86].

The antisecretory effect of rabeprazole has been examined in several randomized, placebo controlled, cross-over studies [87–89]. In a 7-day study of the effect of different doses of rabeprazole on 24-h intragastric acidity, Blanshard et al. found that, on day 7, dosing with rabeprazole 10, 20 and 40 mg significantly decreased 24-h intragastric acidity compared with placebo. However, there was no significant difference among the three doses [87]. In another study involving 19 *H. pylori*-infected asymptomatic volunteers, rabeprazole at doses of 5, 10, 20 and 40 mg once daily was given orally for 7 days [88]. The 24-h intragastric acidity was monitored together with measurement of peptone meal-stimulated acid output. The authors found that BAO and the meal-stimulated acid output were significantly and dose-dependently suppressed by rabeprazole when compared with placebo on days 1 and 7, with the inhibition being pronounced on day 7. They also found that the half time for recovery of acid secretion was about 48 h with the 5-mg dose and longer for higher doses of rabeprazole [88]. In patients with reflux esophagitis, rabeprazole has been shown to be effective in normalizing acid reflux time over 24 h that esophageal pH was <4, with an increasing effect over the duration of treatment [90]. The 24-h intragastric pH increased with rabeprazole 20 mg from 1.86 at baseline to 3.71 on day 1 and 4.17 on day 7. With rabeprazole 40 mg, the intragastric pH increased from 2.01 to 4.37 on day 1 and 4.65 on day 7 [90]. Currently, there is only one published study comparing the antisecretory effect of rabeprazole with omeprazole and placebo in healthy volunteers [91]. The results show that rabeprazole 20 mg given orally in the morning has a faster onset of antisecretory activity than omeprazole 20 mg and produces a significantly greater decrease in 24-h intragastric acidity after a single dose of medication (406 mmol/l/h on day 1 with rabeprazole vs 660 mmol/l/h with omeprazole, $p < 0.001$) [91].

Summary and conclusions

Gastric acid plays an important role in maintaining normal upper gastrointestinal functions. Although the physiological mechanisms which regulate acid secretion are complex and involve many receptors, cells and pathways, the H^+,K^+-ATPase or proton pump is considered the final common pathway for the secretion of acid by the parietal cell. Inhibition of the proton pump markedly reduces gastric acid secretion stimulated by all known stimuli. Currently, four PPIs are available, and all have been proven very effective for suppressing intragastric acidity. However, variations exist in the rapidity of onset of action and the potency of acid inhibition after oral administration at the approved therapeutic doses, and these may speculatively have some clinical implications for the treatment of gastroesophageal reflux disease, and perhaps for eradicating *H. pylori* infection, when a PPI is given with antibiotics. Once-daily dosing in the morning is more effective than dosing in the evening for all the PPIs with respect to suppression of intragastric acidity and daytime gastric acid secretion, in particular, and this may be due to a better bioavailability achieved with morning dosing. When greater acid suppression from higher doses is needed, these drugs must be given twice daily to achieve the optimal suppression of 24-h intragastric acidity.

References

1 Shamburek RD, Schubert ML (1994) Structure and function of the stomach. Role of the proton pump. In: RH Hunt (ed): *Proton pump inhibitors and acid-related diseases*. Adis International, Osaka
2 Fellenius E, Berglindh T, Sachs G, Olbe L, Elander B, Sjostrand SE, Wallmark B (1981) Substituted benzimidazoles inhibit gastric acid secretion by blocking (H^+,K^+) ATPase. *Nature* 290: 159–161
3 Hersey SJ, Sachs G (1995) Gastric acid secretion. *Physiol Rev* 75(1): 155–189
4 Tache Y, Yang H (1990) Brain regulation of gastric acid secretion by peptides. *Ann N Y Acad Sci* 597: 128–145
5 Feldman M, Richardson CT (1986) Role of thought, sight, smell and taste of food in the cephalic phase of gastric acid secretion in humans. *Gastroenterology* 90(2): 428–433
6 DelValle J, Lucey MR, Yamada T (1995) Gastric secretion. In: T Yamada (ed): *Textbook of gastroenterology*, 2nd edn, JB Lippincott, Philadelphia, 295–326
7 Fukuda K, Kubo T, Akiba I, Maeda A, Mishina M, Numa S (1987) Molecular distinction between muscarinic acetylcholine receptor subtypes. *Nature* 327(6123): 623–625
8 Liao CF, Themmen AP, Joho R, Barberis C, Birnbaumer M, Birnbaumer L (1989) Molecular cloning and expression of a fifth muscarinic acetylcholine receptor. *J Biol Chem* 264(13): 7328–7337
9 Kajimura M, Reuben MA, Sachs G (1992) The muscarinic receptor gene expressed in rabbit parietal cells is the m3 subtype. *Gastroenterology* 103(3): 870–875
10 Pfeiffer A, Rochlitz H, Noelke B, Tacke R, Moser U, Mutschler E, Lambrecht G (1990) Muscarinic receptors mediating acid secretion in isolated rat gastric parietal cells are of M3 type. *Gastroenterology* 98(1): 218–222
11 Wilkes JM, Kajimura M, Scott DR, Hersey SJ, Sachs G (1991) Muscarinic responses of gastric parietal cells. *J Membr Biol* 122(2): 97–110
12 Hirschowitz BI, Sachs G (1969) Atropine inhibition of insulin-, histamine- and pentagastrin-stimulated gastric electrolyte and pepsin secretion in the dog. *Gastroenterology* 56(4): 693–702
13 Hirschowitz BI, Keeling D, Lewin M, Okabe S, Parsons M, Sewing K, Wallmark B, Sachs G (1995) Pharmacological aspects of acid secretion. *Dig Dis Sci* 40(2 Suppl): 3S–23S
14 Burland WL, Duncan WA, Hesselbo T, Mills JG, Sharpe PC, Haggie SJ, Wyllie JH (1975) Pharmacological evaluation of cimetidine, a new histamine H_2-receptor antagonist, in healthy man. *Br J Clin Pharmacol* 2(6): 481–486
15 Scholten T, Fritsch WP, Muller JE, Hengels KJ (1982) The inhibition of vagally stimulated acid secretion by pirenzepine and cimetidine. *Scand J Gastroenterol* Suppl 72: 169–171
16 Black JW, Duncan WA, Durant CJ, Ganellin CR, Parsons EM (1972) Definition and antagonism of histamine H_2-receptors. *Nature* 236(5347): 385–390
17 Chew CS, Hersey SJ, Sachs G, Berglindh T (1980) Histamine responsiveness of isolated gastric glands. *Am J Physiol* 238(4): G312–G320
18 Dickenson JM, Hill SJ (1992) Histamine H1-receptor-mediated calcium influx in DDT1MF-2 cells. *Biochem J* 284(Pt 2): 425–431
19 Negulescu PA, Machen TE (1988) Intracellular Ca^+ regulation during secretagogue stimulation of the parietal cell. *Am J Physiol* 254(1 Pt 1): C130–C140

20 Takeuchi K, Speir GR, Johnson LR (1979) Mucosal gastrin receptor. I. Assay standardization and fulfillment of receptor criteria. *Am J Physiol* 237(3): E284–E294

21 Soll AH, Amirian DA, Thomas LP, Reedy TJ, Elashoff JD (1984) Gastrin receptors on isolated canine parietal cells. *J Clin Invest* 73(5): 1434–1447

22 Kopin AS, Lee YM, McBride EW, Miller LJ, Lu M, Lin HY, Kolakowski LF Jr, Beinborn M (1992) Expression cloning and characterization of the canine parietal cell gastrin receptor. *Proc Natl Acad Sci USA* 89(8): 3605–3609

23 Cabero JL, Grapengiesser E, Gylfe E, Li ZQ, Mardh S (1992) Effects of gastrin on cytosolic free Ca^{2+} in individual, acid-secreting rat parietal cells. *Biochem Biophys Res Commun* 183(3): 1097–1102

24 Li ZQ, Mardh S (1996) Interactions between Ca^{2+}- and cAMP-dependent stimulatory pathways in parietal cells. *Biochim Biophys Acta* 1311(2): 133–142

25 Sachs G, Chang HH, Rabon E, Schackman R, Lewin M, Saccomani G (1976) A nonelectrogenic H^+ pump in plasma membranes of hog stomach. *J Biol Chem* 251(23): 7690–7698

26 Richardson CT, Bailey BA, Walsh JH, Fordtran JS (1975) The effect of an H_2-receptor antagonist on food-stimulated acid secretion, serum gastrin and gastric emptying in patients with duodenal ulcers. Comparison with an anticholinergic drug. *J Clin Invest* 55(3): 536–542

27 Sachs G (1997) Proton pump inhibitors and acid-related diseases. *Pharmacotherapy* 17(1): 22–37

28 Jones DB, Howden CW, Burget DW, Kerr GD, Hunt RH (1987) Acid suppression in duodenal ulcer: a meta-analysis to define optimal dosing with antisecretory drugs. *Gut* 28: 1120–1127

29 Burget DW, Chiverton SG, Hunt RH (1990) Is there an optimal degree of acid suppression for healing of duodenal ulcers? A model of the relationship between ulcer healing and acid suppression. *Gastroenterology* 99: 345–351

30 Howden CW, Hunt RH (1990) The relationship between suppression of acidity and gastric ulcer healing rates. *Aliment Pharmacol Ther* 4: 25–33

31 Frislid K, Berstad A (1986) Effect of ranitidine on meal-induced gastric pepsin and acid secretion and the influence of adding ethanol to the meal. *Scand J Gastroenterol* 21: 123–128

32 Gledhill T, Hunt RH (1985) The effect of H_2-receptor antagonists on pepsin secretion in man. *Prog Cli Biol Res* 173: 159–167

33 Goldberg HI, Dodds WJ, Gee S, Montgomery C, Zbroralske FF (1970) Role of acid and pepsin in acute experimental esophagitis. *Gastroenterology* 56(2): 223–230

34 Berstad A (1970) A modified hemoglobin substrate method for the estimation of pepsin in gastric juice. *Scand J Gastroenterol* 5: 343–348

35 Hollander F (1945) What is pH? An explanation of the various measures of acidity employed in gastroenterology. *Gastroenterology* 4: 497–508

36 Kittang E, Aadland E, Schjonsby H (1985) Effect of omeprazole on the secretion of intrinsic factor, gastric acid and pepsin in man. *Gut* 26(6): 594–598

37 Brunner G, Hell M, Hengels KJ, Hennig U, Fuchs W (1995) Influence of lansoprazole on intragastric 24-hour pH, meal-stimulated gastric acid secretion, and concentrations of gastrointestinal hormones and enzymes in serum and gastric juice in healthy volunteers. *Digestion* 56(2): 137–144

38 Wilde MI, McTavish D (1994) Omeprazole: an update of its pharmacology and therapeutic use in acid-related disorders. *Drug* 48(1): 91–132

39 Howden CW, Forrest JA, Meredith PA, Reid JL (1985) Antisecretory effect and oral pharmacokinetics following low dose omeprazole in man. *Br J Clin Pharmacol* 20(2): 137–139

40 Lind T, Cederberg C, Forssell H, Olausson M, Olbe L (1988) Relationship between reduction of gastric acid secretion and plasma gastrin concentration during omeprazole treatment. *Scand J Gastroenterol* 23(10): 1259–1266

41 Prichard PJ, Yeomans ND, Mihaly GW, Jones DB, Buckle PJ, Smallwood RA, Louis WJ (1985) Omeprazole: a study of its inhibition of gastric pH and oral pharmacokinetics after morning or evening dosage. *Gastroenterology* 88: 64–69

42 Andersson T (1996) Pharmacokinetics, metabolism and interactions of acid pump inhibitors: Focus on omeprazole, lansoprazole and pantoprazole. *Clin Pharmacokinet* 31(1): 9–28

43 Chiverton SG, Howden CW, Burget DW, Hunt RH (1992) Omeprazole (20 mg) daily given in the morning or evening: a comparison of effects on gastric acidity, and plasma gastrin and omeprazole concentration. *Aliment Pharmacol Ther* 6: 103–111

44 Lazzaroni M, Sangaletti O, Bianchi Porro G (1992) Gastric acid secretion and plasma gastrin during short-term treatment with omeprazole and ranitidine in duodenal ulcer patients. *Hepato-gastroenterol* 39: 366–370
45 Brummer RJ, Stockbrugger RW (1996) Effect of nizatidine 300 mg at night and omeprazole 20 mg in the morning on 24-hour intragastric pH and bacterial overgrowth in patients with acute duodenal ulcer. *Dig Dis Sci* 41 (10): 2048–2054
46 Huang JQ, Hunt RH (1996) pH, healing rate and symptom relief in acid-related diseases. *Yale J Biol Med* 69: 159–174
47 Hunt RH, Cederberg C, Dent J, Halter F, Howden C, Marks IN, Rune S, Walt RP (1995) Optimizing acid suppression for treatment of acid-related diseases. *Dig Dis Sci* 40 (2 Suppl): 24S–49S
48 Bell NJ, Burget D, Howden CW, Wilkinson J, Hunt RH (1992) Appropriate acid suppression for the management of gastro-oesophageal reflux disease. *Digestion* 51 (Suppl 1): 59–67
49 Verdu EF, Armstrong D, Fraser R, Viani F, Idstrom JP, Cederberg C, Blum AL (1995) Effect of *Helicobacter pylori* status on intragastric pH during treatment with omeprazole. *Gut* 36 (4): 539–543
50 Verdu EF, Armstrong D, Idstrom JP, Labenz J, Stolte M, Dorta G, Borsch G, Blum AL (1995) Effect of curing *Helicobacter pylori* infection on intragastric pH during treatment with omeprazole. *Gut* 37 (6): 743–748
51 Labenz J, Tillenburg B, Peitz U, Idstrom JP, Verdu EF, Stolte M, Borsch G, Blum AL (1996) *Helicobacter pylori* augments the pH-increasing effect of omeprazole in patients with duodenal ulcer. *Gastroenterology* 110 (3): 725–732
52 Verdu EF, Armstrong D, Idstrom JP, Labenz J, Stolte M, Borsch G, Blum AL (1996) Intragastric pH during treatment with omeprazole: role of *Helicobacter pylori* and *H. pylori*-associated gastritis. *Scand J Gastroenterol* 31 (12): 1151–1156
53 Smout AJPM (1998) Is the sensitivity to gastric acid inhibition *Helicobacter pylori* status-dependent? *Scand J Gastroenterol* Suppl 225: 32–35
54 Berčik P, Verdu EF, Armstrong D, Cederberg C, Idstrom JP, Stolte M, Blum AL (1997) Apparent increase in acid output during omeprazole (OME) after cure of *H. pylori* infection (HPI). *Gastroenterology* 112 (4): A70
55 Blum RA (1996) Lansoprazole and omeprazole in the treatment of acid peptic disorders. *Am J Health-Syst Pharm* 53: 1401–1415
56 Delhotal Landes B, Petite JP, Flouvat B (1995) Clinical pharmacokinetics of lansoprazole. *Clin Pharmacokinet* 28 (6): 458–470
57 Gerloff J, Mignot A, Barth H, Heintze K (1996) Pharmacokinetics and absolute bioavailability of lansoprazole. *Eur J Clin Pharmacol* 50 (4): 293–297
58 Bell NJV, Hunt RH (1996) Time to maximize effect of lansoprazole on gastric pH in normal male volunteers. *Aliment Pharmacol Ther* 10: 897–904
59 Nagaya H, Satoh H, Maki Y (1990) Possible mechanism for the inhibition of acid formation by the proton pump inhibitor AG-1749 in isolated canine parietal cells. *J Pharmacol Exp Ther* 252 (3): 1289–1295
60 Satoh H, Inatomi N, Nagaya H, Inada I, Nohara A, Nakamura N, Maki Y (1989) Antisecretory and antiulcer activities of a novel proton pump inhibitor AG-1749 in dogs and rats. *J Pharmacol Exp Ther* 48 (2): 806–815
61 Langtry HD, Wilde MI (1997) Lansoprazole: An update of its pharmacological properties and clinical efficacy in the management of acid-related disorders. *Drugs* 54 (3): 473–500
62 Müller P, Dammann HG, Leucht U, Simon B (1989) Human gastric acid secretion following repeated doses of AG-1749. *Aliment Pharmacol Ther* 3: 193–198
63 Berlin I, Molinier P, Duchier A, Courrel J, Dellatolas F, Duchier J (1992) Dose ranging study of lansoprazole, a new proton pump inhibitor, in patients with high gastric acid secretion. *Eur J Clin Pharmacol* 43: 117–119
64 Fraser AG, Sawyerr AM, Hudson M, Smith MSH, Pounder RE (1996) Morning vs evening dosing of lansoprazole 30 mg daily on twenty-four-hour intragastric acidity in healthy subjects. *Aliment Pharmacol Ther* 10: 523–527
65 Blum RA, Shi H, Karol MD, Greski-Rose PA, Hunt RH (1997) The comparative effects of lansoprazole, omeprazole, and ranitidine in suppressing gastric acid secretion. *Clin Ther* 19 (5): 1013–1023

66 Tolman KG, Sanders SW, Buchi KN, Karol MD, Jennings DE, Ringham GL (1997) The effects of oral doses of lansoprazole and omeprazole on gastric pH. *J Clin Gastroenterol* 24(2): 65–70
67 Takeda H, Hokari K, Asaka M (1995) Evaluation of the effect of lansoprazole in suppressing acid secretion using 24-hour intragastric pH monitoring. *J Clin Gastroenterol* 20(Suppl 1): S7–S9
68 Bruley des Varannes S, Levy P, Lartigue S, Dellatolas F, Lemaire M, Galmiche JP (1994) Comparison of lansoprazole with omeprazole on 24-hour intragastric pH, acid secretion and serum gastrin in healthy volunteers. *Aliment Pharmacol Ther* 8: 309–314
69 Dammann HG, Fuchs W, Richter G, Burkhardt F, Wolf N, Walter TA (1997) Lansoprazole vs omeprazole: influence on meal-stimulated gastric acid secretion. *Aliment Pharmacol Ther* 11: 359–364
70 Cederberg C, Andersson T, Skanberg I (1989) Omeprazole: pharmacokinetics and metabolism in man. *Scand J Gastroenterol* Suppl 166: 33–40
71 Brunner G, Hell M, Hengels KJ, Hennig U, Fuchs W (1995) Influence of lansoprazole on intragastric 24-hour pH, meal-stimulated gastric acid secretion, and concentrations of gastrointestinal hormones and enzymes in serum and gastric juice in healthy volunteers. *Digestion* 56(2): 137–144
72 Timmer W, Ripke H, Kleist P, Ehrlich A, Wieckhorst G, Lucker PW, Fuder H (1995) Effect of four lansoprazole dose levels and one dosage regimen of omeprazole on 24-hour intragastric pH in healthy subjects. *Methods Find Exp Clin Pharmacol* 17(7): 489–495
73 Dammann HG, von zur Muhlen A, Balks HJ, Damaschke A, Steinhoff J, Hennig U, Schwarz JA, Fuchs W (1993) The effects of lansoprazole, 30 or 60 mg daily, on intragastric pH and on endocrine function in healthy volunteers. *Aliment Pharmacol Ther* 7(2): 191–196
74 Fitton A, Wiseman L (1996) Pantoprazole: a review of its pharmacological properties and therapeutic use in acid-related disorders. *Drugs* 51(3): 460–482
75 Huber R, Kohl B, Sachs G, Senn-Bilfinger J, Simon WA, Strum E (1995) Review article: the continuing development of proton pump inhibitors with particular reference to pantoprazole. *Aliment Pharmacol Ther* 9: 363–378
76 Parsons ME (1996) Pantoprazole, a new proton-pump inhibitor, has a precise and predictable profile of activity. *Eur J Gastroenterol Hepatol* 8 (Suppl 1): S15–S20
77 Londong W (1994) Effect of pantoprazole on 24-h intragastric pH and serum gastrin in humans. *Aliment Pharmacol Ther* 8 (Suppl 1): 39–46
78 Koop H, Kuly S, Flüg M, Eissele R, Mönnikes H, Rose K, Lühmann R, Schneider A, Fischer R, Arnold R (1996) Intragastric pH and serum gastrin during administration of different doses of pantoprazole in healthy subjects. *Eur J Gastroenterol Hepatol* 8: 915–918
79 Hannan A, Weil J, Broom C, Walt RP (1992) Effects of oral pantoprazole on 24-hour intragastric acidity and plasma gastrin profiles. *Aliment Pharmacol Ther* 6: 373–380
80 Müssig S, Witzel L, Lühmann R, Schneider A (1997) Morning and evening administration of pantoprazole: a study to compare the effect on 24-hour intragastric pH. *Eur J Gastroenterol Heptaol* 9: 599–602
81 Armbrecht U, Abucar A, Hameeteman W, Schneider A, Stockbrügger RW (1997) Treatment of reflux oesophagitis of moderate and severe grade with ranitidine or pantoprazole comparison of 24-hour intragastric and esophageal pH. *Aliment Pharmacol Ther* 11: 959–965
82 Florent C, Forestier S (1997) Twenty-four-hour monitoring of intragastric acidity: comparison between lansoprazole 30 mg and pantoprazole 40 mg. *Eur J Gastroenterol Hepatol* 9(2): 195–200
83 Prakash A, Faulds D (1998) Rabeprazole. *Drugs* 55(2): 261–326
84 Fujisaki H, Oketani K, Shibata H, Murakami M, Fujimoto M, Wakabayashi T, Yamatsu I, Takeguchi N (1993) Inhibitory action of E3810 on $H^+,K(^+)$-ATPase and gastric acid secretion *in vitro*. *Nippon Yakurigaku Zasshi* 102(6): 389–397 [Article in Japanese]
85 Tomiyama Y, Morii M, Takeguchi N (1994) Specific proton pump inhibitors E3810 and lansoprazole affect the recovery process of gastric secretion in rats differently. *Biochem Pharmacol* 48(11): 2049–2055
86 Yasuda S, Ohnishi A, Ogawa T, Tomono Y, Hasegawa J, Nakai H, Shimamura Y, Morishita N (1994) Pharmacokinetic properties of E3810, a new proton pump inhibitor, in healthy male volunteers. *Int J Clin Pharmacol Ther* 32(9): 466–473

87 Blanshard C, Millson C, Sercombe J, Pounder RE (1996) The effects of rabeprazole on 24-hour intragastric acidity and plasma gastrin concentration in healthy subjects. *Gut* 39 (Suppl 3): A47 (299)

88 Kovacs TOG, Sytnik B, Humphries TJ, Walsh JH (1996) A low dose of a new proton pump inhibitor LY-30764 (E 3810) effectively inhibits acid secretion in humans. *Gastroenterology* 110(4): A161

89 Dammann HG, Burkhardt F, Bell NE, Bjaaland T (1996) Rabeprazole effectively inhibits 24 h H^+ activity and nocturnal acid secretion in healthy subjects. *Gut* 39 (Suppl 3): A47(295)

90 Robinson M, Maton PN, Rodriguez S, Greenwood B, Humphries TJ (1997) Effects of oral rabeprazole on oesophageal and gastric pH in patients with gastro-oesophageal reflux disease. *Aliment Pharmacol Ther* 11: 973–980

91 Williams M, Sercombe J, Pounder RE (1997) Comparison of the effect of rabeprazole and omeprazole on 24-hour intragastric acidity and plasma gastrin concentration in healthy subjects. *Am J Gastroenterol* 92(9): 1627 (abstract)

Proton Pump Inhibitors
ed. by L. Olbe

Consequences of gastric acid inhibition in animals

Enar Carlsson[1] and Niilo Havu[2]

[1] *ASTRA HÄSSLE, Preclinical Research, S-431 83 Mölndal, Sweden*
[2] *ASTRA, Safety Assessment, S-151 36 Södertälje, Sweden*

Introduction

Proton pump inhibitors (PPIs) such as omeprazole, lanzoprazole and pantoprazole are chemically characterized as substituted benzimidazoles. They are chemically relatively stable at neutral pH ($t_{1/2}$ = ~24 h), whereas at acidic pH they are labile and at pH ~ 1 the half-life is ~2 min.

Previous sections of this book have described in detail the mechanisms behind the inhibition of gastric acid secretion. In short, the specificity and selectivity of these products are governed by the following factors.

- The mother compounds are inactive.
- Due to the weak base properties, they are accumulated in the acidic compartments, the secretory cannaliculi of the parietal cell.
- In the acidic secretory cannaliculi the compounds are protonated and transformed to the corresponding sulphenamides.
- The sulphenamides bind covalently to the H^+,K^+-ATPase in the secretory membranes, inhibiting the proton transport.
- The H^+,K^+-ATPase is, except for the kidney, only localized to the parietal cell. *In vivo* the kidney H^+,H^+-ATPase is not inhibited by PPIs, probably due to the fact that there is no acidic milieu in the vicinity of the enzyme and thus no transformation to the active molecule, the sulphenamide.
- The plasma half-lives of the mother compounds are short (1–3 h) in relation to the dose interval (24 h) needed to control acid secretion day and night.

Taken together, their potency, specificity and selectivity make PPIs extremely useful for the treatment of acid-related disorders as well as ideal tools for studying the consequences of long-term acid inhibition both in animals and in humans.

References will mainly be made to omeprazole, the first and most widely documented PPI developed and used in the clinic. In most cases findings have been described and confirmed in studies with lanzoprazole and pantoprazole. Notes about the corresponding findings can be found in prescribing information and investigators' brochures for these products, but there are few publications in the literature.

Long-term studies (≥ 1 year) in dog, rat and mouse with omeprazole

In chronic toxicity studies oral doses of 40, 125 and 400 µmol/kg (14, 43 and 138 µg/kg) have been used in mice and rats, and 2, 16 and 80 µmol/kg (0.7, 5.5 and 28 mg/kg) in dogs [1]. In one additional oncogenicity study in female rats, 5, 10 and 40 µmol/kg (1.8, 3.5 and 14 mg/kg) were used [2]. On repeated daily administration of 40 µmol/kg and above to rats, a complete inhibition of stimulated acid secretion is found 2 h after dosing, whereas 20 to 60% inhibition depending on the dose still remains 24 h after dosing (Fig. 1). With 10 µmol/kg, about 80% inhibition is found 2 h after dosing at steady state during repeated administration.

In the dog, 2 µmol/kg administered orally results in about 90% inhibition of stimulated secretion 2 h after dosing, whereas 35% inhibition remains after 24 h. Doses of 16 and 80 µmol/kg result in 100% inhibition when measured 2 h after administration, and about 80% inhibition remains at 24 h (Fig. 2). With 0.5 µmol/kg administered orally, used in a study over 7 years in dogs, stimulated acid secretion is reduced to 50% 2 h after dosing, and about 20% inhibition remains 24 h later immediately before the next dose at steady state [3].

No tachyphylaxis has been observed in any species at repeated administration. In dogs the effects on acid secretion of daily oral administration have been recorded at intervals for 7 years without any significant change over the years [3]. Thus, these studies are well suited to answer questions about consequences of long-term acid inhibition in animals. The highest doses used in these studies render the test animals almost anacidic for the entire treatment period.

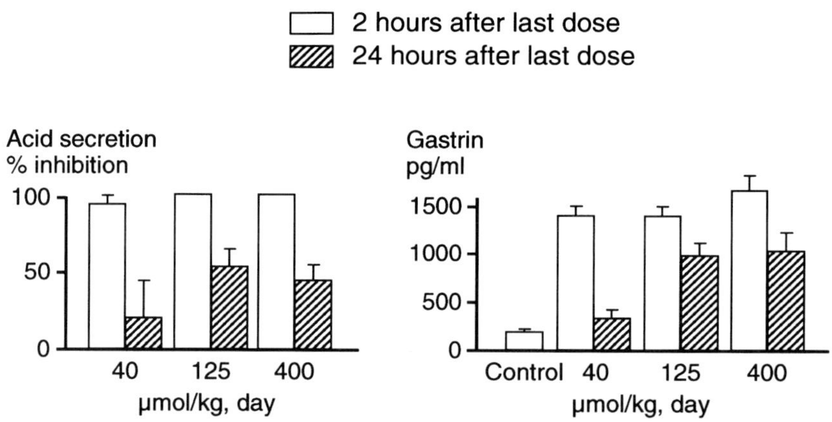

Figure 1. Inhibition of pentagastrin-stimulated acid secretion and plasma gastrin levels in female rats after daily administration of omeprazole ($n = 5$).

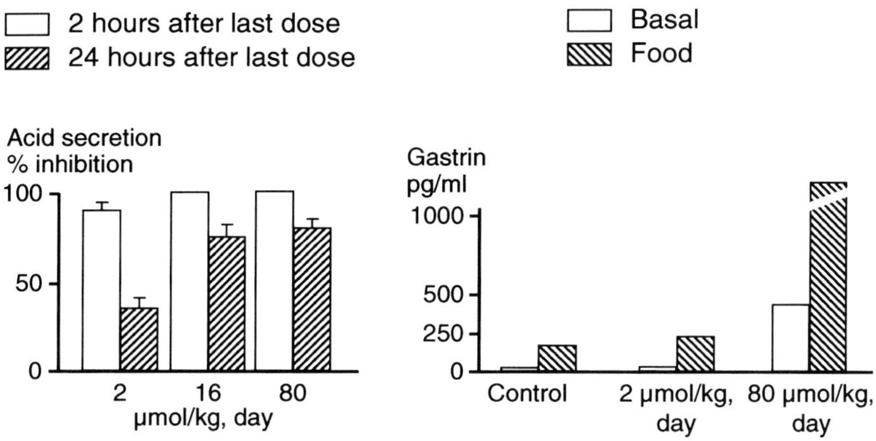

Figure 2. Inhibition of histamine-stimulated acid secretion (2 and 24 h after dosing) and plasma gastrin levels (basal and peak response to feeding 24 h after dosing) in dogs after daily administration of omeprazole ($n = 2–4$).

In the rat no abnormal clinical signs were observed in any of the studies. Food consumption, as well as growth rate and weight gain, was close to normal. Only in rats treated with the highest oral dose, 400 µmol/kg, was a slight but significant retarded growth rate observed. Dogs also showed no significant clinical findings, and food intake and weight gain were normal during treatment [1].

It appears that these animals tolerate situations close to anacidity in the stomach without any major effects on digestion of food or on nutrition.

In this context it is worth mentioning that rabbits seem to be the only species studied where efficient gastric acid inhibition has a significant clinical effect. Oral doses exceeding 80 µmol/kg and above causes decreased food and water intake after only a few days of treatment. These effects were associated with severe constipation. In this species gastric juice secretion, volume as well as acidity probably play an important role for the digestive function.

Gastrointestinal (GI) hormones

Gastrin

Hypergastrinaemia associated with gastric acid inhibition develops in both rats and dogs. Figure 1 shows inhibition of pentagastrin-stimulated acid secretion and plasma gastrin levels 2 and 24 h after dosing in rats. These animals had free access to food. Hypergastrinaemia was recorded after the three doses tested. Two hours after dosing, the lowest dose of omeprazole

40 µmol/kg seemed to induce a maximal gastrin level of about 1500 pg/ml as compared with about 200 pg/ml in controls. One day after dosing the gastrin levels were still significantly above controls in all dosage groups and five times controls after the two highest doses.

Thus it can be concluded that in long-term studies rats have had close to maximal gastrin levels for the entire treatment period – 2 years – which is close to the life span of these animals. Corresponding data regarding gastric acid inhibition and gastrin levels in dogs treated with the doses used in the long-term studies are shown in Figure 2. The inhibitory effects on acid secretion of the doses given to dogs were even more pronounced than the effects produced by the higher doses in rats. The gastrin response pattern in dogs differed from that in the rat. In spite of the pronounced effect on acid secretion with doses of 2 µmol/kg in dogs, neither basal nor food-stimulated gastrin levels differed from controls. Eighty µmol/kg produced pronounced hypergastrinaemia both in the basal state and after food intake. The difference between rats and dogs is most probably explained by the fact that the rat has food in the stomach constantly day and night, whereas dogs have food in the stomach only for a relatively short period of time after a meal. The conditions needed for gastrin release from G cells are high pH in combination with peptides and amino acids from food present in the stomach. This condition is fulfilled constantly day and night in freely fed rats during treatment but only after meals in the dog.

Similar experiments have not been conducted with mice, but analysis of gastrin in blood from treated animals indicates hypergastrinaemia after dosing with omeprazole. However, the duration of the hypergastrinaemia is shorter than in rats and does not cover 24 h. In a 10-week study of oral administration of 400 µmol/kg of omeprazole in rats, the hypergastrinaemia in blood was associated with a fourfold increased tissue concentration of gastrin in the antral mucosa of the animals [4].

Other GI hormones

In long-term studies (1 year or more) only gastrin has been analyzed. However, in the 10-week rat study mentioned above, three other regulatory peptides, enteroglucagon, somatostatin and pancreatic glucagon, were analyzed in blood plasma and in the antral and corpus mucosa tissue. The concentrations of these peptides in plasma did not change significantly, whereas the antral and corporal concentrations of somatostatin were significantly reduced. The content of vasoactive intestinal peptide (VIP), neuropeptide Y (NPY), calcitonine gene-related peptide (CGRP), peptide histidine isoleucine (PHI) and substance P did not change in either antrum or corpus during treatment in this study [4].

Macro- and microscopic findings

All changes related to treatment occurred in the gastric mucosa and were confined to the acid-secreting area.

The oxyntic mucosa showed a dose- and time-dependent hypertrophic gastropathy with mucosal thickening and folding due to the trophic gastrin effect (Fig. 3). The lack of acid stimulation caused disuse atrophy of the chief cells, sometimes with cystic dilation of glands (Fig. 3). Whereas mere mucosal thickening was common in rats, mucosal folding characterized the changes in dogs. These trophic effects explained the increases in stomach weight observed in rats and dogs. All changes were reversible and reverted to normal after treatment.

Except for the enterochromaffin-like (ECL) cells, the density of the different cell types seemed to be mainly unchanged, indicating a balanced, harmonic growth of the different cell types. This is also supported by the finding in the rat that the pepsinogen concentration in the oxyntic hypertrophic mucosa was the same as in the normal control mucosa [2].

The morphology of the different cell types, except for the chief cells in the rat, has also been found to be normal [1]. Some chief cells in rats after long-term treatment contain eosinophilic granules, an observation which has also been reported to occur after treatment with other inhibitors of gastric acid secretion, including H_2-receptor blockers [5].

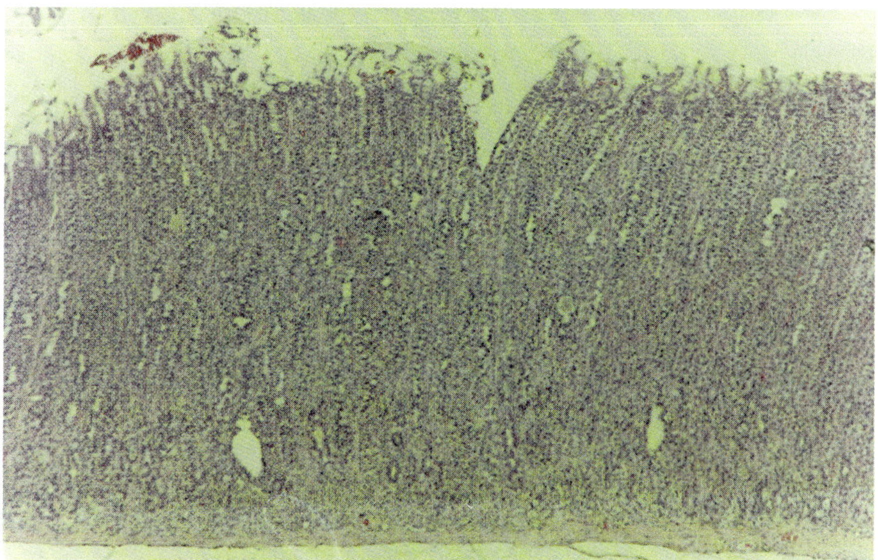

Figure 3. Micrograph of the corpus mucosa in a rat given omeprazole 125 µmol/kg daily for 1 year. HE (Hematoxylin Eosin) staining.

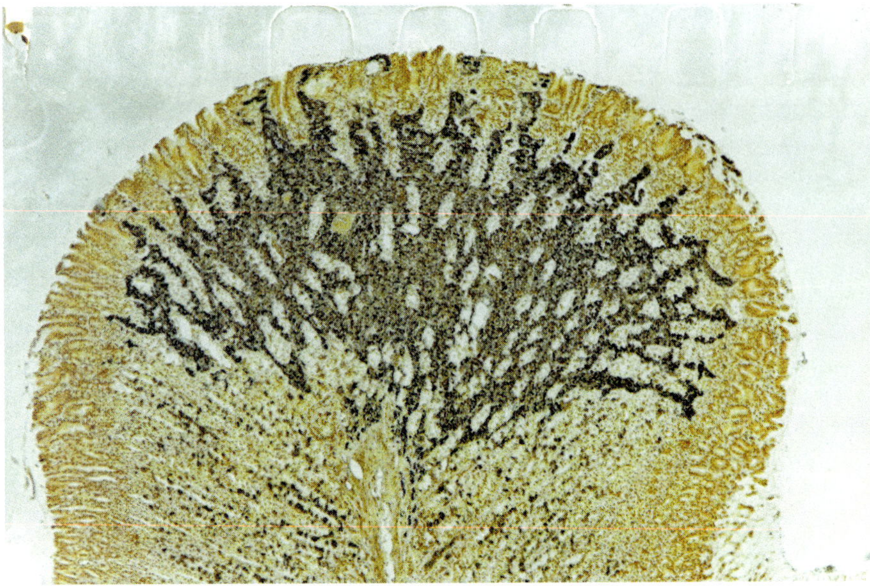

Figure 4. ECL-cell carcinoid in a rat treated with omeprazole 40 µmol/kg daily for 2 years, X53 Grimelius' stain.

Antrectomy prevents the hyperplastic/hypertrophic response in both rats and dogs [2].

ECL-cell hyperplasia and carcinoids

In 24-month rat studies ECL-cell carcinoids were found in the oxyntic mucosa of some rats (Fig. 4). Figure 5 shows the frequency of carcinoids (percentage of carcinoid-bearing rats) plotted against the dose in the two 24-month rat studies performed. There is a clear-cut dose response in both males and females, but the females develop carcinoids at lower doses and significantly more frequently than males. The carcinoids can be characterized as endlife tumours, since the earliest carcinoid was found in a rat treated for 82 weeks. These ECL-cell carcinoids were strictly localized to the oxyntic mucosa of the stomach without any metastases.

Furthermore, in the second of the two 24-month studies, rats treated for 1 year followed by another year without treatment were investigated. The dose was 40 µmol/kg, which after 2 years of treatment results in ECL-cell carcinoids in 25% of the animals. One year of treatment resulted in significant diffuse and also focal ECL-cell hyperplasia (Fig. 6), but no defined carcinoid. After an additional year without treatment, the oxyntic mucosa was normal both in terms of general morphology and in terms of ECL-cells

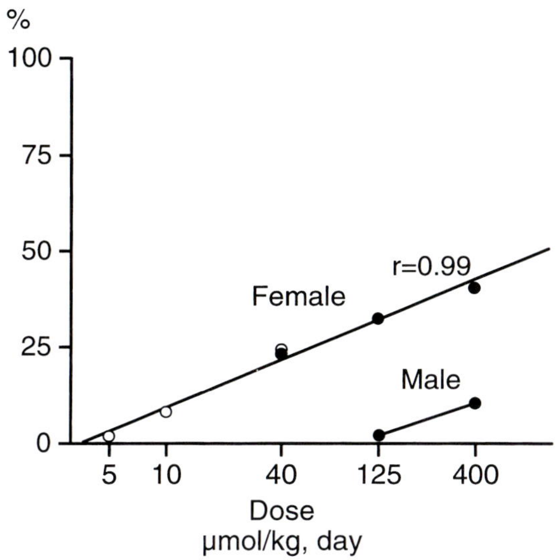

Figure 5. Correlation between frequency of ECL-cell carcinoids and dosage of omeprazole in the two oncogenicity studies (filled circles: first study; open circles: second study).

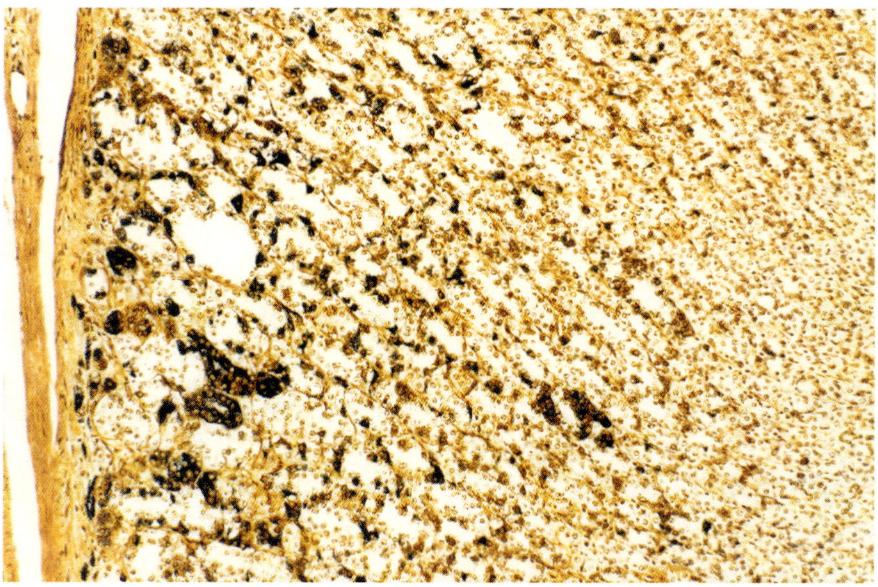

Figure 6. ECL-cell hyperplasia including focal hyperplasia in a rat treated with 40 μmol/kg daily for 1 year, X131 Sevier-Munger stain.

density, demonstrating the reversibility both of the general hypertrophy of the mucosa and of the ECL-cell hyperplasia, including focal changes [6]. It is worth mentioning that old, untreated female rats also demonstrate diffuse ECL-cell hyperplasia, and in rare cases ECL-cell carcinoids have been reported in untreated aged female rats [7]. This hyperplasia in senile animals has not been associated with hypergastrinaemia.

In long-term studies in dogs and mice diffuse ECL-cell hyperplasia has been observed and related to hypergastrinaemia, but carcinoids have not been found in these species following omeprazole treatment [1].

ECL-cell carcinoids in other long-term studies with acid secretion inhibitors and models with reduced acid secretion

In 1985 Poynter et al. reported gastric ECL-cell carcinoids in a lifelong carcinogenicity study of the long-acting H_2-receptor blocker loxtidine [8]. This compound also caused carcinoids in the gastric mucosa of mice treated long-term [9]. Gastric ECL-cell carcinoids have been described with the long-acting H_2-receptor blocker SK&F93479 [10], and the two PPIs lanzoprazole and pantoprazole have been reported to induce carcinoids as has the most widely used H_2-receptor blocker, ranitidine [5, 6]. Partially corpectomized rats (75% of the oxyntic mucosa removed) show significantly reduced acid secretion associated with hypergastrinaemia and development of both ECL-cell hyperplasia and ECL-cell carcinoids in the remaining part of the oxyntic mucosa [11]. The common feature of all these studies has been reduced acid secretion with secondary hypergastrinaemia. Antrectomy prevents ECL-cell hyperplasia [12] and probably carcinoid formation as well, although no lifelong studies have been performed in antrectomized rats.

In summary, long-term efficient reduction of acid secretion results in continuous, high concentrations of gastrin in the rat and periods of hypergastrinaemia after a meal in the dog. In both species hypergastrinaemia leads to general hypertrophy of the gastric mucosa. Both in rats and dogs diffuse ECL-cell hyperplasia has been observed. In addition, rats develop gastric ECL-cell carcinoids, characterized as end-of-life tumours.

All these changes except for the carcinoids have been shown to be reversible upon withdrawal of treatment and normalization of gastrin levels [6]. Whether carcinoids are also reversible has not been studied, since they occur very late during the life span of the rat.

Effect of hypergastrinaemia in other organs

Johnson et al. found mitotic effects of pentagastrin administration in several GI organs, including pancreas and colon [13]. None of the studies with high doses of omeprazole resulting in hypergastrinaemia have led to hypertrophic changes in these organs. Furthermore, omeprazole treatment and hypergastrinaemia did not influence either the growth rate or frequency of colonic tumours that developed after treatment with a carcinogen [14, 15]. These data are consistent with the findings of Oscarsson et al. demonstrating lack of effect of hypergastrinaemia beyond the oxyntic mucosa [16].

Observation *in vitro* indicates that pentagastrin might bind to colonic cell receptors and activate cell growth [17]. The discrepancy might be explained by the fact that the effects of endogenously released gastrin differ from those of pentagastrin [18]. On the other hand, progastrin-derived peptides have been found in human colonic carcinomas and may act as an autocrine trophic factor [19].

Does oxyntic mucosal hyperplasia result in hypersecretion of acid after withdrawal of treatment?

This question has been carefully studied in the dog. One year of treatment at a high dose of omeprazole (80 μmol/kg daily) resulted in hypertrophy of the oxyntic mucosa related to hypergastrinaemia that developed after the high dose [20, 21]. A moderate dose, 2 μmol/kg, had no histological effect. Acid secretion and morphology of the gastric mucosa were studied before the 1-year treatment period and then followed for 18 months after discontinued treatment. During this period basal as well as pentagastrin-stimulated secretion and morphology of the gastric mucosa were followed monthly.

Basal acid secretion returned to pretreatment values after 1 week and did not change significantly thereafter. On the other hand, the pentagastrin response in the high-dose group increased and reached a level significantly above the response before the 1-year treatment period, but gradually returned to the control level during the follow-up period. Morphology also returned to normal during the corresponding time. There was no increased response to pentagastrin in the low-dose group.

Thus, hypertrophy that develops secondary to pronounced acid inhibition and hypergastrinaemia was associated with an increased capacity to produce acid upon maximal stimulation. However, basal acid secretion is unchanged in spite of the increased hypertrophy and increased parietal cell mass. The changes were fully reversible.

Summary

Long-term studies with omeprazole and other long-acting inhibitors of gastric acid secretion have revealed the consequences of pronounced reduction of gastric acid secretion.

1. High doses rendering the experimental animals almost anacidic during the treatment period, 1–2 years, are well tolerated and have practically no effect on food intake or nutritional status.
2. The experimental animals develop hypergastrinaemia, but the pattern differs between rats and dogs. Rats demonstrate continuously high gastrin levels over 24 h whereas dogs show plasma gastrin peaks with high levels after food intake only. The tissue concentration of gastrin in antrum is increased, whereas a reciprocal decrease of somatostatin is found.
3. Hypergastrinaemia results in hypertrophy of the oxyntic mucosa, manifested in the rat mainly as increased mucosal height and in the dog also by increased folding.
4. Hypergastrinaemia also results in ECL-cell hyperplasia in rats, dogs and mice. In the rat this ECL-cell hyperplasia proceeds to ECL-cell carcinoids in some animals.
5. Both general mucosal hypertrophy and ECL-cell hyperplasia are fully reversible after normalization of acid secretion and gastrin levels.
6. In the dog hypertrophy of the oxyntic mucosa has been found to be associated to an increased capacity to secrete acid upon maximal stimulation with pentagastrin. Unstimulated, basal levels were not influenced.
7. The gastrin effects were all confined to the oxyntic mucosa without any effects in other organs, such as colon or pancreas.

References

1 Ekman L, Hansson E, Havu N, Carlsson E, Lundberg C (1985) Toxicological studies on omeprazole. *Scand J Gastroenterol* 20(Suppl 108): 53–69

2 Carlsson E (1989) A review of the effects of long-term acid inhibition in animals. *Scand J Gastroenterol* 24(Suppl 166): 19–23

3 Säfholm C, Havu N, Forssell H, Sundell G, Mattson H (1994) Effect of 7 years' daily oral administration of omeprazole to beagle dogs. *Digestion* 55: 139–147

4 Allen JM, Bishop AE, Daly MJ, Larsson H, Carlsson E, Polak JM, Bloom SR (1986) Effect of inhibition of acid secretion on the regulatory peptides in the rat stomach. *Gastroenterology* 90: 970–977

5 Havu N, Mattsson H, Ekman L, Carlsson E (1990) Enterochromaffin-like cell carcinoids in the rat gastric mucosa following long-term administration of ranitidine. *Digestion* 45: 189–195

6 Carlsson E, Havu N, Mattsson H, Ekman L, Ryberg B (1991) Gastric carcinoids in rats treated with inhibitors of gastric acid secretion. In: R Håkanson, F Sundler (eds): *The stomach as an endorcine organ*. Elsevier, Amsterdam, 461–471

7 Majka J, Sher S (1989) Spontaneous gastric carcinoid tumor in an aged Sprague-Dawley rat. *Vet Pathol* 26: 88–90

8 Poynter D, Pick CR, Harcourt RA, Selway SAM, Ainge G, Harman IW, Spurling NW, Fluck PA, Cook JL (1985) Association of long lasting unsurmountable histamine H_2-blockade and gastric carcinoid tumours in the rat. *Gut* 26: 1284–1295

9 Poynter D, Selway SAM, Papworth SA, Riches SR (1986) Changes in the gastric mucosa of the mouse asociated with long lasting unsurmountable histamine H_2 blockade. *Gut* 27: 1338–1346

10 Harleman JH, Betton GR, Dormer C, McCrossan M (1987) Gastric neuroendocrine cell hyperplasia after treatment with the long-acting, potent H_2-receptor antagonist SK&F 93479. *Scand J Gastroenterol* 22: 595–600

11 Mattsson H, Havu N, Bräutigam J, Carlsson K, Lundell L, Carlsson E (1991) Partial gastric corpectomy results in hypergastrinaemia and development of gastric ECL-cell carcinoids in the rat. *Gastroenterology* 100: 311–319
12 Larsson H, Carlsson E, Mattsson H et al (1986) Plasma gastrin and gastric enterochromaffin-like cell activation and proliferation. Studies with omeprazole and ranitidine in intact and antrectomized rats. *Gastroenterology* 90: 391–399
13 Johnson LR (1981) Regulation of gastrointestinal growth. In: LR Johnson (ed): *Physiology of the gastrointestinal tract*: Raven Press, New York, 169–196
14 Pinson DM, Havu N, Sztern MI, Mattsson H, Looney GA, Kimler BF, Hurwitz A (1995) Drug-induced hypergastrinemia: absence of trophic effects on colonic carcinoma in rats. *Gastroenterology* 108: 1068–1074
15 Graffner H, Singh G, Chaudry I, Milson JW (1992) Omeprazole-induced hypergastrinaemia does not influence growth of colon carcinoma. *Dig Dis Sci* 37: 485–489
16 Oscarsson J (1979) Variated serum gastrin concentration: trophic effects on the gastrointestinal tract of the rat. *Acta Physiol Scand Suppl* 475: 1–27
17 Hoosein NM, Kiener PA, Curry RC (1988) Antiproliferative effects of gastrin receptor antagonists and antibodies to gastrin on human colon carcinoma cell lines. *Cancer Res* 48: 7179–7183
18 McGregor DB, Jones RD, Karlin DA, Romsdahl MM (1983) Comparison of effects of pentagastrin and gastrin on rat colon mucosa. *J Surg Res* 34: 325–331
19 McWilliams DF, Watson SA, Crosbee DM, Michaeli D, Seth R (1998) Coexpression of gastrin and gastrin receptors (CCK-B and ΔCCK-B) in gastrointestinal tumour cell lines. *Gut* 42: 795–798
20 Forsell H, Helander HF, Sundell GW (1986) Structure and function of the dog gastric mucosa during and after a 1-year treatment with omeprazole. I. Macro- and microscopic findings. *Scand J Gastroenterol* Suppl 118: 79–81
21 Sundell GW, Nilsson G (1986) Structure and function of the dog gastric mucosa during and after a 1-year treatment with omeprazole. II. Effects on gastric acid secretion and blood levels of gastric hormones. *Scand J Gastroenterol* Suppl 118: 82–85

Proton Pump Inhibitors
ed. by L. Olbe

Consequences of gastric acid inhibition in man

Werner Creutzfeldt

Department of Medicine, Georg-August-University, Robert-Koch-Straße 40, D-37075 Göttingen, Germany

Introduction

For more than 100 years it has been known that gastric acid secretion is not the only but an essential causative factor in the pathogenesis of acid-related diseases. Thus reduction of acid secretion became a major therapeutic goal. For most of this century, effective acid reduction could be achieved only by surgery (gastric resection and vagotomy). The introduction of potent inhibitors of acid secretion, that is the H_2-receptor blocking agent cimetidine and its analogues in the late seventies and the even more potent proton pump inhibitor (PPI) omeprazole and its analogues in the late eighties have revolutionized therapy. Surgery became superfluous for benign oesophagogastric diseases, except in case of perforation or haemorrhage. However, soon after the introduction of the H_2-receptor blockers concern was expressed about the risk of hypochlorhydria or achlorhydria. This concern originates in the conviction that gastric acid is needed for normal life and that achlorhydria will cause serious problems. But do we really know how much gastric acid we need?

This chapter will discuss the consequences of gastric acid inhibition in humans such as hypergastrinaemia or bacterial overgrowth. Both are considered as possible risk factors for the development of gastritis and gastrointestinal tumours. In recent years several reviews have dealt with the theoretical arguments against long-term treatment with potent acid-suppressing drugs and the available clinical observations and epidemiological data [1–7].

Hypergastrinaemia

In 1970, after the development of a radioimmunoassay for gastrin, hypergastrinaemia was described and related to achlorhydria in nonantral atrophic gastritis [8]. Pernicious anaemia became a model for gastrin-acid-feedback regulation in humans and the possible consequences of long-lasting excessive hypergastrinaemia due to achlorhydria [2, 3]. Accordingly, an increase in gastrin plasma levels could be expected in patients treated with inhibitors of gastric secretion.

However, the elevation of plasma gastrin levels during therapy with H_2-receptor blockers or PPI were found to be an order of magnitude smaller than in patients with perncious anaemia and achlorhydria due to type A gastritis. During short and long-term treatment with omeprazole 20 mg daily, fasting gastrin levels remained in the upper normal range [9, 10]. However, postprandial gastrin levels increased significantly: 24-h integrated gastrin levels rose 5-fold during treatment with 20 mg omeprazole and 2.4-fold with 150 mg ranitidine twice daily [10]. The elevations are in the range of integrated gastrin levels after vagotomy and are correlated with the reduction of gastric secretion [11].

During long-term maintenance treatment with high doses of PPI (40 mg omeprazole, 60 mg lansoprazole and 80 mg pantoprazole), mean fasting gastrin levels rose to three times normal values in the first 3 months of treatment and did not increase further despite treatment for several years [12–17]. Only in about 20% of patients treated with high doses of PPI did fasting gastrin levels exceed four times the upper normal limit [14]. Elevated gastrin levels normalized within 10 days of cessation of treatment [4, 18]. In antrectomized patients, low gastrin levels remained unchanged during long-term treatment with high doses of PPI [14, 15, 17].

The finding of hypergastrinaemia (albeit smaller than in pernicious anaemia) in some patients treated long term with potent inhibitors of gastric acid secretion has generated concern, because gastrin stimulates not only gastric acid secretion but also the growth of some gastrointestinal cells and their tumours. Whether this concern is supported by clinical and anatomical observations or epidemiological facts will be investigated in the following sections.

ECL cell hyperplasia and gastric carcinoids

Gastrin dependence of the growth of histamine-producing endocrine cells of the oxyntic mucosa (the so-called enterochromaffin-like or ECL-cells) has been demonstrated in numerous animal experiments (see previous chapter). ECL cell hyperplasia has been found in rats made hypochlorhydric and hypergastrinaemic by either feeding H_2-receptor blocking agents and PPIs or by operative means, such as antrum exclusion or subtotal corpectomy. After 2 years even gastric carcinoids developed under these conditions.

In humans, the occurrence of endocrine cell proliferation and occasionally of carcinoids in achlorhydric patients with nonantral atrophic gastritis has been known for decades [19] and has been related to their excessive hypergastrinaemia [20–22]. However, according to recent studies the achlorhydria carcinoid sequence in humans is more complicated [2]. Nonantral gastric endocrine growths have been classified in hyperplasia, dysplasia and neoplasia [23]. Dysplasia (precarcinoid) and neoplasia (carcinoid) were found in hypergastrinaemic patients only in association with type A autoimmungastritis and pernicious anaemia and with gastrinoma as part of a multiple endocrine neoplasia type I (MEN-I syndrome) [24]. Long-lasting excessive hypergastrinaemia alone, as in case of the more frequent sporadic Zollinger-Ellison syndrome, leads only to nonantral endocrine hyperplasia, mostly of the diffuse and linear type. Benign micronodular hyperplasia hardly occurs, and carcinoids have never been observed in patients with sporadic Zollinger-Ellison syndrome, who usually have no gastritis [25].

To answer the question whether during long-term treatment with PPIs similar changes occur as in animals and patients with pernicious anaemia or MEN-I syndrome, the growth of antral and nonantral gastric endocrine cells was monitored in serial gastric biopsies of patients with ranitidine-resistant peptic ulceration treated with omeprazole [14, 26, 27] and lansoprazole [16] for up to 8 and 5 years, respectively. The antral G- and D-cell volume density did not significantly change during therapy with omeprazole [14], whereas a significant increase in antral G-cell density during lansoprazole treatment was described [16]. Also after proximal selective vagotomy, which increases the plasma gastrin levels to the same extent as long-term omeprazole treatment [11], a significant increase in antral G cells was reported [27a]. Simultaneously, the volume density of the endocrine cells in the oxyntic mucosa was significantly elevated 4 years after vagotomy [27a]. This corresponds to the finding in the nonantral gastric mucosa in the three omeprazole studies and the group treated with lansoprazole. Quantitative morphometry revealed a doubling of the oxyntic endocrine (mostly ECL) cells after 5 years [14, 16]. Qualitatively, linear and micronodular hyperplasia increased in all long-term studies [14, 16, 26, 27]. However, no dysplasia or neoplasia (carcinoids) have been observed in these ongoing systematic prospective studies or in any other endoscopic or histological surveillance. The increase of oxyntic endocrine cells was positively correlated to elevated fasting serum gastrin levels and an increase of focal preatrophic and atrophic gastritis in the oxyntic mucosa.

Because hypergastrinaemia and atrophic gastritis are closely related, it is difficult to assess their respective role in the process of ECL cell hyperplasia observed in these long-term studies with high dosages of omeprazole or lansoprazole. However, the occurrence of micronodular hyperplasia predominantly in biopsies containing areas of preatrophic and atrophic gastritis was obvious [28, 29] (Fig. 1). From this result it follows that PPIs and/or drug-induced hypergastrinaemia are less important than the concomitant atrophic gastritis for endocrine cell growth in human oxyntic mucosa. This conclusion is supported by the frequently hypotrophic and regressive pattern of cells composing the micronodules in atrophic areas of oxyntic mucosa and the demonstration that they have no proliferative capacity when labeled with 5-bromodeoxyuridine [30].

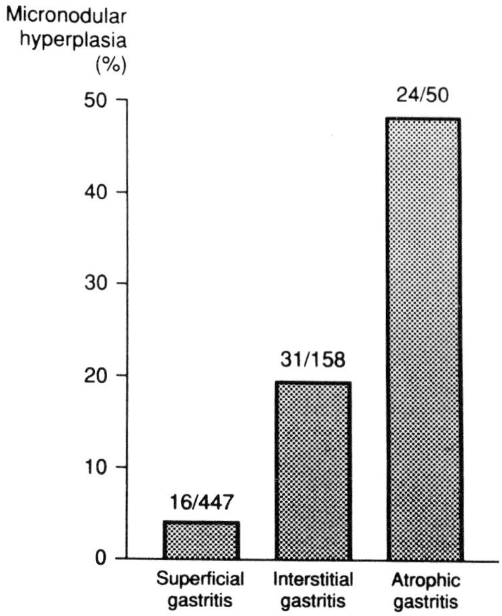

Figure 1. Prevalence of micronodular hyperplasia of argyrophil cells in 655 gastric biopsy dates (4–6 biopsies per date) of 74 patients treated long term with omeprazole, 40 mg daily. Absolute numbers are given above the columns. From ref. 28 with permission.

Only in one of the long-term studies monitoring gastric endocrine cell growth was the *Helicobacter pylori* status of patients systematically investigated [16]. The authors found a close relation between *H. pylori* infection, chronic atrophic gastritis and micronodular endocrine cell growth in oxyntic mucosa. They concluded that *H. pylori* represents an important factor for the progression of fundic gastritis and the development of endocrine cell hyperplasia during long-term lansoprazole treatment [16].

Gastric acid inhibition and the course of gastritis

The finding of a close correlation between gastric endocrine cell growth and chronic gastritis described in the previous section and of a progression of atrophic gastritis during long-term treatment with PPIs [14, 16, 26, 27] raises the question whether this reflects only the natural course of gastritis or whether acid suppression increases the risk of atrophic corpus gastritis. Recent papers have concluded that long-term acid suppression with omeprazole [31] or lansoprazole [16, 32] accelerates the development of chronic atrophic gastritis, especially in *H. pylori*-infected patients, and that therefore eradication of *H. pylori* should be considered before long-term treatment of reflux oesophagitis is begun. Moreover, antisecretory therapy with PPIs has been shown to improve living conditions for *H. pylori* in the oxyntic mucosa while deteriorating conditions for growth in the antral mucosa [33]. This could explain intragastric distribution changes in *H. pylori* [34] and gastritis [14, 29] during treatment with omeprazole.

However, these observations have not been regarded by the Food and Drug Administration (FDA) Gastrointestinal Drugs Advisory Committee as sufficient evidence that PPIs are unsafe in patients with *H. pylori* infection [7]. Indeed, the natural history of chronic gastritis is poorly understood. It varies in different countries and is dependent on a series of unknown factors (including virulence of different *H. pylori* strains) and concomitant gastric diseases as well as on different treatment and individual response (see Tabs 1 and 2). Thus, the annual increment of atrophic corpus gastritis in patients with peptic ulceration varies in different geographical areas between 1.5 and 10.4% and in the general population between 1.25 and 3.3%. From this it follows that controlled randomized intervention

Table 1. Natural history of atrophic corpus gastritis: prevalence and annual increment (cohorts without gastric disease)

Author*	Country	*n*	Follow-up (years)	Prevalence (%) First (Biopsy)	Prevalence (%) Last (Biopsy)	Annual increment (%)
Correa et al. (1976) (1)	Columbia (Narino)	286	–	56.3		–
	Columbia (Cartagena)	30	–	13.4		–
Correa et al. (1990) (2)	Columbia (Narino)	1422	5	45.2	62.0	3.3
Ihamäki et al. (1978) (3)	Finland (normal mucosa)	78	25	0	14	0.6
	(superficial gastritis)	50	25	0	42	1.7
Maaros et al. (1985) (4)	Estonia	56 35	4 7	22 22	27 37	1.3 2.1
Villako et al. (1991) (5)	Estonia	142	6		21	1.25
Kuipers et al. (1995) (6)	Netherlands					
	HP +	58	11.5	24	45	1.8
	HP –	49	11.5	14	18	0.3

* References: (1) *J Natl Cancer Inst* 57: 1027–1025
(2) *Cancer Res* 50: 4737–4740
(3) *Scand J Gastroenterol* 13: 771–775
(4) *Scand J Gastroenterol* 20: 198–204
(5) *Scand J Gastroenterol* 26(Suppl 186): 135–141
(6) *Lancet* 345: 1525–1528.

Table 2. Natural history of atrophic corpus gastritis: prevalence and annual increment (cohorts with peptic ulceration and different treatment)

Author*	Country	Condition and treatment[a]	*n*	Follow-up (years)	Prevalence (%) First (Biopsy)	Prevalence (%) Last (Biopsy)	Annual increment (%)
Maaros et al. (1985) (1)	Estonia	GU antacids	60	4	26	50	6.0
			39	7	26	79	7.6
Jönsson et al. (1988) (2)	Sweden	juxta pyloric ulcer					
		cimetidine maint	37	2.5	10.8	18.9	3.2
		proximal vag X	23	2.5	4.3	30.4	10.4
Peetsalu et al. (1991) (3)	Estonia	DU					
		medical treatment	187[b]			1	
		1. complete vag X	129	8		29	3.6
		2. incomplete vag X	130	8		12	1.5
Solcia et al. (1992) (4)	Scandinavia	DU, GU, GERD					
		omeprazole maint	203	1.5	1.0	6	3.3
			98	2.5	1.0	15	5.6
			57	3.5	1.0	19	5.1
Lamberts et al. (1993) (5)	Germany	DU, GU, GERD					
		omeprazole maint	42	4	1.8	7.2	1.4
			24	5	1.8	20.8	3.8
Klinkenberg-Knol et al. (1994) (6)	Netherlands	GERD					
		omeprazole maint	25	4	0	20	5.0
Kuipers et al. (1996) (7)	Netherlands	GERD					
		omeprazole	HP + 59	5	0	31	6.2
		maint (62 years)	HP – 46	5	0	4	0.8
	Sweden	fundoplication	HP + 31	5	3	3	0
		(53 years)	HP – 41	5	0	0	0

Table 2 (continued)

Author*	Country	Condition and treatment[a]	*n*	Follow-up (years)	Prevalence (%) First (Biopsy)	Prevalence (%) Last (Biopsy)	Annual increment (%)
Eissele et al. (1997) (8)	Germany	DU, GU, GERD					
		lansoprazole maint	33	2	10.5	30.3	9.9
			24	5	10.5	37.5	5.4
			(HP + 14		21	64	
			HP − 20		5	14)	
Lundell et al. (1997) (9)	Sweden	GERD					
		omeprazole	HP + 65	3	4.6	14	3.1
		maint (54 years)	HP − 85	3	1.2	0	0
		fundoplication	HP + 70	3	5.7	12.5	2.3
		(51 years)	HP − 75	3	0	0	0

* References:
(1) *Scand J Gastroenterol* 20: 198–204
(2) *Scand J Gastroenterol* 23: 433– 441
(3) *Scand J Gastroenterol* 26(Suppl. 186): 77–83
(4) *Digestion* 51(Suppl 1): 82–92
(5) *Gastroenterology* 104: 1356–1370
(6) *Ann Intern Med* 121: 161–167
(7) *N Engl J Med* 334: 1018–1022
(8) *Gastroenterology* 112: 707–717
(9) *Gastroenterology* 112: A28

[a] GU, gastric ulcer; DU, duodenal ulcer; GERD, gastro-esophageal reflux disease; maint, maintenance therapy; HP ±, *Helicobacter pylori*-positive, resp. negative; vag X, vagotomy.

[b] The non-operated patients were 6 years younger than the operated; 32% were female compared with 14% of the operated patients; ulcer history varied from 1 to 20 years, mean 3.5 ± 4 years.

studies are needed to evaluate the need for *H. pylori* eradication before any long-term treatment with PPIs (for instance in patients with reflux oesophagitis).

None of the studies mentioned above which have suggested this approach [16, 31, 32] included a matched control group. Thus a more recent study [35] is of interest in which 309 Swedish patients with gastrooesophageal reflux disease were randomized either to antireflux surgery or to treatment with omeprazole, followed by yearly gastric biopsies for 3 years. Gastric glandular atrophy developed only in *H. pylori*-positive patients, but was equally frequent in both treatment groups (omeprazole, 9; surgery, 8). Intestinal metaplasia was not observed in the two treatment groups. This is in agreement with a low (5%) incidence of intestinal metaplasia (complete type only) found in two previous studies, in which patients were treated with omeprazole for more than 5 years and no [14] or no significant [31] annual increment of intestinal metaplasia was observed. This is an important finding, because, intestinal metaplasia, *not atrophic gastritis*, is a possible precursor to cancer [36, 37]. Finally, it should be mentioned that poor agreement among pathologists about the definition and diagnosis of atrophic gastritis [38, 39] is a handicap that must be considered. Hopefully, this will change with the acceptance of the Classification and Grading of Gastritis (updated Sydney system) [40]. On the other hand, the best classification can hardly eliminate the inevitable sampling error which occurs in multifocal atrophic gastritis.

Three studies have been excluded from Table 2 because their results are far outside the range of those listed in the Tables 1 and 2. It is unclear whether this is due to uncertainty about the diagnostic criteria for atrophic fundic gastritis or to our incomplete knowledge of the natural history of chronic gastritis in different populations and/or diseases: two studies showed no atrophic gastritis after treatment for 3 years in France [41] and 1 year in Asia [42] with omeprazole, while in one uncontrolled study from Norway an increase of atrophic gastritis (grade 1 only) from 2.3 to 20.5% was observed after 1 year of lansoprazole treatment in *H. pylori*-positive patients with gastro-esophageal reflux disease (GERD) [32].

From these contradictory reports we can only conclude that the available data do not prove the contention that long-term treatment with PPIs facilitates the development of atrophic gastritis in the oxyntic mucosa. A recent publication supports this view [42a]. In a cross sectional study with 534 GERD patients in France (mean age 60 years) treated for 23 ± 1.4 months with omeprazole or for 35.7 ± 3.7 months with H_2-receptor antagonists the prevalence of moderate and severe corpus atrophic gastritis was 9% (omeprazole), 15.4% (H_2-receptor antagonists) and 15.9% (controls), respectively. In all groups moderate and severe atrophic gastritis was 3–4 times more frequent in *H. pylori* positive than negative patients. Further controlled studies in different geographical areas are indicated to definitively assess this important issue.

Bacterial overgrowth of the stomach and intestine

Gastric acid is regarded as an important barrier against bacterial colonization of the stomach and duodenum, thus protecting against gastrointestinal infections [43, 44]. Below pH 4.0, that is in the normal acid stomach, the bacterial flora is sparse (with the exception of *H. pylori*) while above pH 5.0 a resident gastric flora exists, including faecal-type organisms such as *Streptococcus faecalis* and *Bacteroides fragilis*. These data have been collected in patients with pernicious anaemia and complete type A atrophic gastritis. But similar changes have also been found in some patients after gastric surgery (partial gastrectomy or vagotomy). They have also been reported during treatment with H_2-receptor antagonists [45, 46], omeprazole [47–49] and lansoprazole [50].

What is the clinical significance of these findings? A recent epidemiological study of 170,000 users of antiulcer drugs does not support the long-standing hypothesis that suggests a major role for acid reduction in the development of bacterial gastroenteritis (especially from *Campylobacter* and *Salmonella* species) [51]. There was only a small increased risk in omeprazole users compared with users of H_2-receptor blocking agents, but no dose or treatment duration response was observed [51]. This may be due to the fact that acid inhibition by H_2-receptor-blocking agents and even PPIs seldom maintains gastric pH above 4.0 for the whole 24-h period and that a 15-min exposure to gastric pH below 3.0 is known to be bactericidal [43].

In a comparative study of 4 weeks of treatment of duodenal ulcer patients with either nizatidine (300 mg at night) or omeprazole (20 mg), 24-h acid secretion was significantly more reduced by omeprazole than by nizatidine, especially during the day; however, the difference in gastric bacterial colonization after either omeprazole or nizatidine did not reach significance [52]. Another study comparing treatment with omeprazole (20 mg) and cimetidine (800 mg) daily for 4 weeks resulted in a significantly higher incidence of gastric and duodenal bacterial overgrowth after omeprazole (53%) than after cimetidine (17%) [53]. Since overgrowth of both colonic-type bacteria and bacteria normally found in the mouth, pharynx and respiratory tract (including potential pathogens such as *Klebsiella* and *Pseudomonas*) is found in the gastric juice after gastric acid inhibition [44, 49, 52], concern has been raised in relation to the possible effects of antisecretory therapies in intensive care medicine. An increased incidence of nosocomial pneumonias in some reports [54, 55] is not a general finding [56], and could not be confirmed in prospective randomized trials [57, 57a].

It has been speculated that bacterial overgrowth in the jejunum during acid inhibition may produce malabsorption, similar to the blind-loop syndrome. However, despite elevated concentrations of colonic-type bacteria in the duodenum during omeprazole therapy [48, 49, 58], malabsorption of fat and carbohydrates could not be demonstrated [48, 58]. Also, serum concentrations of vitamins (B_{12}, β-carotene) and of albumin, ferritin, calcium and other minerals have been found in the normal range even after treatment for several years [53, 59–61]. It is of interest that despite decreased absorption of protein-bound cyanocobalamin during omeprazole treatment [61, 62] serum B_{12} levels remained normal [53, 59–61].

One recent report showed increased bile acid deconjugation (demonstrated by ^{14}C-glycocholic acid breath test) by bacterial overgrowth in the jejunum after treatment of healthy volunteers or patients with gastric ulcer for 5 weeks with 20 mg of omeprazole daily which normalized after tetracycline treatment [63]. Increased steatorrhea has also been claimed in this study but is poorly documented by the semiquantitative ^{14}C-triolein breath test [63] and is in contradiction to the negative finding of another study which measured 72 h of fat excretion quantitatively after treatment with 40 mg of omeprazole daily [48].

A keystone in the theory of gastric carcinogenesis inaugurated by Correa [64] is the formation of potentially noxious *N*-nitroso compounds in the stomach. The frequent occurrence of hypo- or achlorhydria in patients with gastric cancer, for instance 31% in a large study from the Mayo Clinic [65], is considered as evidence for the suggestion that low gastric acid favours increased production of *N*-nitroso compounds via bacterial overgrowth. However, this hypothesis has not yet been convincingly validated. It is also not supported by observations in patients with gastric bacterial overgrowth during treatment with drugs inhibiting acid secretion. In fact, there are serious doubts about the relative contribution of chemical and bacterial nitrosation. Chemical nitrosation is favoured by acid rather than neutral pH [66, 67]. Furthermore, different methods used for measuring in vivo nitrosation yielded contradictory results [68–70]. The best method for measuring *N*-nitroso compounds seems to be the method of Pignatelli [44]. It is therefore of interest that low levels of *N*-nitroso compounds have been found with this method in patients with achlorhydria [69]. The controversies in this field have been extensively discussed in a recent review [70]. Meanwhile, the concentration of *N*-nitroso compounds has also been measured in the gastric juice of subjects with gastric bacterial overgrowth, including nitrate-reducing bacteria during treatment with omeprazole. However, there was no increase in the concentration of nitrates or nitrites or of *N*-nitroso compounds in the gastric juice [53, 71], confirming earlier observations with cimetidine [72].

It can thus be concluded that bacterial overgrowth frequently occurs as a consequence of acid inhibition in humans but that this event is of little clinical significance. General studies have shown that during treatment with H_2-receptor-blocking agents or PPIs gastrointestinal infections and the incidence of nosocomial pneumonia in intensive care medicine are not markedly increased. There is also no indication that long-term gastric inhibition with omeprazole leads to malabsorption of nutrients, vitamins or minerals. Finally, increased formation of *N*-nitroso compounds in the stomach as a consequence of bacterial overgrowth after inhibition of acid secretion by omeprazole has not been found. Therefore, an important step in the Correa hypothesis of gastric carcinogenesis is lacking. Obviously, achlorhydria as an isolated factor is not enough to initiate gastric carcinoma [73].

Gastrointestinal malignancy

Gastric tumours

The most serious problem of long-lasting gastric acid inhibition in humans is the question whether it promotes the development and growth of gastrointestinal malignancies [76]. This suggestion originates from the clinical observation that hypo- or achlorhydria are frequent in patients with gastric cancer [65].

Achlorhydria due to atrophic corpus gastritis (type A) is an essential part of pernicious anaemia. The observed threefold excess risk of developing gastric carcinoma of the intestinal type found in large cohorts of patients with pernicious anaemia [74, 75] and also, albeit less frequently, after reduction of gastric secretion by vagotomy or gastric resection (Tab. 3) has created concern about the safety of gastric acid inhibition by H_2-receptor-blocking agents or PPIs [76, 77]. Two factors have been suggested to be responsible for this increased risk: bacterial overgrowth and hypergastrinaemia. However, these hypotheses are only partly consistent with the clinical and epidemiological data summarized in Table 3. Excessive hypergastrinaemia is present in pernicious anaemia, and moderately elevated plasma gastrin levels also occur after vagotomy, while lower than normal plasma gastrin levels are found after distal gastrectomy (Billroth I and II). While in pernicious anaemia and after vagotomy elevated plasma gastrin levels seem to correlate with an especially high risk for gastric carcinoma, this could also be explained by the preserved distal stomach, where the majority of cancers originate.

Whether bacterial overgrowth plays a significant aetiopathogenetic role under the three conditions summarized in Table 3 is doubtful, because it can be expected in all three groups of patients and thus would hardly explain the variable cancer risk, especially the difference between duodenal and gastric ulcer patients.

Three conclusions are obvious from Table 3. First, increased gastric cancer risk depends on the duration of the state of reduced acid secretion and is significant only 20 years after the gastric operation (when hypochlorhydria in autoimmune gastritis starts is unknown; however, it is thought to begin many years before the anaemia is diagnosed). Second, increased cancer risk depends on the type of operation and is greater after Billroth II than after Billroth I gastrectomy [78], and most cancers start close to the stoma; this implies that factors common to the whole gastric remnant, like

Table 3. Standardized incidence ratio (SIR) and 95% confidence interval of cancer at different sites in patients with achlorhydria or decreased acid secretion

Author*	Size of cohort (*n*)	Follow-up (years)	Site of carcinoma: stomach	pancreas	colon	rectum	oesophagus	lung
I. Pernicious anaemia								
Brinton et al. (1989) (1) (USA) Men:	5161	6.8 (mean)	3.21[a] (2.2–4.6)	0.72 (0.3–1.5)	1.05 (0.7–1.5)	0.95 (0.5–1.6)	1.47 (0.7–2.6)	0.8 (0.6–1.0)
Hsing et al. (1993) (2) (Sweden)	4517	5.9 (mean)						
Men:	2021		2.8 (2.0–3.6)	*1.7* (1.0–2.8)	1.0 (0.5–1.6)	*1.7* (1.0–2.7)	*3.1* (1.3–6.1)	0.9 (0.5–1.5)
Women:	2496		3.1 (2.3–4.1)	*1.8* (1.1–2.8)	1.1 (0.7–1.7)	0.9 (0.4–1.8)	*3.3* (1.3–6.7)	1.2 (0.5–2.3)
II. Vagotomy								
Watt et al. (1984) (3) (Northern Ireland)[b]	735	15–20	3.3	*2.0*	*2.3*		3.0	*3.53*
Caygill et al. (1986) (4) (England)[b]	518	20–40						
< 20 years after operation			0.7					
20 + years after operation			*7.8*					
Lundegardh et al. (1994) (5) (Sweden)	7198	10–18	1.33 (0.92–1.86)					
vagotomy with drainage	1863		1.1 (0.57–2.03)					
vagotomy without drainage	5335		1.5 (0.92–2.17)					
Fisher et al. (1993) (13) (USA) (1994) (14) vagotomy with drainage	3535	18–20	*1.6* (1.1–2.6)		0.83 (0.6–1.2)			

Table 3 (continued)

Author*	Size of cohort (n)	Follow-up (years)	Site of carcinoma: stomach	pancreas	colon	rectum	oesophagus	lung
III. Gastric resection[c]								
Tokudome et al. (1984) (6) (Japan)	3827	10–33	*0.34* (0.23–0.47)					
Caygill et al. (1986) (4) (England) (1987) (7)	4466	20–40	*1.58* (1.25–1.96)					
< 20 years after operation			1.04[d]	0.7	0.7		0.8	*1.3*
20 + years after operation			*4.39*	*3.8*	*1.6*		*2.3*	*3.9*
Viste et al. (1986) (8) (Norway)	3470	25–45	*2.1* (1.68–2.59)					
Lundegardh et al. (1988) (9) (Sweden) (1990) (15)	6459	20–33	*1.66* (1.27–2.13)		0.87 (0.73–1.03)			
< 20 years after operation	Billroth I		0.37 (0.15–0.77)		0.75 (0.58–0.96)			
	Billroth II		0.63 (0.43–0.89)					
20 + years after operation	Billroth I		0.44 (0.12–1.13)		1.02 (0.79–1.29)			
	Billroth II		*2.06* (1.56–2.66)					
Tersmette et al. (1991) (10) (Netherlands)	2633	15–59	*1.4*		1.0			*1.6*

Table 3 (continued)

Author*	Size of cohort (n)	Follow-up (years)	Site of carcinoma stomach	pancreas	colon	rectum	oesophagus	lung
Gastric resection[c] (continued)								
Möller, Toftgaard (1991) (11) (Sweden)	4107	15–32	1.07	1.18	0.92	1.02	1.41	*1.66*
< 20 years after operation			0.85	1.05	0.75	1.06	1.49	*1.59*
20 + years after operation			*1.80*	1.44	1.22	0.92	1.21	*1.80*
Macintyre, O'Brien (1994) (12) (Scotland) only duodenal ulcer	2241	20–40	1.07 (0.72–1.53)	1.22 (0.67–2.05)	1.25 (0.9–1.7)		1.48 (0.79–2.53)	*1.37* (1.45–1.61)
< 20 years after operation			0.94 (0.57–1.47)		1.39 (0.85–2.15)			*1.25* (1.03–1.5)
20 + years after operation			1.19 (0.51–2.35)		0.99 (0.36–2.16)			*1.5* (1.16–1.91)

* References: (1) *Brit J Cancer* 59: 810–813
(2) *Cancer* 71: 745–750
(3) *Brit Med J* 288: 1335–1338
(4) *Lancet* i: 929–931
(5) *Gut* 35: 946–949
(6) *Cancer Res* 44: 2208–2212
(7) *Gut* 28: 924–928
(8) *Lancet* ii 502–505
(9) *N Engl J Med* 319: 195–200
(10) *Gastroenterology* 101: 148–153
(11) *Gut* 32: 740–744
(12) *Gut* 35: 451–454
(13) *J Natl Cancer Inst* 85: 1303–1310
(14) *Am J Epidemiol* 139: 684–692
(15) *Ann Surgery* 212: 714–719

[a] Significant differences ($p < 0.05$ and less) are underlined.
[b] Vagotomy plus drainage procedure, duodenal ulcer only.
[c] Only cohort studies with more than 2000 gastric resections for peptic ulcer; patients with gastric and duodenal ulcer are pooled if not stated otherwise.
[d] Duodenal ulcer ($n = 2577$): < 20 years after operation SIR 0.4 and 20 years + after operation 3.6; gastric ulcer ($n = 1385$): < 20 years after operation SIR 2.7 and 20 years + after operation 5.5.

acidity and bacterial contents, are less important, and that reflux might be the key factor. Third, increased risk of gastric stump cancer is reduced or absent in patients with gastric resection for duodenal ulcer. The latter observation is not quite obvious from Table 3 because the data of the two ulcer types are pooled. However, in a large meta-analysis of published cohort studies the increased risk of gastric cancer was only seen in patients after surgery for gastric, not for duodenal ulcer [79].

While hypergastrinaemia does not explain the increased cancer risk in all three patient groups in Table 3, and bacterial overgrowth with consecutive formation of N-nitroso compounds as a single causal factor has been questioned, diffuse or focal atrophic gastritis with intestinal metaplasia is common to all states of reduced acid secretion. Atrophic gastritis is most prominent in pernicious anaemia, but also present after vagotomy (see Tab. 2) and after distal gastrectomy, especially with bile reflux after the Billroth II procedure.

Thus, the epidemiological data do not favour the contention that long-lasting achlorhydria or reduced acid secretion as such increase gastric cancer risk; the risk is best explained by the presence or development of atrophic gastritis in pernicious anaemia and in the operated stomach. Progression from chronic gastritis to intestinal metaplasia to dysplasia and cancer is slow [64a]. Thus, the relative cancer risk is low for 15 to 20 years after operation but increases steadily thereafter to 1.5 to 3.0 [79]. However, since the absolute figures for cancer development after gastric surgery are small, routine endoscopic screening does not appear to be justified [77]. Also, screening for gastric tumours in patients with pernicious anaemia has been repeatedly discussed. However, the data (relative cancer risk 3.0) do not support the need for regular endoscopic surveillance.

Table 4 shows, that 5 (1.5%) gastric carcinomas and 11 (3.2%) carcinoids have been found by endoscopic screening of 342 patients with pernicious anaemia. Thus endoscopy is advised after the diagnosis of perni-

Table 4. Prevalence of gastric tumors in pernicious anaemia (results of endoscopic screening)

Author*	*n*	Carcinoid (*n*)	Adenocarcinoma (*n*)
Elsborg et al. (1977) (1) (Denmark)	68	0	0
Stockbrügger et al. (1983) (2) (England)	80	1	1
Borch (1986) (3) (Sweden)	123	5	4
Follow up (mean 2.8 years)	61	0	0
Kokkola et al. (1998) (4) (Finland)	71	5	0
Follow up (mean 5.8 years)	42	8[a]	2

* References: (1) *Scand J Gastroenterol* 12: 49–52
(2) *Gut* 24: 1141–1147
(3) *Scand J Gastroenterol* 21: 21–30
(4) *Scand J Gastroenterol* 33: 88–92

[a] three new cases and five recurrences.

cious anaemia has been made in a patient but further surveillance only in case of precancerous lesions or if a carcinoid has been found and removed [80]. In the latter case intervals of 3 years are sufficient.

Gastric carcinoids are rare. In a large series of 1867 carcinoids, only 2.3% were located in the stomach, and only 0.3% of gastric tumours were carcinoids [81]. It is now well established that of these only ECL carcinoids are gastrin-dependant. ECL-carcinoids have been observed exclusively in patients with long-lasting pernicious anaemia (prevalence about 3.0%, see Tab. 4) or with MEN-I syndrome with gastrinoma [82]. They arise in the oxyntic mucosa and are benign (i.e., not metastasizing) tumours [82, 83], while the rare sporadic gastric carcinoids are found in normogastrinaemic patients. The latter are multihormonal, located in the gastric antrum or corpus and may metastasize and behave like endocrine carcinomas [82, 83]. The claim that diffuse gastric carcinomas are also neuroendocrine gastrin-dependent tumours ("ECL-omas") [84] is pure speculation, because ECL cells have not been identified in diffuse gastric carcinomas [85].

Gastrin dependence of gastric adenocarcinomas has not been established. Earlier studies described binding of gastrin-17 to human gastric carcinoma cell lines [86] and growth stimulation of gastric cancer cell lines by gastrin [87, 88]. However, more recent studies on gastrin gene receptor expression found gastrin receptor messenger RNA (mRNA) only in one of two small cell gastric carcinoma cell lines, but not in 12 gastric adenocarcinoma cell lines tested or in 8 gastric adenocarcinoma tissues tested [89]. This negative finding is important, because the increased gastric cancer risk of hypergastrinaemic patients with pernicious anaemia is due to an increase in adenocarcinoma of the intestinal type only [77]. From this it follows that hypergastrinaemia is probably not responsible for the threefold excess risk of stomach cancer in pernicious anaemia.

The effect of the long-term use of gastric acid-inhibiting drugs on the development of gastric malignancies is difficult to evaluate. To date only reports on post-marketing surveillance of the H_2-blocking agents cimetidine and ranitidine for up to 10 years have been published [90–93]. Except for an initial rise in the occurrence of gastric cancer and several other tumours in the first years no increased risk of cancer development could be detected (except smoking-related cancers). Selection bias rather than use of the drug is likely to be the explanation; examples are medication of anti-ulcer drugs in the late stages of many diseases and also to counter the adverse gastric effects of other drugs used in the treatment of serious disorders [92, 93].

No large-scale surveillance reports are yet available for omeprazole or other PPIs. However, neither gastric carcinoids nor carcinomas have been observed in several prospective long-term studies for up to 10 years with omeprazole, nor has dysplasia of the gastric endocrine cells or the mucosa been found in multiple biopsies. Also, no increase in intestinal metaplasia occurred [14, 31, 35].

Neoplastic gastric polyps have not been found during long-term follow-up of patients treated with omeprazole. However, the occurrence of gastric glandular cysts ("fundic gland polyps") has been observed in several prospective surveillance studies [94, 95]. These harmless cystic polyps are the most frequent gastric polyps and are unrelated to the PPI treatment and to *H. pylori* infection [94]. The same applies to the "hyperplastic polyps" which have been found during long-term omeprazole treatment [95]. They also are benign and are apparently related to *H. pylori* infection, because they disappear after eradication of *H. pylori* [96].

Colorectal and pancreas tumours

Since the observation of gastric carcinoids in rats after long-term treatment with acid-inhibiting drugs and the demonstration of their gastrin dependence, it has been speculated that growth of tumours at other sites might also be promoted by drug-induced hypergastrinaemia [3]. Colorectal tumours especially were expected to be sensitive to such hormone effects, because gastrin dependence of colon cancer cell lines and of tumour transplants have been described [97–101] as well as gastrin binding by colon carcinoma cells [89, 100, 102]. In addition, higher plasma gastrin levels than in matched controls have been reported in patients with colon polyps and colon cancer [103].

However, several important facts do not support such speculations. Omeprazole-induced hypergastrinaemia did not influence the growth of a mouse colon carcinoma expressing gastrin receptors [100] and did not promote but rather inhibited the induction and growth of methylazoxymethanol-induced colonic carcinomas in rats [104, 105]. Binding of gastrin by colon carcinoma cells occurs via a 78-kDa gastrin-binding protein [106], while gastrin receptor mRNA was detected only in a minority (11% of 56) of colorectal carcinoma samples [89, 107]. There is also growing evidence that the gastrin gene is expressed in the colon and that progastrin and glycine-extended gastrin are products of the normal colon mucosa and of colon carcinomas [108–110]. These findings are considered to be evidence for a role of gastrin and its precursors as local autocrine growth factors in the colon and in colon carcinomas [99, 111, 112].

Nonamidated gastrin is even secreted into the circulation, and elevated total gastrin plasma levels have been found in some patients with colon carcinoma whose amidated gastrin levels were normal [113]. This could perhaps help to understand the varying results of clinical studies on fasting and postprandial plasma gastrin levels in patients with colorectal tumours: some authors found more patients with elevated total gastrin levels in the tumour group than in the respective control group [103, 114–116], whereas other authors measured identical fasting gastrin levels in patients with colon tumours and controls [3, 117–120]. An occasionally observed decrease of elevated plasma gastrin levels after resection of the tumour [114–116] could also be explained by production of gastrin or its precursors by the tumour.

In contrast to the experimental studies, which are still controversial, the epidemiological data are indisputable. They clearly show that in large cohorts of patients with significant endogenous hypergastrinaemia due to pernicious anaemia [74, 75] the prevalence of colorectal carcinomas is not increased (see Tab. 3). Also, the prevalence of pernicious anaemia in a Danish cohort of 1777 patients with colorectal carcinoma corresponded with 0.2% to the frequency of the general population [121].

In 97 patients with Zollinger-Ellison syndrome, a fasting gastrin level 31 times above normal and a mean disease duration of 10 years, the degree of colonic neoplasia (polyps or cancer) discovered by colonoscopy was in the range of control groups [122]. Clearly, these epidemiological data do not support the contention that elevated gastrin levels promote the development and growth of colon tumours. An increased incidence ratio of carcinomas of the oesophagus and pancreas has been found (Tab. 3) only in the Swedish cohort of male and female patients with pernicious anaemia [74], not however in male patients from USA [75]. This difference is difficult to explain, but must be due to a confounding factor unrelated to hypergastrinaemia or achlorhydria.

Bacterial overgrowth is said to increase the concentration of *N*-nitroso compounds in the stomach, but it has also been suggested that in the operated stomach a circulating carcinogen is produced which acts at distant sites and increases cancer risk in multiple organs [123]. Another hypothesis relates carcinogenesis in the large bowel to the effect of altered bacterial flora on bile acids (deconjugation and 7-dehydroxylation to deoxycholic acid and lithocholic acid), which act as tumour promoters in colorectal cancer [124]. Some animal experiments and epidemiological studies on the concentration of faecal bile acids and colon cancer incidence in different populations support this theory [124]. Since hypochlorhydria and bacterial overgrowth with consecutive bile acid deconjugation occur after gastric surgery (vagotomy with drainage and distal gastrectomy) [125], the relative risk of colorectal cancer after gastric surgery was investigated. While several small studies found a significantly higher incidence of large bowel cancer after gastrectomy or vagotomy and drainage [123, 125–127], more recent large cohort studies have not confirmed this finding (see Tab. 3) and have clearly shown that the relative risk for colorectal cancer after vagotomy [128] and gastric resection [129–132] was not increased. Only cancer of the lung and other smoking- and alcohol-related cancers were more frequent (see Tab. 3).

We conclude from this that gastric acid reduction by gastric surgery does not result in increased risk for colorectal tumours [133].

Summary

1. Long-lasting profound gastric acid inhibition may lead to hypergastrinaemia and bacterial overgrowth of the stomach and proximal bowel. This chapter summarizes the hypothetical consequences of these events as well as the available experimental data and clinical observations in patients with reduced acid secretion, that is pernicious anaemia, gastric resection, vagotomy and long-term treatment with drugs inhibiting gastric acid secretion.
2. Hypergastrinaemia in humans is excessive in pernicious anaemia and moderate after vagotomy and during treatment with H_2-receptor-blocking agents and PPIs. The gastrin levels usually correspond with the reduction of gastric secretion.
3. Moderate hypergastrinaemia after vagotomy or during long-term treatment with PPIs induces slight hyperplasia of the ECL cells in the oxyntic mucosa and no dysplasia. The occurrence of micronodular hyperplasia correlated with the presence of atrophic gastritis. Gastric carcinoids in humans have only been found in patients with pernicious anaemia and gastrinoma as part of the MEN-I syndrome.
4. The contention that long-term treatment with PPIs facilitates the development of atrophic gastritis in *H. pylori*-infected patients is not supported by the available epidemiological data and could not be confirmed in a prospective controlled study.
5. Bacterial overgrowth frequently occurs as consequence of acid inhibition in humans but is of little clinical consequence. Neither gastrointestinal infections nor nosocomial pneumonia in intensive care medicine are significantly increased. Increased formation of *N*-nitroso compounds in the stomach after omeprazole treatment has not been found.
6. Analysis of epidemiological data shows that the increased risk of gastric cancer more than 20 years after gastric resection or vagotomy and in patients with pernicious anaemia is due to chronic atrophic gastritis and is not a consequence of decreased acid secretion or hypergastrinaemia.
7. The claim that achlorhydria alone or together with hypergastrinaemia as in pernicious anaemia or reduced acid secretion after gastric surgery lead to increased cancer risk at distant sites, especially the colon, has not been confirmed in large cohort studies.
8. The occasional finding of increased plasma gastrin levels in patients with colorectal tumours can be explained by production of nonamidated gastrin by some tumours. The growth response to gastrin of colon cancer transplants or cell lines is probably due to the role of gastrin as an autocrine growth factor in colon tissue as documented by the presence of mRNA for gastrin and gastrin receptors in colon cancer cells.

References

1 Frontiers in digestive diseases: omeprazole. *Dig Dis Sci* (1995); 40(Suppl): 1S–131S
2 Creutzfeldt W (1988) The achlorhydria-carcinoid sequence: role of gastrin. *Digestion* 39: 61–79
3 Creutzfeldt W, Lamberts R (1991) Is hypergastrinaemia dangerous to man? *Scand J Gastroenterol* 26(Suppl 180): 179–191
4 Creutzfeldt W (1994) Risk-benefit assessment of omeprazole in the treatment of gastrointestinal disorders. *Drug Safety* 10: 66–82
5 Yeomans ND (ed) (1993) Inhibition of gastric acid secretion. *Baillière's Clinical Gastroenterology* 1: 1–194
6 Modlin IM, Goldenring JR, Lawton GP, Hunt R (1994) Aspects of the theoretical basis and clinical relevance of low acid states. *Am J Gastroenterol* 89: 308–318
7 Freston JW (1997) Long-term acid control and proton pump inhibitors: interactions and safety issues in perspective. *Am J Gastroenterol* 92(Suppl): 51S–57S
8 Yalow RS, Berson SA (1970) Radioimmunoassay of gastrin. *Gastroenterology* 58: 1–14
9 Lundell L, Backman L, Ekström P et al (1991) Prevention of relapse of reflux esophagitis after endoscopic healing: efficacy and safety of omeprazole compared with ranitidine. *Scand J Gastroenterol* 26: 248–256
10 Lanzon-Miller S, Pounder RE, Hamilton MR et al (1987) Twenty-four-hour intragastric acidity and plasma gastrin concentration before and during treatment with either ranitidine or omeprazole. *Aliment Pharmacol Ther* 1: 239–251
11 Lind T, Cederberg C, Olausson M, Olbe L (1990) 24-hour intragastric acidity and plasma gastrin after omeprazole treatment and after proximal gastric vagotomy in duodenal ulcer patients. *Gastroenterology* 99: 1593–1598
12 Brunner G, Creutzfeldt W, Harke U, Lamberts R (1989) Efficacy and safety of long-term treatment with omeprazole in patients with acid related diseases resistant to ranitidine. *Can J Gastroenterol* 3(Suppl A): 72–76
13 Jansen JBMJ, Klinkenberg-Knol EC, Meuwissen SGM et al (1990) Effect of long-term treatment with omeprazole on serum gastrin and serum group A and C pepsinogens in patients with reflux esophagitis. *Gastroenterology* 99: 621–628
14 Lamberts R, Creutzfeldt W, Strüber HG et al (1993) Long-term omeprazole therapy in peptic ulcer disease: gastrin, endocrine cell growth, and gastritis. *Gastroenterology* 104: 1356–1370
15 Brunner G, Arnold R, Hennig U, Fuchs W (1993) An open trial of long-term therapy with lansoprazole in patients with peptic ulceration resistant to extended high-dose ranitidine treatment. *Aliment Pharmacol Ther* 7(Suppl 1): 51–55
16 Eissele R, Brunner G, Simon B et al (1997) Gastric mucosa during treatment with lansoprazole: *Helicobacter pylori* is a risk factor for argyrophil cell hyperplasia. *Gastroenterology* 112: 707–717
17 Brunner G, Harke U (1994) Long-term therapy with pantoprazole in patients with peptic ulceration resistant to extended high-dose ranitidine treatment. *Aliment Pharmacol Ther* 8(Suppl 1): 59–64
18 Klinkenberg-Knol EC, Jansen JBMJ, Lamers CBHW et al (1990) Temporary cessation of long-term maintance treatment with omeprazole in patients with H_2-receptor-antagonist-resistant reflux oesophagitis. Effects on symptoms, endoscopy, serum gastrin, and gastric acid output. *Scand J Gastroenterol* 25: 1144–1150
19 Wilander E (1981) Achylia and the development of gastric carcinoids. *Virch Arch Abt A Path Anat* 394: 151–160
20 Carney JA, Go VLW, Fairbanks VF, Moore SB, Alport EC, Nora FE (1983) The syndrome of gastric argyrophil carcinoid tumors and nonantral gastric atrophy. *Ann Intern Med* 99: 761–766
21 Borch K, Renvall H, Liedberg G (1985) Gastric endocrine cell hyperplasia and carcinoid tumors in pernicious anemia. *Gastroenterology* 88: 638–648
22 Borch K, Renvall H, Liedberg G, Andersen BN (1986) Relations between circulating gastrin and endocrine cell proliferation in the atrophic gastric fundic mucosa. *Scand J Gastroenterol* 21: 357–363
23 Solcia E, Bordi C, Creutzfeldt W et al (1988) Histopathological classification of nonantral gastric endocrine growth in man. *Digestion* 41: 185–200

24 Solcia E, Capella C, Fiocca R et al (1990) Gastric argyrophil carcinoidosis in patients with Zollinger-Ellison syndrome due to type 1 multiple endocrine neoplasia. A newly recognized association. *Am J Surg Pathol* 14: 503–513
25 Maton PN, Lack EE, Collen MJ et al (1990) The effect of Zollinger-Ellison syndrome and omeprazole therapy on gastric oxyntic endocrine cells. *Gastroenterology* 99: 943–950
26 Solcia E, Rindi G, Havu N, Elm G (1989) Qualitative studies of gastric endocrine cells in patients treated long-term with omeprazole. *Scand J Gastroenterol* 24(Suppl 166): 129–137
27 Klinkenberg-Knol EC, Festen HPM, Jansen JBMJ et al (1994) Long-term treatment with omeprazole for refractory reflux esophagitis: efficacy and safety. *Ann Intern Med* 121: 161–167
27a Koop H, Frank M, Kuly S et al (1993) Gastric argyrophil (enterochromaffin-like), gastrin, and somatostatin cells after proximal selective vagotomy in man. *Dig Dis Sci* 38: 295–302
28 Creutzfeldt W, Lamberts R (1992) Inter-relationship between serum gastrin levels, gastric mucosal histology and gastric endocrine cell growth. *Digestion* 51(Suppl 1): 76–81
29 Solcia E, Fiocca R, Havu N et al (1992) Gastric endocrine cells and gastritis in patients receiving long-term omeprazole treatment. *Digestion* 51(Suppl 1): 82–92
30 Solcia E, Fiocca R, Villani L et al (1991) Morphology and pathogenesis of endocrine hyperplasias, precarcinoid lesions, and carcinoids arising in chronic atrophic gastritis. *Scand J Gastroenterol* 26(Suppl 180): 146–159
31 Kuipers EJ, Lundell L, Klinkenberg-Knol EC et al (1996) Atrophic gastritis and *H. pylori* infection in patients with reflux esophagitis treated with omeprazole of fundoplication. *N Engl J Med* 334: 1018–1022
32 Berstad AE, Hatlebakk JG, Maartmann-Moe H et al (1997) *H. pylori* gastritis and epithelial cell proliferation in patients with reflux oesophatitis after treatment with lansoprazole. *Gut* 41: 740–747
33 Sachs G (1997) Gastritis, *Helicobacter pylori*, and proton pump inhibitors. *Gastroenterology* 112: 1033–1036
34 Logan RPH, Walker MM, Misiewicz JJ et al (1995) Changes in the intragastric distribution of *H. pylori* during treatment with omeprazole. *Gut* 36: 12–16
35 Lundell L, Havu N, Andersson A et al (1997) Gastritis development and acid suppression therapy revisited. Results of a randomised clinical study with long-term follow-up. *Gastroenterology* 112: A28
36 Lechago J, Correa P (1993) Prolonged achlorhydria and gastric neoplasia: is there a causal relationship? *Gastroenterology* 104: 1554–1557
37 Rubin CE (1997) Are there three types of *Helicobacter pylori* gastritis? *Gastroenterology* 112: 2108–2110
38 El-Zimaity HMT, Graham DY, Al-Assi MT et al (1996) Interobserver variation in the histopathological assessment of *Helicobacter pylori* gastritis. *Hum Pathol* 27: 35–41
39 Genta RM (1997) *Helicobacter pylori*, inflammation, mucosal damage, and apoptosis: pathogenesis and definition of gastric atrophy. *Gastroenterology* 113: S51–S55
40 Dixon MF, Genta RM, Yardley JH et al (1996) Classification and grading of gastritis. *Am J Surg Pathol* 20: 1161–1181
41 Guillaume C, Vissuzaine C, Pospai D et al (1995) Influence des traitements prolongés par inhibiteurs de la pompe à protons sur la gastrinémie et la muqueuse fundique. *Gastroenterol Clin Biol* 19: 811–817
42 Goh KL, Boonyapisit S, Lai KH et al (1995) Prevention of duodenal ulcer relapse with omeprazole 20 mg daily: a randomized double-blind, placebo-controlled study. *J Gastroenterol Hepatol* 10: 92–97
42a Diebold MD, Richardson S, Duchateau A, Bigard MA, Colin R, Cortot A, Fauchere JL, Zeitoun P (1998) Factors influencing corpus argyrophil cell density and hyperplasia in reflux esophagitis patients treated with antisecretory drugs and controls. *Dig Dis Sci* 43: 1629–1635
43 Howden CW, Hunt RH (1987) Relationship between gastric secretion and infection. Gut 28: 96–107
44 Heatley RV, Sobala GM (1993) Acid suppression and the gastric flora. *Baillière's Clin Gastroenterol* 7: 167–181

45 Stockbruegger RW (1985) Bacterial overgrowth as a consequence of reduced gastric acidity. *Scand J Gastroenterol* (Suppl 111): 7–16
46 Thomas JM, Misiewicz JJ, Cook AR et al (1987) Effects of one year treatment with ranitidine and of truncal vagotomy on gastric contents. *Gut* 28: 726–738
47 Sharma BK, Santana IA, Wood EC (1984) Intragastric bacterial activity and nitrosation before, during and after treatment with omeprazole. *Br Med J* 280: 717–719
48 Saltzman JR, Kowdley KV, Pedrosa MC et al (1994) Bacterial overgrowth without clinical malabsorption in elderly hypochlorhydric subjects. *Gastroenterology* 106: 615–623
49 Fried M, Siegrist H, Frei R et al (1994) Duodenal bacterial overgrowth during treatment in outpatients with omeprazole. *Gut* 35: 23–26
50 Colin-Jones DG (1993) Safety of lansoprazole. *Aliment Pharmacol Ther* 7 (Suppl 1): 56–60
51 Rodriguez LAG, Ruigomez A (1997) Gastric acid, acid-suppressing drugs, and bacterial gastroenteritis: how much of a risk? *Epidemiology* 8: 571–574
52 Brummer RJM, Stockbrügger RW (1996) Effect of nizatidine 300 mg at night and omeprazole 20 mg in the morning on 24-hour intragastric pH and bacterial overgrowth in patients with acute duodenal ulcer. *Dig Dis Sci* 41: 2048–2054
53 Thorens J, Froehlich F, Schwizer W et al (1996) Bacterial overgrowth during treatment with omeprazole compared with cimetidine: a prospective randomized double blind study. *Gut* 39: 54–59
54 Daschner F, Kappstein I, Engels I et al (1988) Stress ulcer prophylaxis and ventilation pneumonia: prevention by antibacterial cytoprotective agents? *Infection Control and Hospital Epidemiol* 9: 59–65
55 Lehot JJ, Deleat-Besson R, Bastien O et al (1990) Should we inhibit gastric acid secretion before cardiac surgery? *Anesth Analg* 70: 185–190
56 Driks MR, Craven DE, Celli BR et al (1987) Nosocomial pneumonia in intubated patients given sucralfate as compared with antacids or histamine type 2 blockers. *N Engl J Med* 317: 1376–1382
57 Simms HH, DeMaria E, McDonald L et al (1992) Role of gastric colonization in the development of pneumonia in critically ill trauma patients: results of a prospective randomized trial. *J Trauma* 31: 531–536
57a Cook D, Guyatt G, Marshall J et al (1998) A comparison of sucralfate and ranitidine for the prevention of upper gastrointestinal bleeding in patients requiring mechanical ventilation. *N Engl J Med* 338: 791–797
58 Lewis SJ, Franco S, Young G et al (1996) Altered bowel function and duodenal bacterial overgrowth in patients treated with omeprazole. *Aliment Pharmacol Ther* 10: 557–561
59 Koop H: Review article: metabolic consequences of long-term inhibition of acid secretion by omeprazole. *Aliment Pharmacol Ther* 1992; 6: 399–406
60 Koop H, Bachem MG (1992) Serum iron, ferritin, and Vitamin B_{12} during prolonged omeprazole therapy. *J Clin Gastroenterol* 14: 288–292
61 Festen H, Klinkenberg-Knol E, Kuipers E et al (1993) Cobalamin absorption during omeprazole treatment: short and long-term studies. *Gastroenterology* 104: A77
62 Marcuard SP, Albemaz L, Khazanie PG (1994) Omeprazole therapy causes malabsorption of cyanocobalamin (Vitamin B_{12}). *Ann Intern Med* 120: 211–215
63 Shindo K, Machida M, Fukumura M et al (1998) Omeprazole induces altered bile acid metabolism. *Gut* 42: 266–271
64 Correa P, Haenszel W, Cuello C et al (1975) A model for gastric cancer epidemiology. *Lancet* 2: 58–60
64 a Correa P (1988) A human model of gastric carcinogenesis. *Cancer Res* 48: 3554–3560
65 Küster G, Remine W, Dockerty M (1972) Gastric cancer in pernicious anaemia and in patients with and without achlorhydria. *Ann Surg* 175: 783–789
66 Hall CN, Darkin D, Brimblecombe R, Cook AJ, Kirkham JS, Northfield TC (1986) Evaluation of the nitrosamine hypothesis of gastric carcinogenesis in precancerous conditions. *Gut* 27: 491–498
67 Hall CN, Kirkham JS, Northfield TC (1987) Urinary N-nitrosoproline excretion: a further evaluation of the nitrosamine hypothesis of gastric carcinogenesis in precancerous conditions. *Gut* 28: 216–220
68 Houghton PWJ, Leach S, Owen RW et al (1989) Use of a modified N-nitrosoproline test to show intragastric nitrosation in patients at risk of gastric cancer. *Br J Cancer* 60: 231–234

69 Sobala GM, Pignatelli B, Schorah CJ et al (1991) Levels of nitrite, nitrate, n-nitroso compounds, ascorbic acid and total bile acids in gastric juice of patients with and without precancerous conditions of the stomach. *Carcinogenesis* 2: 193–198
70 Yeomans ND, Brimblecombe RW, Elder J et al (1995) Effects of acid suppression on microbial flora of upper gut. *Dig Dis Sci* 40: 81S–95S
71 Verdu E, Viani F, Armstrong D (1994) Effect of omeprazole on intragastric bacterial counts, nitrates, nitrites and nitroso compounds. *Gut* 35: 455–460
72 Milton-Thompson GJ, Lightfoot NF, Ahmet Z et al (1982) Intragastric acidity, bacteria, nitrite and N-nitroso compounds before and after cimetidine treatment. *Lancet* i: 1091–1095
73 Lechago J, Correa P (1993) Prolonged achlorhydria and gastric neoplasie: is there a causal relationship? *Gastroenterology* 104: 1554–1557
74 Brinton LA, Gridley G, Hrubec Z et al (1989) Cancer risk following pernicious anaemia. *Br J Cancer* 59: 810–813
75 Hsing AW, Hansson LE, McLaughlin JK et al (1993) Pernicious anemia and subsequent cancer. *Cancer* 71: 745–750
76 Houben GMP, Stockbrügger RW (1995) Bacteria in the aetio-pathogenesis of gastric cancer: a review. *Scand J Gastroenterol* 30(Suppl 212): 13–18
77 Fuchs CS, Mayer RJ (1995) Gastric carcinoma. *N Engl J Med* 333: 32–41
78 Lundegardh G, Adami HO, Helmick C et al (1988) Stomach cancer after partial gastrectomy for benign ulcer disease. *N Engl J Med* 319: 195–200
79 Tersmette AC, Offerhaus GJA, Termette KWF et al (1990) Meta-analysis of the risk of gastric stump cancer: detection of high risk patient subsets for stomach cancer after remote partial gastrectomy for benign conditions. *Cancer Res* 50: 6486–6489
80 Kokkola A, Sjöblom SM, Haapiainen R, Sipponen P et al (1998) The risk of gastric carcinoma and carcinoid tumours in patients with pernicious anaemia. *Scand J Gastroenterol* 33: 88–92
81 Godwin DJ (1975) Carcinoid tumors: an analysis of 2837 cases. *Cancer* 36: 560–569
82 Rindi G, Luinetti O, Cornaggia M, Capella C, Solcia E (1993) Three subtypes of gastric argyrophil carcinoid and the gastric neuroendocrine carcinoma: a clinicopathologic study. *Gastroenterology* 104: 994–1006
83 Rappel S, Altendorf-Hofmann A, Stolte M (1995) Prognosis of gastric carcinoid tumours. *Digestion* 56: 455–462
84 Waldum HL, Haugen OA, Isaksen C et al (1991) Are diffuse gastric carcinomas neuroendocrine tumours (ECL-omas)? *Eur J Gastroenterol Hepatol* 3: 245–249
85 Creutzfeldt W, Solcia E (1991) Are diffuse gastric carcinomas neuroendocrine tumours ECL-omas? *Eur J Gastroenterol Hepatol* 3: 179–191
86 Weinstock J, Baldwin GS (1988) Binding of gastrin-17 to human gastric carcinoma cell lines. *Cancer Res* 48: 932–937
87 Watson S, Durrant L, Morris D (1989) Gastrin: growth enhancing effect on human gastric and colonic tumor cells. *Br J Cancer* 59: 554–558
88 Ishizuka J, Martinez J, Townsend CM, Thompson JC (1992) The effect of gastrin on growth of human stomach cancer cells. *Ann Surg* 215: 528–534
89 Matsushima Y, Kinoshita Y, Nakata H et al (1994) Gastrin receptor gene expression in several human carcinomas. *Jpn J Cancer Res* 85: 819–824
90 Möller H, Lindvig K, Lefter R et al (1989) Cancer occurrence in a cohort of patients treated with cimetidine. *Gut* 30: 1558–1562
91 La Vecchia C, Negri E, D'Avanzo B, Franceschi S (1990) Histamine-2-receptor antagonists and gastric cancer risk. *Lancet* 36: 355–357
92 Colin-Jones DG, Langman MJS, Lawson DH et al (1992) Postmarketing surveillance of the safety of cimetidine: 10 year mortality report. *Gut* 33: 1280–1284
93 Möller H, Nissen A, Mosbech J (1992) Use of cimetidine and other peptic ulcerdrugs in Denmark 1977–1990 with analysis of the risk of gastric cancer among cimetidine users. *Gut* 33: 1166–1169
94 Stolte M, Bethke B, Seifert E et al (1995) Observation of gastric glandular cysts in the corpus mucosa of the stomach under omeprazole treatment. *Z Gastroenterol* 33: 146–149
95 Schenk BE, Kuipers EJ, Klinkenberg-Knol EC et al (1997) Gastric polyps during long-term omeprazole treatment for gastroesophageal reflux disease. *Gastroenterology* 112: A281

96 Sugano K, Fukushima, Yazaki Y (1997) Regression of hyperplastic polyps of the stomach by eradication of *helicobacter pylori*. *Gastroenterology* 112: A300
97 Beauchamp RD, Townsend CM, Singh P et al (1985) Proglumide, a gastrin receptor antagonist, inhibits growth of colon cancer and enhances survival in mice. *Ann Surg* 202: 303–309
98 Hoosein NM, Kiener PA, Curry RC et al (1988) Antiproliferative effects of gastrin receptor antagonists and antibodies to gastrin on human colon carcinoma cell lines. *Cancer Res* 48: 7179–7183
99 Hoosein NM, Kiener PA, Curry RC, Brattein MG (1990) Evidence for autocrine growth stimulation of cultured colon tumor cells by a gastrin/cholecystokinin-like peptide. *Exp Cell Res* 186: 15–21
100 Graffner H, Singh G, Chaudry I, Milson JW (1992) Omeprazole-induced hypergastrinemia does not influence growth of colon carcinoma. *Dig Dis Sci* 37: 485–489
101 Smith JP, Kramer ST, Demers LM (1993) Effects of gastrin and difluoromethylornithine on growth of human colon cancer. *Dig Dis Sci* 38: 520–528
102 Singh P, Townsend CM, Thompson JC et al (1990) Gut hormones in colon cancer: past and prospective studies. *Cancer J* 3: 28–33
103 Smith JP, Wood JG, Solomon TE (1989) Elevated gastrin levels in patients with colon cancer or adenomatous polyps. *Dig Dis Sci* 34: 171–174
104 Penman ID, El-Omar E, McGregor JR et al (1993) Omeprazole inhibits colorectal carcinogenesis induced by azoxymethane in rats. *Gut* 34: 1559–1565
105 Pinson DM, Havu N, Sztern MI et al (1995) Drug-induced hypergstrinemia: absence of trophic effects on colonic carcinoma in rats. *Gastroenterology* 108: 1068–1074
106 Baldwin GS (1994) Anti-proliferative gastrin/cholecystokinin receptor antagonists target the 78 kDa gastrin-binding protein. *Proc Natl Acad Sci USA* 91: 7593–7597
107 Imdahl A, Mantamadiotis T, Eggstein S et al (1995) Expression of gastrin, gastrin/CCK-B and gastrin/CCK-C receptors in human colorectal carcinomas. *J Cancer Res Clin Oncol* 121: 661–666
108 Finley GG, Koski RA, Melhem MF et al (1993) Expression of the gastrin gene in the normal human colon and colorectal adenocarcinoma. *Cancer Res* 53: 2919–2926
109 Luttichau HR, Van Solinge WW, Nielsen FC, Rehfeld JF (1993) Developmental expression of the gastrin and cholecystokinin genes in rat colon. *Gastroenterology* 104: 1092–1098
110 Van Solinge WW, Nielsen FC, Friis-Hansen L et al (1993) Expression but incomplete maturation of progastrin in clorectal carcinomas. *Gastroenterology* 104: 1099–1107
111 Rehfeld JF (1995) Gastrin and colorectal cancer: a never ending dispute? *Gastroenterology* 108: 1307–1310
112 Hollande F, Imdahl A, Mantamadiotis T et al (1997) Glycine-extended gastrin acts as an autocrine growth factor in a nontransformed colon cell line. *Gastroenterology* 113: 1576–1588
113 Ciccotosto GD, McLeish A, Hardy KJ, Shulkes A (1995) Expression, processing and secretion of gastrin in patients with colorectal carcinoma. *Gastroenterology* 109: 1142–1153
114 Seitz JF, Giovannini M, Gouvernet J, Gauthier AP (1991) Elevated serum gastrin levels in patients with colorectal neoplasia. *J Clin Gastroenterol* 13: 541–545
115 Wong K, Beardshall K, Waters CM et al (1991) Postprandial hypergastrinaemia in patients with colorectal cancer. *Gut* 32: 1352–1354
116 Penman ID, El-Omar E, Ardill JES et al (1994) Plasma gastrin concentrations are normal in patients with colorectal neoplasia and unaltered following tumor resection. *Gastroenterology* 106: 1263–1270
117 Suzuki H, Matsumoto K, Terashima H (1988) Serum levels of gastrin in patients with colorectal neoplasia. *Dis Colon Rectum* 31: 716–717
118 Kaufmann HP, Ottenjann R (1991) Serum-Nüchtern-Gastrin-Werte bei Kolonadenomen und kolorektalen Karzinomen. *Z Gastroenterol* 29: 527–528
119 Yapp R, Modlin IM, Kumar RR et al (1992) Gastrin and colorectal cancer evidence against an association. *Dig Dis Sci* 37: 481–484
120 Kikendall JW, Glass AR, Sobin LH, Bowen PE (1992) Serum gastrin is not higher in subjects with colonic neoplasia. *Am J Gastroenterol* 87: 1394–1397
121 Elsborg L, Mosbech J (1979) Pernicious anaemia as a risk factor in gastric cancer. *Acta Med Scand* 206: 315–318

122 Orbuch M, Venzon DJ, Lubensky IA et al (1996) Prolonged hypergastrinemia does not increase the frequency of colonic neoplasia in patients with Zollinger-Ellison syndrome. *Dig Dis Sci* 41: 604–613
123 Caygill CPJ, Hill MJ, Hall CN et al (1987) Increased risk of cancer at multiple sites after gastric surgery for peptic ulcer. *Gut* 28: 924–928
124 Hill MJ (1983) Bile, bacteria and bowel cancer. *Gut* 24: 871–875
125 Mullan FJ, Wilson HK, Majury CW et al (1990) Bile acids and the increased risk of colorectal tumours after truncal vagotomy. *Br J Surg* 77: 1085–1090
126 Watt PCH, Patterson CC, Kennedy TL (1984) Late mortality after vagotomy and drainage for duodenal ulcer. *Br Med J* 288: 1335–1338
127 Bundred NJ, Whitfield BCS, Stanton E et al (1985) Gastric surgery and the risk of subsequent colorectal cancer. *Br J Surg* 72: 618–619
128 Fisher SG, Davis F, Nelson R et al (1994) Large bowel cancer following gastric surgery for benign disease: a cohort study. *Am J Epidemiol* 139: 684–692
129 Lundegardh G, Adami HO, Helmick C, Zack M (1990) The risk of large bowel cancer after partial gastrectomy for benign ulcer disease. *Ann Surgery* 212: 714–719
130 Möller H, Toftgaard C (1991) Cancer occurrence in a cohort of patients surgically treated for peptic ulcer. *Gut* 32: 740–744
131 Tersmette AC, Offerhaus GJA, Giardiello FM et al (1991) Long-term prognosis after partial gastrectomy for benign conditions. *Gastroenterology* 101: 148–153
132 Macintyre IMC, O'Brien F (1994) Death from malignant disease after surgery for duodenal ulcer. *Gut* 35: 451–454
133 Munnangi S, Sonnenberg A (1997) Colorectal cancer after gastric surgery: a meta-analysis. *Am J Gastroenterol* 92: 109–113

Proton Pump Inhibitors
ed. by L. Olbe

The acid tolerance of *Helicobacter pylori*

George Sachs [1], David Scott [1], David Wecks [1] and Klaus Melchers [2]

[1] *UCLA and Wadsworth VA, Los Angeles, CA 90073, USA*
[2] *Byk Gulden, D-78467 Konstanz, Germany*

Introduction

For millions of years prokaryotes have orchestrated their genetic players to produce survival strategies that overcome almost all ills that bacterial flesh is heir to. Infection of mammalian gastric mucosae by *Helicobacter* spp. is due to this organism's insistence on habitation of probably the most unfriendly environment in the mammalian body, the inside of the stomach. The eradication of *H. pylori* for treatment of peptic ulcer disease not associated with non-steroidal anti-inflammatory drugs (NSAIDs), steroids or severe stress is now accepted as part of medical treatment of this set of illnesses. Whether the infection should always be treated with violence is a point of discussion [1].

Therapy with proton pump inhibitors and two antibiotics is the most frequently prescribed medication, with perhaps bismuth along with ranitidine and two antibiotics as other possible therapy [2]. The rationale for the need for the former combination is becoming clearer but monotherapy would be more desirable, simplifying treatment and avoiding the use of antibiotics necessary for treatment of other infections. Most feel that a general antibiotic is inappropriate for global eradication and an *H. pylori*-specific compound would be preferable. In order to understand the biological basis of this infection and pave the way for treatment to take advantage of the characteristics of this gastric pathogen, the biology of *H. pylori* is of pivotal interest.

Since the discovery of the association of gastric infection by *H. pylori* [3], the major emphasis of research in this area has naturally been focussed on eradication [4], epidemiology [5] and pathogenesis [6]. It was recognized early on that bacterial production of urease was significant factor in bacterial survival in the stomach [7], and the urease operon was among the first set of genes that was sequenced [8]. Rather little attention has been paid to the biological details surrounding the organism's use of urease for gastric survival [9]. Bacteria have adapted remarkably to a variety of environments, acidic, neutral or alkaline. Bacteria surviving and growing in acidic media are classified as acidophiles, either obligatory or facultative, those able to survive and grow in neutral media are neutralophiles, and those able to survive and grow in alkaline media are classified as alkalophiles. *H. pylori* uses its urease activity to be an acid-tolerant neutralophile.

The way *H. pylori* does this is likely to be interesting, since several microorganisms display urease activity but do not survive even gastric passage [10]. An organism that has adopted a urease mechanism for gastric passage but not for gastric colonization is *Yersinia enterocolitica*. This organism has a cytoplasmic urease with a sharp pH optimum at 5 that is activated when cytoplasmic pH falls [11]. At a cytoplasmic pH of 5, however, protein synthesis is sharply curtailed; thus this urease does not allow *Yersinia* to colonize the stomach, just to survive gastric transit.

The urease produced by *Helicobacter* spp. is a neutral pH optimum enzyme [12]; therefore, a fall of cytoplasmic pH is not an adaptive mechanism for this organism. The inhabitation of the gastric mucosa by *Helicobacter* such as *H. pylori* requires specialization of properties of this microaerophilic bacterial species in order to enable survival and growth on the gastric surface and within antral glands. It should be noted that there are also *Helicobacter* that do not inhabit the stomach, although why some of them have gastric adapted and some not is as yet unknown [13].

Bacterial bioenergetics

Aerobic bacteria (including microaerophilic bacteria) synthesize ATP by coupling oxidation of substrates to the generation of an electrochemical

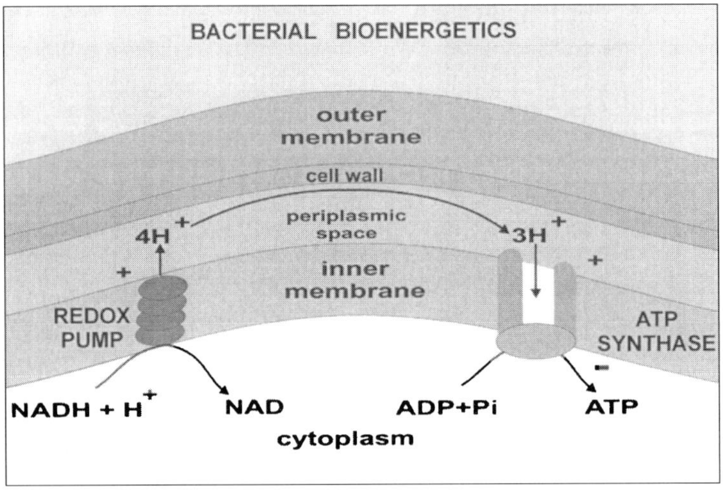

Figure 1. The general mechanism for ATP synthesis by aerobes and microaerobhiles. The environmental pH that is tolerated is pH 4 to 7. This pH is the same as that found in the periplasmic space unless there are specialized mechanisms for pH regulation such as urease. Over the range of pH from 4 to 7, various substrates are oxided via a series of electron acceptors which in turn are reoxidized by oriented redox complexes so that protons are exported electrogenically across the cytoplasmic membrane. This generates an interior negative potential and an inward pH gradient to provide the proton motive force for aerobic ATP synthesis and H^+ gradient linked uptake or export of ions or solutes.

proton gradient across their cytoplasmic membrane and then dissipation of this proton gradient through the cytoplasmic membrane's ATP synthase to generate ATP from ADP and P_i. The proton gradient is composed of two components, an actual pH gradient and a potential difference across the membrane which results in an electrochemical driving force for H^+ across the ATP synthesis complex. A balance of these two constituents of the proton energy charge of the membrane enables bacterial survival over a range of pH 2 to 11 depending on whether they are acidophiles, neutralophiles or alkalophiles. It is the pH of the periplasmic space or the transmembrane potential that is regulated to adapt to conditions of varying pH.

The circulation of protons across the bacterial cytoplasmic membrane is electrogenic, that is to say export of protons by the redox pumps oxidizing substrate generates current and voltage and uptake of protons through the F_1F_0 ATPase also generates current and voltage in the opposite direction. The gradient of hydrogen ions is expressed as a function of the chemical and electrical potential where the electrochemical gradient of hydrogen ions is the driving force for ATP generation by the chemiosmotic mechanism first recognized by Peter Mitchell in 1961 [14]. The thermodynamic equation describing the electrochemical gradient for H^+, namely

$$\begin{aligned} \text{p.m.f (in mV)} &= \Delta \bar{\mu}_{H}^{+} = -RT/F \ln [H^{+}_{out}]/[H^{+}_{in}] + \Delta \psi \\ &= -61\, \Delta pH + PD \end{aligned}$$

where $\Delta \bar{\mu}_{H}^{+}$ is the electrochemical gradient for protons, R is the gas constant, T the temperature in degrees Kelvin, F is the Faraday constant and $\Delta \psi$ is the transmembrane potential, referred to in text as *PD*

predicts that there is a reciprocal relationship between the pH gradient and the potential difference, that is as the inward pH gradient increases, the PD decreases and vice versa in order to maintain a relatively constant proton motive force. The chemiosmotic mechanism for ATP generation by a neutralophile is illustrated in Figure 1.

Structure of *H. pylori*

H. pylori is a motile, Gram-negative organism that can be cultured in microaerophilic (low O_2) conditions, although it adapts to high O_2 at higher culture densities. It has an outer membrane, the outer leaflet of which is lipopolysaccharide, a cell wall and periplasmic space, an inner membrane and cytoplasm. The bioenergetic survival of the organism depends on the maintenance of an adequate proton motive force between the periplasmic space and the cytoplasm across its inner or cytoplasmic membrane. The organism is helical or spiral in shape, and possesses six to eight flagella at one end. Flagellar function depends on the activity of a flagellar motor that also is driven by the proton motive force generated across the cytoplasmic membrane of the organism. Control of periplasmic pH is vital for survival and growth of the organism in its gastric environment. The organism also has a set of stringency response genes that control, for example, cell wall biosynthesis, preventing cell division in unfriendly environments.

The Bacterial genome

The genome contains about 1500 genes, 300 of which encode membrane proteins, many with as yet unknown functions [15]. The sequences encoding for membrane proteins comprise genes such as the F_1F_0 ATP synthase complex and various oxido-reductases such as cytochrome o, several transporters and a variety of two-component signaling systems (the equivalent of eukaryotic receptors). Some of the recognized transporters are illustrated in Figure 2.

The organism contains enzymes for glucose metabolism, lacks β galactosidase (hence is unable to metabolize lactose), some of the enzymes of the Krebs cycle (no isocitrate dehydrogenase), and most important, the urease gene cluster encoding ureA and ureB (urease) and ureE,F,G,H and I

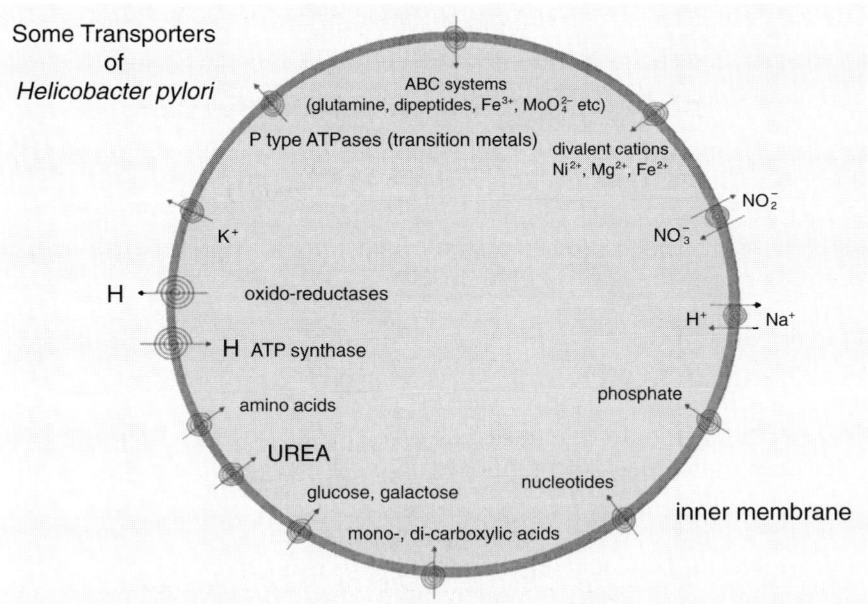

Figure 2. Some of the transporters identified in the *H. pylori* genome. There are several other integral membrane proteins that are as yet functionally unclassified. The urea transporter is postulated based on data presented below.

as part of the ure operon. Synthesis of urease is constitutive, accounting for as much as 15% of the organism's protein. The genome also encodes for several outer membrane proteins (OMPs) some of which are porins, able to transport a variety of molecules into or out of the periplasmic space. Some of these have a higher isoelectric point than that of neutralophiles such as *Escherichia coli* or *Bacillus subtilis*. Perhaps this higher isoelectric point is useful in transient resistance to a fall of pH but cannot be used for chronic protection against acid.

Survival and growth characteristics of *H. pylori*

The survival and growth of organisms as a function of medium pH is diagnostic of their bioenergetic profile. For example, neutralophiles such as *E. coli* characteristically are able to survive between pH 4 and 8 and grow well between pH 6 and 8. When these properties of *H. pylori* are measured as shown in Figure 3, it seems that this organism shares survival and growth characteristics with *E. coli*. Here organisms are placed at various pH levels and then put on agar plates at pH 7 to determine colony forming units for survival, or are kept in growth medium at fixed pH and colony forming units counted for growth [16, 17].

From the measurement of survival which is found at a medium pH of only greater than 4, it is obvious that without specialized acid-adaptive mechanisms *H. pylori* would not be found in the stomach. It is also clear

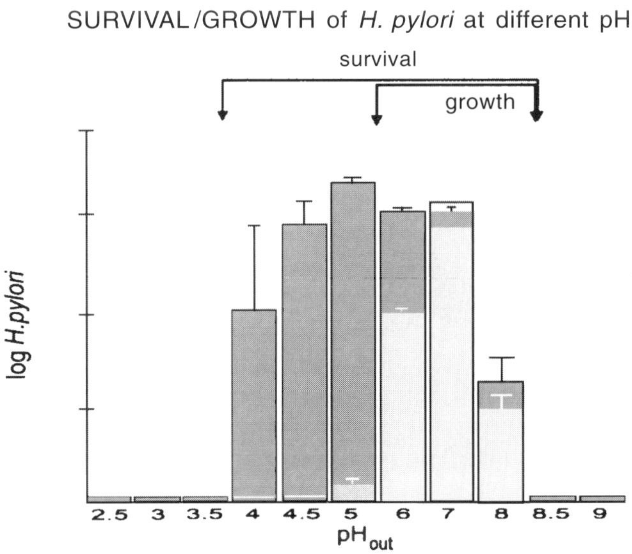

Figure 3. Survival of *H. pylori* in the absence of urea and growth in the absence of urea as a function of fixed medium pH.

that any colonization without adaptive mechanisms would be impossible given the pH characteristics of growth. A similar conclusion can be derived from measurements of protein synthesis *in vitro*, where a correlation is found between protein synthesis and growth.

Metabolism of *H. pylori* at different pH

Bacterial metabolism should also correlate with survival. There are various ways of measuring metabolism, such as oxygen consumption, CO_2 production from labeled glucose or incorporation of radioactivity into protein. A particularly convenient means that is also adaptable to monitoring of urease activity is the measurement of pH changes induced by a bacterial suspension. A microphysiometer is an instrument capable of very sensitive measurement of pH changes in a flow-through system, which avoids the use of strong buffers to maintain a constant pH environment. A light-addressable pH sensor is computer-controlled to measure the pH within eight chambers simultaneously that contain about 10^5 agar-immobilized bacteria through which solution at different pH is pumped. The pH change is read out in µV/s for 16 s when the pump stops for 16 s in a 40 s pump cycle.

The bacteria are able to acidify the medium at neutral pH or greater due to the production of metabolic acid and alkalinize the medium below pH 5.5 due to reabsorption of H^+ for ATP synthesis, as shown in Figure 4. The pH range of metabolism displayed here corresponds to what was found using standard survival measurements, again attesting to the neutralophile properties of the gastric organism. The presence of glutamine stimul-

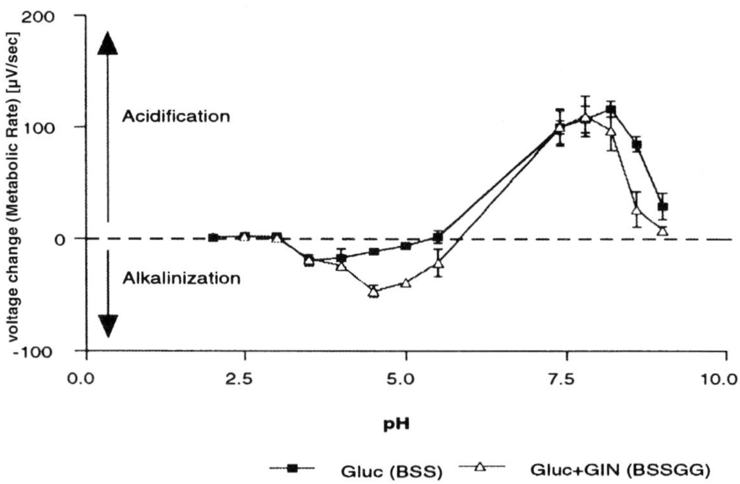

Figure 4. Metabolism of *H. pylori* measured by changes of chamber pH as a function of medium pH in the absence of urea in a lightly buffered glucose medium or glucose + glutamine medium

ates alkalinization slightly at pH < 6, perhaps due to NH_3 production by glutaminase [18].

Bioenergetic profile of *H. pylori*

The potential difference and pH gradient across the cytoplasmic membrane of *H. pylori* as a function of medium pH also enable conclusions as to the nature of the membrane homeostatic machinery necessary for gastric habitation by this organism. The organism is too small for microelectrode measurements of pH or potential difference, and less direct methods using dye probes of these parameters have proved successful.

For measurement of cytoplasmic pH a fluorescent pH dye, BCEFC, is loaded into the organisms by incubation with a nonfluorescent ester, BCECF-AM, that is hydrolyzed by bacterial esterase inside the organism and stays trapped due to the three negative charges produced by removal of the AM groups. For measurement of membrane potential, a cationic lipid permeable dye, $diS^- C_3^-(5)$ is used that decreases fluorescence as it accumulates inside the organism due to a negative interior potential.

With these dyes it is possible to calibrate the fluorescence signal as a function of pH or membrane potential. It was found that at a medium pH of 7, the internal pH was 8.4 and the transmembrane potential –131 mV. A pH gradient of 1.4 inward corresponds to a potential of –90 mV, and hence, from the equation above, the driving force for entry of H^+ across the ATP synthase at neutral pH is –221 mV, similar to that found in other aerobic bacteria.

When membrane potential was measured as a function of medium pH, the presence of a PD was found between pH 4 and pH 8, exactly the pH range over which the organism survives, as shown in Figure 5. As predicted by the proton motive force equation, as medium pH became more acidic, the potential difference decreased, since the inward pH gradient increased, and as medium pH became more alkaline, the potential difference increased to compensate for the decrease in inward pH gradient, to maintain a relatively constant driving force for ATP synthesis.

The absence of a membrane potential below pH 4 was irreversible if the organism was kept at this pH for longer than 5–10 min and the absence of a membrane potential above pH 8 was also irreversible if this pH was maintained for longer than 30 min [19].

Overall, therefore, *H. pylori* behaves as a neutralophile and displays no evidence for direct adaptive mechanisms that would enable survival at the highly acidic pH that gastric contents must reach several times during the day. It is regulation of the periplasmic environment that is important for the organism rather than that of environmental pH, and for survival in stomach acid, rapid adaptive mechanisms must be present. The most important of these is urease activity.

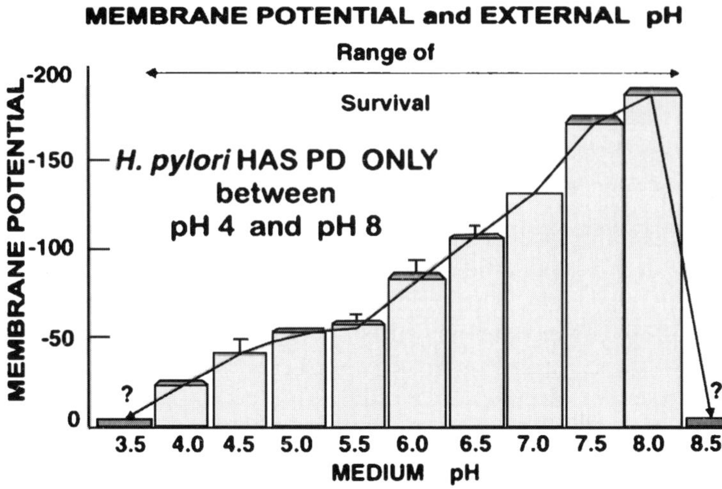

Figure 5. Inner-membrane potential of *H. pylori* as a function of fixed medium pH.

Acid adaptation by *H. pylori* via urease activity

The action of urease is the hydrolysis of urea to ammonia and carbamic acid followed by spontaneous cleavage of carbamate to ammonia and carbon dioxide thus:

$$CO(NH_2)_2 + H_2O \rightarrow NH_3HCO_2NH_2 \rightarrow NH_3 + CO_2$$

resulting in strong alkalinization of the medium. In the absence of strong buffering, the pH of the medium will reach the pK_a of the NH_4^+/NH_3 couple, namely 9.5. Urease is composed of two subunits, ureA and ureB and contains Ni^{2+} as an essential ion. It is the major protein synthesized by *H. pylori*.

Urease activity was recognized as an important parameter enabling acid survival early on in research on the gastric mechanisms of *H. pylori*. The enzyme is found both in the cytoplasm and is loosely associated with the cell surface, presumably due to binding to the lipopolysaccharide of the outer leaflet of the outer membrane [20, 21].

It has been considered for some time that this external urease is responsible for elevating the microenvironment of the organism to a level compatible not only with life but with growth. This is probably an oversimplification, given the measurement of the pH activity curve of the external enzyme as compared with the activity of the cytoplasmic enzyme as displayed in Figure 6.

Here urease activity present in the intact organism was measured, and urease activity that was removed by washing the surface was measured as a function of fixed medium pH using $^{14}CO_2$ liberated from labeled urea.

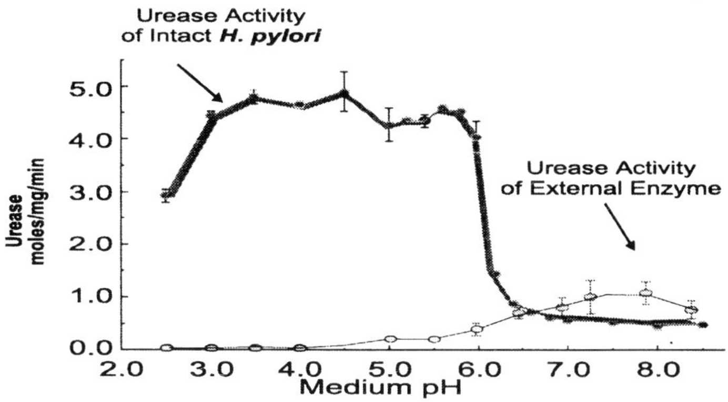

Figure 6. pH optimum of urease on the bacterial surface and in intact bacteria. After 24 h-culture 5% of urease is found on the surface and 95% inside the organism.

The vast majority of the urease was found in intact bacteria, but was inactive until a medium pH of 6.5 was reached. As medium pH was lowered, there was a >10-fold increase in urease activity that was maintained until a pH of 2.5 was obtained. A simple interpretation of these data is that there is activation of a urea transport at about pH 6.5 with an EC_{50} of pH 6 and that activation of this transport enables constant internal urease activity until a pH of 2.5 is reached [22].

It is also clear that the pH activity profile of the surface urease says that this urease is unable to affect the pH outside the organism at a pH below 4. Hence, internal urease must be used to permit survival when gastric pH falls to 4 or below!

These studies were done using strong buffering to prevent any change of pH. Strong buffering of gastric contents is unusual, so the examination of urease activity was repeated in the microphysiometer, where weakly buffered glucose medium was superfused over 10^5 bacteria with urea and urease activity assessed by alkalinization of the medium.

There is about a 20-fold activation of urease activity as the pH falls to below 4 (Fig. 7). At higher pH in the small volume of the chamber, internal urease activity is able to elevate chamber pH very rapidly; hence, urease activity is only transient. At a pH of 3, the level of acid is sufficient to require significant levels of urease activity in order to attempt to elevate pH. These data also show that internal urease is activated by acidification of the medium but stays inactive at neutral pH [18].

When experiments are carried out to measure the effect of urease activation on periplasmic pH or transmembrane potential, it is found that the addition of urea at pH 3, 4 or 5 brings periplasmic pH to a value of 6.2 and the transmembrane potential to a value of –105 mV. The driving force for entry of H^+ across the ATP synthase is therefore maintained constant at about –220 mV.

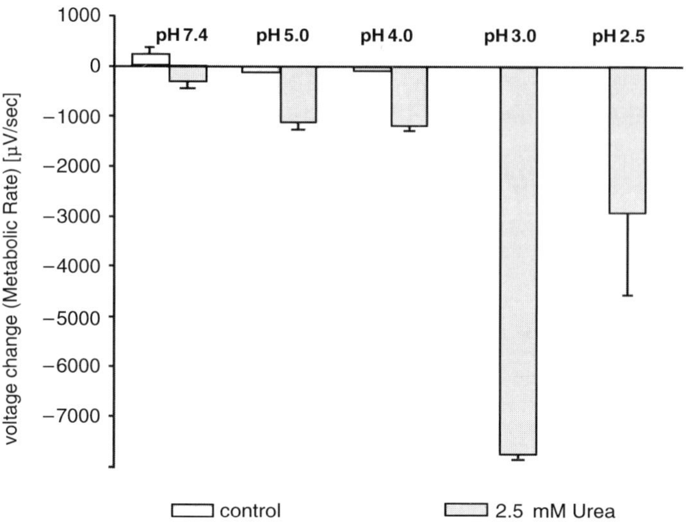

Figure 7. Urease activity as a function of perfusion pH in the microphysiometer. Urease activity is seen at pH 5 and 4, and a large increase is seen at pH 3 and 2.5.

These data show that the presence of urea and activation of urease by acidic medium pH enable acid survival of *H. pylori*. A model for the activation of internal urease by activation of a urea transport system is shown in Figure 8.

At a medium pH > 6.5, the urea transporter is inactive, and only surface urease modifies pH. Below pH 6.2, the transporter is activated and urea

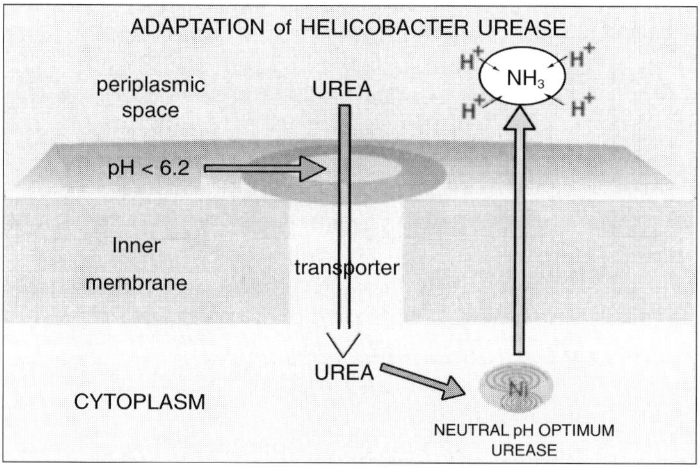

Figure 8. A model for regulation of urea transport by *H. pylori* as a function of medium pH. Urea transport is activated at pH < 6.2, and internal urease activity results in NH_3 production, diffusion into the periplasmic space and buffering of H^+.

accesses internal urease. Internal urease activity results in the export of NH_3 and elevation of periplasmic pH to 6.2. Above this periplasmic pH internal urease is inactivated; below this pH internal urease is activated, enabling the set point of pH 6.2 to be reached down to a pH of 2.5 at mM levels of urea.

Urease is essential for *H. pylori*

The elimination of urease activity by either growth selection for urease negative mutants or intentional removal of one of the urease enzyme genes results in strains that are unable to infect animal models [23, 24]. It is possible to obtain some infection if acid is severely inhibited by omeprazole, but the infection does not persist after removal of the drug.

A model that is substantiated by the above data for the adaptation of *H. pylori* to the gastric environment is shown in Figure 9.

In summary, all current data suggest that *H. pylori* is an acid-tolerant neutralophile rather than a facultative acidophile and that its acid tolerance derives from an acid-activated urea transporter allowing urea access to the cytoplasmic urease present in the organism. Is it possible to demonstrate this activation of urease in a direct experiment?

In order to do this, *H. pylori* were cocultured with a gastric cell line, AGS, and viewed in a superfusion chamber in a confocal microscope. Present in the medium was BCECF, a dye that increases its fluorescence between a pH of 5 and 8. This dye is excited at 488 nM, and emission is read at > 530 nM. As pH increases from a perfusion pH of 4.5, an increase in green fluorescence is seen, indicating alkalinization of the region sensed by the dye. BCECF is impermeant, and hence in this experiment will measure only changes in medium pH. In a separate series of experiments, cell pH and cell calcium were measured by videoimaging.

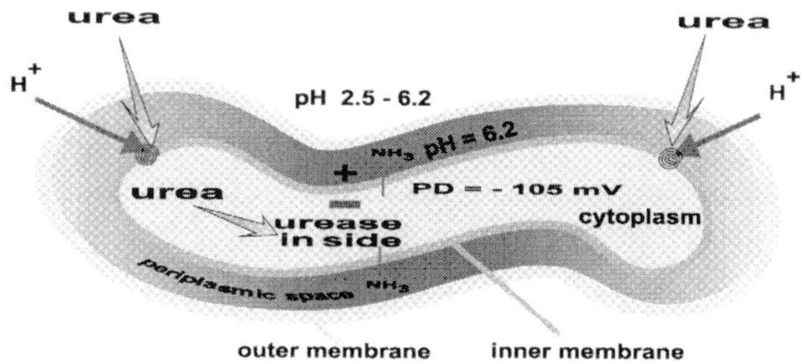

Figure 9. A model of the regulation of periplasmic pH by *H. pylori*, showing acid-dependent activation of a uea transporter, activation of internal urease activity at a pH < 6.2 and thus maintenance of periplasmic pH at 6.2 and membrane potential at – 105 mV.

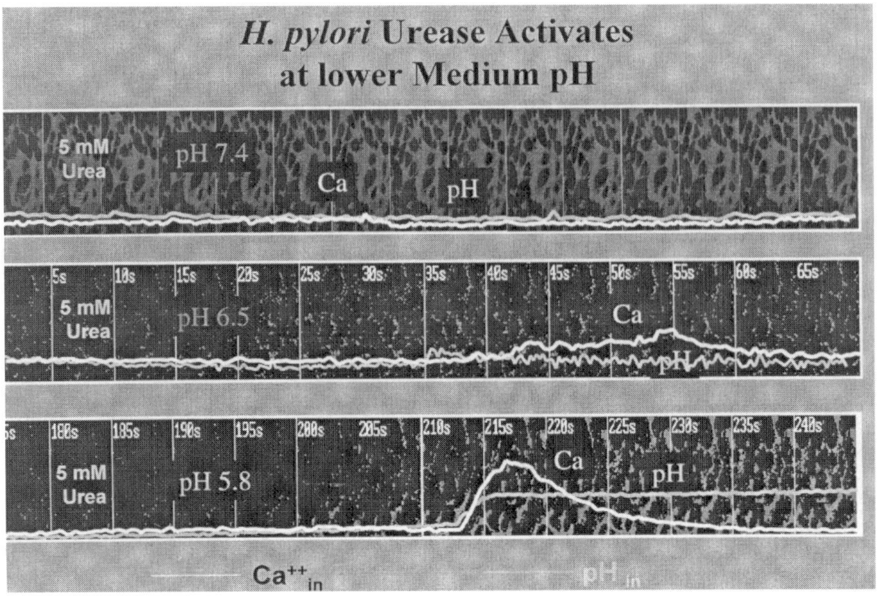

Figure 10. A combination of confocal and videomicroscopy of AGS cells cocultured with *H. pylori*. The medium pH is as indicated, and urea was added where shown. In a separate series of experiments, pH_i and Ca_i were measured under identical conditions. Each frame of the confocal images is a 5 s interval.

Figure 10 shows that with the addition of urea at pH 7.4, there is no change in medium pH or cellular calcium or pH. At pH 6.5, there is a slight increase in medium pH and cell pH with a slow rise in cell calcium. However, at pH 5.8, where internal bacterial urease is activated, there is a rapid rise in medium pH, cell pH and cell calcium. These data are consistent with the expectation that internal bacterial urease is responsible for elevation of medium pH by activation of a urea transporter. Further, the increase of medium NH_3 results in cell alkalinization and elevation of cell calcium, which may eventually result in cell damage or apoptosis.

The idea that acid activation of bacterial urease occurs in the human stomach may account for the occurrence of duodenal ulcer even though it is difficult to find bacteria dwelling in the duodenum. Antral habitation by the organism appears to correlate with the occurrence of duodenal ulcer. Under the acidic conditions of the stomach the bacterial urease is active and there is production of NH_3. However, in acid most of this is NH_4^+, and this cation does not penetrate the cell. However, when gastric juice flows into the duodenum, the juice is neutralized, and there is now a much higher concentration of NH_3. This, as shown in the experiment of Figure 11, can penetrate the duodenal cell and there elevate pH_i and Ca_i. This can result in damage to the duodenal cell in the absence of bacterial habitation in the area of an ulcer as suggested in Figure 11.

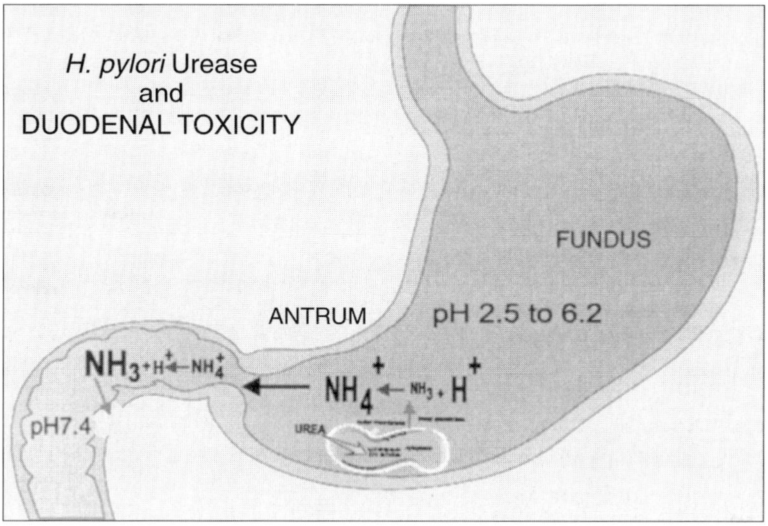

Figure 11. A hypothetical model of the causation of duodenal ulcer. Gastric acid activates bacterial urease in antral organisms, but most of the NH_3 is converted to NH_4^+. When the juice empties into the duodenum, more NH_3 is present due to the higher pH. This permeant gas can then rapidly enter duodenal cells and can result in increased cell apoptosis and ulceration.

This hypothesis suggests that induction of apoptosis in the duodenum may be associated with infection [25] and may require a concerted effect of urease activity in the stomach and products of the pathogenicity island [1].

References

1 Blaser MJ (1998) *Helicobacter pylori* and gastric disease. *Brit Med J* 316: 1507–1510
2 McGowan CC, Cover TL, Blaser MJ (1996) *Helicobacter pylori* and gastric acid: biological and therapeutic implications. *Gastroenterology* 110: 926–938
3 Warren JR, Marshall B (1983) Unidentified curved bacilli on gastric epithelium in acitve chronic gastritis. *Lancet* i, 1273–1275
4 Walsh JH, Peterson WL (1995) The treatment of *Helicobacter pylori* infection in the management of peptic ulcer disease. *N Engl J Med* 333: 984–991
5 Graham DY (1989) *Campylobacter pylori* and peptic ulcer disease. *Gastroenterology* 96: 615–625
6 Dunn BE, Cohen H, Blaser MJ (1997) *Helicobacter pylori*. *Clin Microbiol Rev* 10: 720–741
7 Marshall BJ, Barrett LJ, Prakash C, McCallum RW, Guerrant RL (1990) Urea protects *Helicobacter (Campylobacter) pylori* from the bactericidal effect of acid. *Gastroenterology* 99: 697–702
8 Labigne A, Cussac V, Courcoux P (1991) Shuttle cloning and nucleotide sequences of *Helicobacter pylori* genes responsible for urease activity. *J Bacteriol* 173: 1920–1931
9 Ferrero RL, Lee A (1996) The importance of urease in acid protection for the gastric colonizing bacteria, *Helicobacter pylori* and *Helicobacter felis*. *Microb Ecol Health Dis* 4: 121–134
10 Mobley HLT, Island MD, Hausinger RP (1995) Molecular biology of microbial ureases. *Microbiol Rev* 59: 451–480

11 Young GM, Amid D, Miller VR (1996) A bifunctional urease enhances survival of pathogenic *Yersinia enterocolitica* and *Morganella morganii* at low pH. *J Bacteriol* 178: 6487–6495
12 Dunn BE, Camphell GP, Perez-Perez GI, Blaser MJ (1990) Purification and characterization of urease from *Helicobacter pylori*. *J Biol Chem* 265: 9464–9469
13 Fox JG, Lee A (1997) Role of *Helicobacter* species in newly recognized gastrointestinal tract disease of animals. *Lab Animal Science* 47: 222–255
14 Mitchell P (1966) Chemiosmotic coupling in oxidative and photosynthetic phosphorylation. *Biol Rev* 41: 445–502
15 Tomb JF, White O, Kerlavage AR, Clayton RA, Sutton GG et al (1997) The complete genome sequence of the gastric pathogen *Helicobacter pylori*. *Nature* 388: 539–547
16 Clyne M, Labigne A, Drumm B (1995) *Helicobacter pylori* requires an acidic environment to survive in the presence of urea. *Infect Immun* 63: 1669–1673
17 Morgan DR, Freedman F, Depew CE, Kraft WG (1987) Growth of *Campylobacter* in liquid media. *J Clin Microbiol* 25: 2123–2125
18 Rektorschek M, Weeks D, Sachs G, Melchers K. Influence of pH on metabolism and urease activity of *Helicobacter pylori*. *Gastroenterology; in press*
19 Meyer-Rosberg K, Scott DR, Rex D, Melchers K, Sachs G (1996) The effect of the environmental pH on the proton motive force of *Helicobacter pylori*. *Gastroenterology* 111: 886–900
20 Phadnis SH, Parlow MH, Levy M, Ilver D, Caulkins CM, Connors JB, Dunn BE (1995) Surface localization of *Helicobacter pylori* urease and a heat shock protein homolog requires bacterial autolyis. *Infect Immun* 64: 905–912
21 Hawtin PR, Stacey AR, Newell DG (1990) Investigation of the structure and localization of the urease of *Helicobacter pylori* using monoclonal antibodies. *J Gen Microbiol* 136: 1995–2000
22 Scott DR, Weeks D, Hong C, Postius S, Melchers K, Sachs G (1998) The role of internal urease in acid resistance of *Helicobacter pylori*. *Gastroenterology* 114: 58–70
23 Eaton KA, Morgan DR, Brooks CL, Krakowka S (1991) Essential role of urease in the pathogenesis of gastritis induced by *Helicobacter pylori* in gnotobiotic piglets. *Infect Immun* 59: 2470–2475
24 Tsuda M, Karita M, Morshed MG, Okita K, Nakazawa TA (1994) Urease negative mutant of *Helicobacter pylori* constructed by allelic exchange mutagenesis lacks the ability to colonize the nude mouse stomach. *Infect Immun* 62: 3586–3589
25 Chen G, Sordillo EM, Ramey WG, Reidy J, Holt PR, Krajewski S, Reed JC, Blaser MJ, Moss SF (1997) Apoptosis in gastric epithelial cells is induced by *Helicobacter pylori* and accompanied by increased expression of BAK. *Biochem Biophys Res Comm* 239: 626–632

Proton Pump Inhibitors
ed. by L. Olbe

Interactions of proton pump inhibitors and *Helicobacter pylori in vivo*

Andre Louis Blum and Jan Martínek

Division de Gastro-Enterologie, Chuv, Lausanne, Switzerland

Introduction

There are multiple interactions between proton pump inhibitors (PPIs) and *Helicobacter pylori in vivo*. This chapter deals with two aspects: First, we discuss the effect of *H. pylori* on pH control by PPIs and on the clinical effectiveness of these drugs. Second, we focus on the effect of PPIs on *H. pylori* and on gastritis. Of special interest is the question whether long-term treatment with PPIs leads, in *H. pylori*-infected subjects, to the development of atrophic gastritis and associated changes, considered by some authors to represent a precancerous condition.

Effect of *H. pylori* on the pH control by PPIs

In infected subjects, we have observed a higher intragastric pH with a given dose of a PPI than in noninfected subjects. This observation was first made when comparing *H. pylori*-positive and *H. pylori*-negative subjects and later confirmed when the same subjects were examined before and after cure of the infection [1–3; Fig. 1]. The effect is significant and amounts to a difference of 2 pH units over a 24-h period. Without omeprazole, the intragastric pH of infected subjects was similar to the pH of noninfected subjects [1–4]. We have observed the same phenomenon in otherwise healthy subjects and in patients with duodenal ulcer disease. Thus, the higher pH during PPI administration is not due to a lower overall acidity of the infected stomach. Our observations have been confirmed by other authors. Without omeprazole, and depending on the experimental conditions, others have described lower, increased or unchanged acid output after cure of the infection.

Several possible mechanisms may account for the *H. pylori*-omeprazole interaction. It might be related to the pharmacokinetic properties of PPIs, to the changes induced by *H. pylori*-related gastritis or to a direct product of *H. pylori* such as ammonia.

We first tested whether our observation could be explained by an effect of infection on pharmacokinetics of PPIs. For example, activation to sul-

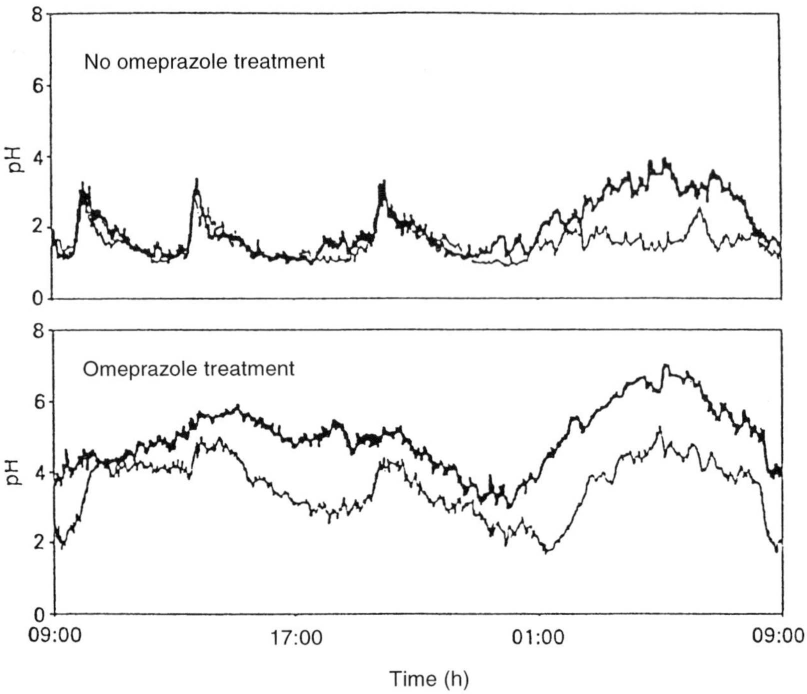

Figure 1. Median 24-h pH curves before (thick lines) and 4 weeks after cure of *H. pylori* infection (thin lines). In a double-blind and cross-over study, 18 asymptomatic volunteers received omeprazole 20 mg/day for 1 week. A 24-h intragastric pH metry was performed the day before omeprazole treatment was started (upper panel) and on day 8 of omeprazole treatment (lower panel). The difference between the two omeprazole curves, but not between baseline curves, was statistically significant ($p = 0.005$). From ref. 2.

fenamide could be more rapid. However, in a first study, we found similar serum levels of omeprazole in infected and noninfected individuals. Subsequently, we used a reversible pump blocker with a different mode of action – pumaprazole – and compared it with omeprazole. Pumaprazole had the same inhibitory effect on gastric acidity as omeprazole and, like omeprazole, had a much more pronounced effect on gastric acidity before than after cure of the infection [4]. Since pumaprazole is not activated in the parietal cell and binds reversibly to the proton pump, and since the half-life of omeprazole is not affected by cure of the infection, the hypothesis that PPIs lose their apparent effectiveness after cure of the infection because of different pharmacokinetics can be discarded [5].

We have also tested the hypothesis that the apparent increase of effectiveness of omeprazole in *H. pylori*-positive subjects is due to ammonia production of *H. pylori* and thus to the neutralizing effect of ammonia. In subjects with *H. pylori* infection, we found high ammonia concentrations in gastric juice. After cure of the infection, ammonia concentrations fell to very low levels [6]. We then investigated the effect of *H. pylori* infection on acid output, intragastric pH and ammonia concentration during omeprazole treatment. The measured pH values were corrected for the neutralizing effect of ammonia present in gastric juice. The corrected pH was much lower than the measured pH, and corresponded to the pH measured during omeprazole treatment after cure of the infection. Thus, we have provided evidence that, in subjects with *H. pylori* infection, omeprazole leads to a higher pH in gastric juice mainly because ammonia produced by *H. pylori* has a neutralizing effect [7]. In contrast, bile and duodenal contents entering the stomach by duodenogastric reflux as well as proteins appear to contribute little to this high intragastric pH. Other authors came to differing conclusions, not finding a link between elevated pH and ammonia production [8]; they attribute the high pH to decreased acid output as a consequence of corpus gastritis, which develops during omeprazole treatment. In our own study, we were unable to find such an effect of gastritis on the pH control of omeprazole [2, 4].

The "ammonia hypothesis" as well as the "gastritis hypothesis" need to be tested in further studies. It should also be noted that the effectiveness of omeprazole and, to a lesser degree, of other PPIs, depends on the *S*-mephenytoin 4′-hydroxylase (CYP2C19) genotype [9, 10]. Subjects with CYP2C19 mutations metabolize omeprazole slowly and have higher intragastric pH values during omeprazole treatment than subjects without such mutations. This fact has not been taken into account in previous investigations.

Effect of PPIs on *H. pylori in vivo*

PPI treatment leads to dose-dependent inhibition of *H. pylori* in the stomach [11, 12]. The explanation for this effect comes from *in vitro* observations. At high pH values, in the presence of urea and a weak buffer, urease activity produces very high periplasmatic pH values which are bactericidal [13–16]. The detailed explanation of this mechanism is given in the chapter dealing with interactions between PPIs and *H. pylori in vitro*. This inhibition is, in our view, the major explanation of the adjuvant effect of PPIs during anti-*H. pylori* therapy. Other effects, such as a PPI-induced increase of antibiotic secretion by the gastric epithelium [17] and a diminished inactivation of antibiotics by lowered gastric acid [18], may play a less important role. The suppressive effect of PPIs on *H. pylori* is the basis for anti-*Helicobacter* therapies with a PPI plus one or, preferably, two antibiotics [19, 20].

PPI treatment changes the distribution of *H. pylori* in the stomach. Even after short-term treatment, *H. pylori* density decreases in the antrum and increases in the corpus [12, 21]. We speculate that this effect is due to pH changes within the ecological niche of the bacteria. The rising pH during PPI treatment renders the antrum – previously ideal for *H. pylori* growth – too alkaline, while the corpus, too acid in untreated patients without mucosal atrophy, is now hospitable to the microorganism.

It is unlikely that PPI-induced redistribution of *H. pylori* is due to a direct drug effect. PPIs and sulfenamides do not specifically bind to *H. pylori* or to its ATPases [22]. Also, there is no evidence that PPIs with an antibacterial effect *in vitro* have a more pronounced effect in this respect than PPIs with a weak antibacterial effect [23–26].

Changes in *Helicobacter* density are paralleled by changes of the severity of gastritis. Gastritis improves in the antrum and worsens in the corpus and fundus [12, 21]. This fact has practical implications: when attempting to diagnose *H. pylori* infection by endoscopic biopsies, both antral and corpus biopsies must be studied, particularly when PPIs are taken, in order to prevent false negative results [27–30].

While monotherapy with PPIs is not recommended as treatment of *H. pylori* infection, short- to medium-term PPI treatment is still associated with a cure of both infection and gastritis, in 0–14% of patients treated, significantly more often than placebo treatment [23, 31–34].

Effect of long-term administration of PPIs on *Helicobacter* gastritis and the development of precancerous lesions

Atrophic gastritis

H. pylori-infected patients suffering from gastrooesophageal reflux disease may need PPI maintenance therapy over many years in an attempt to prevent recurrences or the development of complications such as Barrett's oesophagus. No clinically relevant adverse events were reported in a first series of long-term studies [35–37]. Subsequently, however, it was claimed that patients with *H. pylori* infection treated with omeprazole over several years are at a higher risk to develop atrophic gastritis in the corpus than patients without *H. pylori* infection [38]. In an open, nonrandomized prospective study two differing cohorts of patients were treated for gastro-oesophageal reflux disease either by omeprazole or by fundoplication and were followed for 3 to 8 years. Among *H. pylori*-infected patients treated with omeprazole, an increased incidence of atrophic gastritis was observed as compared with patients treated with fundoplication. No such effect was observed when subjects not infected by *H. pylori* were studied. As atrophic gastritis has traditionally been thought to be a precancerous condition [39, 40], the question was raised whether long-term treatment with PPIs in *H. pylori*-positive patients increases the risk of developing gastric cancer. In two other studies, atrophy of oxyntic mucosa developed more frequently in *H. pylori*-infected individuals treated for 1 to 5 years with lansoprazole than in lansoprazole-treated individuals without *H. pylori* infection [41, 42]. Again, these studies were nonrandomized, and differing cohorts of patients were compared. In addition, the diagnostic criteria of atrophy used in these studies are controversial. Moreover, it is unknown whether the type of corpus atrophic gastritis in PPI-treated patients with *H. pylori* infection is a risk factor for developing cancer. Finally, these observations were not corroborated in other studies. Schenk et al. observed similar degrees of mucosal atrophy before and after 1 year of omeprazole treatment in *H. pylori*-positive patients [43]. Another study comparing 12 months of treatment with either lansoprazole or omeprazole confirmed these results [21]. An uncontrolled long-term study with pantoprazole yielded to similar conclusions [44]. Most important, in a large randomized prospective 3-year clinical trial comparing the efficacy of omeprazole with fundoplication for gastrooesophageal reflux disease, there was a much higher incidence of atrophic gastritis in the corpus of individuals infected by *H. pylori* but a similar incidence among those treated with and without omeprazole [45]. Additional adequately designed studies with an even longer follow-up will be needed before the safety of long-term PPI treatment of *H. pylori*-infected subjects is established.

One of the most important problems in the past, in our view, was inappropriate diagnosis of atrophic gastritis. Gastric mucosal atrophy has been defined as a "gland loss", without specifying the structures between the glands. The histological diagnosis of "loss" may be erroneous when the gastric glands appear sparse, because they are separated by an inflammatory infiltrate [46]. A strict and meaningful definition of atrophy is prerequisite for further studies.

Intestinal metaplasia

While there is a close correlation between intestinal metaplasia and gastric mucosal atrophy, it is yet unclear whether *H. pylori* is a risk factor for the development of intestinal metaplasia [46, 47]. There is no evidence that omeprazole produces intestinal metaplasia in *H. pylori*-negative subjects [21, 35, 37, 38, 41–45, 48]. Most importantly, the question whether omeprazole accelerates the appearance of intestinal metaplasia in *H. pylori*-infected subjects remains unanswered. Preliminary data of a randomized clinical trial comparing omeprazole maintenance treatment and fundoplication in *H. pylori*-infected patients with reflux oesophagitis would indicate that long-term omeprazole treatment does not favour intestinal metaplasia [45]. Other studies are difficult to interpret [21, 35, 38, 41, 42].

Other potentially premalignant lesions allegedly induced by omeprazole treatment in H. pylori-infected subjects

Table 1 gives a list of a series of phenomena which some authors consider to represent premalignant conditions. The only phenomena closely associated with *H. pylori* infection and more pronounced during omeprazole treatment are hypergastrinaemia and enterochromaffine like (ECL)-hyperplasia [49–51]. The role of hypergastrinaemia as a premalignant condition

Table 1. Premalignant conditions other than atrophic gastritis and intestinal metaplasia

Phenomenon	Specifications	Premalignant condition?	PPIs[a]	*H. pylori*[b]	PPIs + *H. pylori*[c]	Ref.
• Autoimmune gastritis	special form of *H. pylori* gastritis	probable	no	possible	not known	52
• Genotoxicity	e.g., p53 mutation of mucosal cells	conceivable	no	conceivable	probably no	53–56
• Hyper-gastrinemia	due to *H. pylori* gastritis and/or hypoacidity	controversial	yes	yes	yes	49–51
• ECL-hyperplasia	in gastric corpus/fundic region	conceivable	no	yes	yes	41, 45, 51
• Free radicals	increased production	conceivable	no	yes	probably no	57, 58
• Antioxidant mechanisms	e.g., diminished vitamin C levels in gastric juice	conceivable	conceivable	yes	conceivable	57–59
• *N*-nitroso compounds	increased concentrations in gastric juice	controversial	no	not known	probably no	58, 60–62
• Apoptosis	diminished or increased in gastric epithelium	controversial	no	yes	probably no	57, 58, 63
• Epithelial proliferation	of gastric mucosa	controversial	no	yes	conceivable	42, 46
• COX 1 up-regulation	prostaglandin E2 synthesis	controversial	not known	conceivable	not known	64
• Bacterial overgrowth	in the gastric lumen	no	yes	no	not known	58, 60–62
• Nitrates	increased concentrations in gastric juice	no	controversial	no	not known	58–60

[a] Phenomenon induced by PPIs.
[b] Phenomenon induced by *H. pylori* (or by host response to the infection).
[c] Phenomenon is more pronounced in *H. pylori*-infected subjects when PPIs are given.

is controversial. ECL-hyperplasia may well play a role in the development of carcinoids. However, carcinoids have never been observed as a consequence of omeprazole treatment in *H. pylori*-infected patients [48–51]. All other phenomena mentioned in Table 1 such as autoimmune gastritis, genotoxicity, increased production of free radicals, alteration of antioxidant mechanisms, increased concentrations of nitrates and N-nitroso compounds, alteration of apoptosis, increased epithelial proliferation of gastric mucosa and bacterial overgrowth are either very rare or not more frequent in *H. pylori*-infected subjects receiving omeprazole, or are not clinically relevant. However, more studies will have to be conducted in order to evaluate the precise role of these phenomena in the development of gastric malignancies.

Clinical consequences of the effect of *H. pylori* on PPI efficacy of PPIs

In *H. pylori*-infected patients with reflux oesophagitis, maintenance treatment with PPIs has a better effect in preventing recurrences than in non-infected subjects [65]. It might be argued that this is not due to a direct interaction between PPI and *H. pylori*, but to PPI-induced mucosal atrophy in the presence of *H. pylori*. This controversial mechanism, if it occurs at all, takes more time than a few months to a year. In addition, PPIs appear, at least in some studies, to be more effective in curative treatment when oesophagitis patients are infected with *H. pylori* than when they are not infected [65, 66; Fig. 2]. In this short period of a few weeks, atrophy cannot develop.

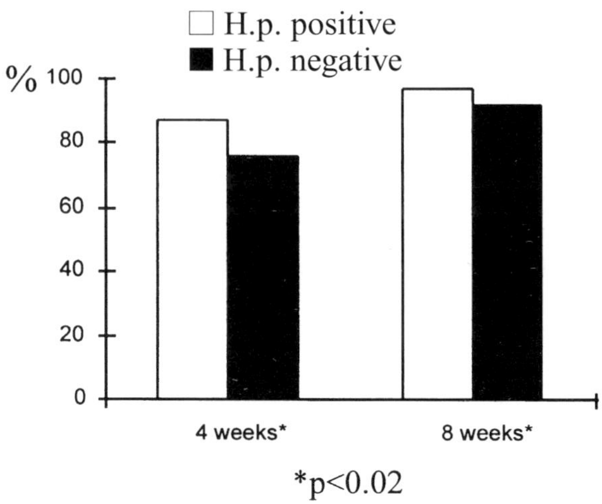

Figure 2. Healing rates for *H. pylori*-positive (white bars, $n = 335$) and *H. pylori*-negative (black bars, $n = 511$) patients with reflux esophagitis after 4 and 8 weeks of treatment with pantoprazole 40 mg once daily. From ref. 66.

Another interesting example where an *H. pylori* infection appears to augment the effectiveness of PPIs is the prevention and treatment of non-steroidal anti-inflammatory drug (NSAID)-induced ulcers. In a large controlled clinical trial, both duodenal and gastric ulcers in NSAID consumers healed more rapidly when PPIs were given to infected patients than when the patients were not infected with *H. pylori*. The healing of NSAID-related ulcers at 8 weeks with omeprazole was 83% in *H. pylori*-positive and 75% in *H. pylori*-negative patients; the difference being statistically significant [67]. This difference was even more marked with ranitidine. In the case of secondary prevention of NSAID-induced ulcers, similar observations have been reported. Seventy nine percent of *H. pylori*-positive subjects, but only 60% of *H. pylori*-negative subjects, remained in remission on omeprazole when continuing NSAID intake [67]. Thus, *H. pylori* infection seems to be beneficial to NSAID users, but a formal, prospective randomized study will be necessary to firmly establish this point.

In the case of NSAID gastropathy, the explanation for the *H. pylori*-PPI interaction is not as clear as in reflux oesophagitis, which is a pure acid-induced disorder (a minor role of alkaline reflux is controversial [68]. In NSAID consumers *H. pylori* may, at least under certain conditions, increase prostaglandin synthesis, whereas NSAIDs are thought to be gastrotoxic mainly by inhibition of gastric prostaglandin synthesis [64, 69]. Future studies will be needed to evaluate which of the two mechanisms, stronger pH control or increased prostaglandin synthesis, is a better explanation for the favourable effect of *H. pylori* on omeprazole treatment in NSAID consumers.

References

1 Verdú EF, Armstrong D, Fraser R, Viani F, Iström J-P, Cederberg C, Blum AL (1995) Effect of *Helicobacter pylori* status on intragastric pH during treatment with omeprazole. *Gut* 36: 539–543

2 Verdú EF, Armstrong D, Idström J-P, Labenz J, Stolte M, Dorta G, Börsch G, Blum AL (1995) Effect of curing *Helicobacter pylori* infection on intragastric pH during treatment with omeprazole. *Gut* 37: 743–748

3 Labenz J, Tillenburg B, Peitz U, Idström J-P, Verdú EF, Stolte M, Börsch G, Blum AL (1996) *Helicobacter pylori* augments the pH-increasing effect of omeprazole in patients with duodenal ulcer. *Gastroenterology* 110: 725–732

4 Martínek J, Blum AL, Stolte M, Wiesel P (1997) Effect of BY841 (INN: pumaprazole) and of omeprazole on intragastric acidity before and after cure of *Helicobacter pylori* infection. *Gut* 41: A35

5 Wurst W, Hartmann M (1996) Current status of acid pump antagonists (reversible PPIs). *Yale J Biol Med* 69: 233–243

6 Verdú EF, Armstrong D, Sabovcikova L, Idström J-P, Cederberg C, Blum AL, Bercik P (1998) High concentrations of ammonia, but not volatile amines, in gastric juice of subjects with *Helicobacter pylori* infection. *Helicobacter*; *in press*

7 Bercik P, Verdú EF, Armstrong D, Cederberg C, Idström J-P, Stolte M, Blum AL (1997) Apparent increase in acid output during omeprazole after cure of *H. pylori* infection. *Gastroenterology* 112: A70

8 Gillen D, Wirz A, Neithercut W, Ardill J, McColl KEL (1998) Neutralization by ammonia cannot explain *H. pylori's* potentiation of omeprazole's efficacy. *Gastroenterology* 114: A132

9 Furuta T, Ohashi K, Takashima M, Hanai H, Kubota T, Ishizaki T, Kaneko E (1998) CYP2C19 genotype status and effect of omeprazole on intragastric pH. *Gastroenterology* 114: A127
10 Tucker GT (1994) The interaction of proton pump inhibitors with cytochromes P450. *Aliment Pharmacol Ther* 8 (Suppl 1): 33–38
11 Weil J, Bell GD, Powell K, Morden A, Harrison G, Gant PW, Jones PH, Trowell JE (1991) Omeprazole and *Helicobacter pylori*: temporary suppression rather than true eradication. *Aliment Pharmacol Ther* 5: 309–313
12 Logan RP, Walker MM, Misiewicz JJ, Gummett PA, Karim QN, Baron JH (1995) Changes in the intragastric distribution of *Helicobacter pylori* during treatment with omeprazole. *Gut* 36: 12–16
13 Iwahi T, Satoh H, Nakao M, Iwasaki T, Yamazaki T, Kubo K, Tamura T, Imada A (1992) Lansoprazole, a novel benzimidazole proton pump inhibitor, and its related compounds have selective activity against *H. pylori*. *Antimicrob Agents Chemother* 35: 490–496
14 Sjöstrom JE, Kühler T, Larsson H (1997) Basis for the selective antibacterial activity in vitro of proton pump inhibitors against *Helicobacter spp*. *Antimicrob Agents Chemother* 41: 1797–1801
15 Sjöstrom JE, Fryklund J, Kühler T, Larsson H (1997) *In vitro* antibacterial activity of omeprazole and its selectivity for *Helicobacter spp*. are dependent on incubation conditions. *Antimicrob Agents Chemother* 40: 621–626
16 Stoschus B, Dominguez-Munoz JE, Kalhori N, Sauerbruch T, Malfertheiner P (1996) Effect of omeprazole on *Helicobacter pylori* urease activity *in vivo*. *Eur J Gastroenterol Hepatol* 8: 811–813
17 Goddard AF, Jessa MJ, Barrett DA, Shaw PN, Idstrom JP, Cederberg C, Spiller RC (1996). Effect of omeprazole on the distribution of metronidazole, amoxicillin and clarithromycin in human gastric juice. *Gastroenterology* 111: 358–367
18 Debets-Ossenkopp YJ, Namavar F, MacLaren DM (1995) Effect of an acidic environment on the susceptibility of *H. pylori* to trospectomycin and other antimicrobial agents. *Eur J Microbiol Infect Dis* 14: 353–355
19 Anonymous (1994) NIH concensus conference. *Helicobacter pylori* in peptic ulcer disease. NIH concensus development panel on *Helicobacter pylori* in peptic ulcer disease. *JAMA* 272: 65–69
20 Anonymous (1997) Current European concepts in the management of *Helicobacter pylori* infection. The Maastricht Consensus Report. *Gut* 41: 8–13
21 Stolte M, Meining A, Schmitz JM, Alexandridis T, Seifert E (1998) Changes in *Helicobacter pylori*-induced gastritis in the antrum and corpus during 12 months of treatment with omeprazole and lansoprazole in patients with gastro-oesophageal reflux disease. *Aliment Pharmacol Ther* 12: 247–253
22 Peterson WL (1997) The role of antisecretory drugs in the treatment of *Helicobacter pylori* infection. *Alimet Pharmacol Ther* 11 (Suppl 1): 21–25
23 Wilde MI, McTavish D (1994) Omeprazole: an update of its pharmacology and therapeutic use in acid-related disorders. *Drugs* 48: 91–132
24 Misiewicz JJ, Harris AW, Bardhan KD, Levi S, O'Morain C, Cooper BT, Kerr GD, Dixon MF, Langworthy H, Piper D (1997) One-week triple therapy for *Helicobacter pylori*: a multicentre comparative study. Lansoprazole *Helicobacter* Study Group. *Gut* 41: 735–739
25 Fukuda Y (1996) Suppression of *Helicobacter pylori* colonisation with omeprazole. *Scand J Gastroenterol* 31 (Suppl 214): 54–55
26 Midolo PD, Turnidge JD, Lambert JR (1997) Bactericidal activity and synergy studies of proton pump inhibitors and antibiotics against *Helicobacter pylori in vitro*. *J Antimicrobial Chemother* 39: 331–337
27 Mion F, Delecluse HJ, Rousseau M, Berger F, Brazier JL, Minaire Y (1994) ^{13}C-urea breath test for the diagnosis of *Helicobacter pylori* infection. Comparison with histology. *Gastroenterol Clin Biol* 18: 1106–1111
28 Goddard AF, Logan RPH (1997) Review article: urea breath tests for detecting *Helicobacter pylori*. *Aliment Pharmacol Ther* 11: 641–649
29 Rollan A, Giancaspero R, Arrese M, Figueroa C, Vollrath V, Schultz M, Duarte I, Vial P (1997) Accuracy of invasive and noninvasive tests to diagnose *Helicobacter pylori* infection after antibiotic treatment. *Am J Gastroenterol* 92: 1268–1274

30 Wyatt JI, Gray SF (1992) Detection of *Helicobacter pylori* by histology. In: BJ Rathbone, RV Heatley (eds) *Helicobacter pylori and gastroduodenal disease*. Blackwell Science Ltd, Oxford, 51–57
31 Lind T, Veldhuyzen van Zanten S, Unge P, Spiller RC, Bayerdörffer E, O'Morain C, Bardhan KD, Bradette M, Chiba N, Wrangstadh M et al (1996) Eradication of *Helicobacter pylori* using one-week triple therapies combining omeprazole with two antimicrobials: the MACH 1 study. *Helicobacter* 1: 138–144
32 Talley NJ, Janssens J, Lauritsen K, Racs I (1998) Cure of *H. pylori* does not abolish symptoms in non-ulcer dyspepsia: a randomized double-blind placebo controlled trial with 12 months follow-up. *Aliment Pharmacol Ther; in press*
33 Blum AL, Arnold R, Koelz HR et al (1997) Treatment of functional dyspepsia (FD) with omeprazole and ranitidine. *Gastroenterology* 110: A73
34 Penston JG, McColl KE (1997) Eradication of *Helicobacter pylori*: an objective assessment of current therapies. *Br J Clin Pharmacol* 43: 223–243
35 Lamberts R, Creutzfeldt W, Strüber HG, Brunner G, Solcia E (1993) Long-term omeprazole therapy in peptic ulcer disease: gastrin, endocrine cell growth and gastritis. *Gastroenterology* 104: 1356–1370
36 Solcia E, Fiocca R, Havu N, Dalväg A, Carlsson R (1992) Gastric endocrine cells and gastritis in patients receiving long-term omeprazole treatment. *Digestion* 51 (Suppl 1): 82–92
37 Klinkenberg-Knol EC, Festen HPM, Jansen JBMJ, Lamers CBHW, Nelis F, Snel P, Lückers A, Dekkers CPM, Havu N, Meuwissen SGM (1994) Long-term treatment with omeprazole for refractory reflux esophagitis: efficacy and safety. *Ann Intern Med* 121: 161–167
38 Kuipers EJ, Lundell L, Klinkenberg-Knol EC, Havu N, Festen HPM, Liedman B, Lamers CBHW, Jansen BMJ, Dalenbäck J, Snel P et al (1996) Atrophic gastritis and *Helicobacter pylori* infection in patients with reflux esophagitis treated with omeprazole or fundoplication. *N Engl J Med* 334: 1018–1022
39 Tatsuta M, Iishi H, Nakaizumi A, Okuda S, Taniguchi H, Hiyama T et al (1993) Fundal atrophic gastritis as a risk factor for gastric cancer. *Int J Cancer* 53: 70–74
40 Cheli R, Santi L, Ciancarmerla G, Canciani G (1973) A clinical and statistical follow-up study of atrophic gastritis. *Am J Dig Dis* 18: 1061–1065
41 Eissele R, Brunner G, Simon B, Solcia E, Arnold R (1997) Gastric mucosa during treatment with lansoprazole: *Helicobacter pylori* is a risk factor for argyrophil cell hyperplasia. *Gastroenterology* 113: 2018–2019
42 Berstad AE, Hatlebakk JG, Maartmann-Moe H, Bestad A, Brandtzaeg P (1997) *Helicobacter pylori* gastritis and epithelial cell proliferation in patients with reflux oesophagitis after treatment with lansoprazole. *Gut* 41: 740–747
43 Schenk BE, Kuipers EJ, Nelis GF, Thijs JC, Bloemena E, Snel P, Luckers P, Klinkenberg-Knol EC, Festen PP, Viergever PP et al (1998) *H. pylori* eradication for chronic gastritis during omeprazole therapy for GERD. *Gastroenterology* 114: A279
44 Brunner G, Harke U (1994) Long-term therapy with pantoprazole in patients with peptic ulceration resistant to extended high-dose ranitidine treatment. *Aliment Pharmacol Ther* 8 (Suppl 1): 59–64
45 Lundell L, Havu N, Andersson A, Miettienen P, Myrvold HE, Pedersen SA, Thor K (1997) Gastritis development and acid suppression therapy revisited. Results of a randomised clinical study with long-term follow-up. *Gastroenterology* 112: A28
46 Genta RM (1997) *Helicobacter pylori*, inflammation, mucosal damage and apoptosis: pathogenesis and definition of gastric atrophy. *Gastroenterology* 113: S51–S55
47 Filipe MI, Muñoz N, Matko I, Pompe-Kirn V, Jutersek A, Teuchmann S, Benz M, Prijon T (1994) Intestinal metaplasia types and the risk of gastric cancer: a cohort study in Slovenia. *Int J Cancer* 57: 324–329
48 Havu N (1998) Gastric morphology during long-term omeprazole therapy. *Gastroenterology* 114: A145
49 Martínek J, Koelz HR, Blum AL (1997) Säureforschung und Ulkustherapie. *Arzneim-Forsch/Drug Res* 47 (II): 1424–1435
50 Pantoflickova D, Martínek J, Blum AL. Safety and potential hazards of long-term inhibition of gastric acid secretion. *Drug Safety; in press*
51 Freston JW, Borch K, Brand SJ, Carlsson E, Creutzfeldt W, Hakanson R, Olbe L, Solcia E, Walsh JH, Wolfe MM (1995) Effects of hypochlorhydria and hypergastrinemia on structure and function of gastrointestinal cells. *Dig Dis Sci* 40: 50S–62S

52 Appelmelk BJ, Negrini R (1997) *Helicobacter pylori* and gastric autoimmunity. *Curr Opin Gastroenterol* 13: 31–34

53 Sachs G, Wallmark B (1989) Biological basis of omeprazole therapy. *J Gastroenterol Hepatol* 4 (Suppl 2): 2–18

54 Sachs G, Scott D (1990) Cell digestion and genotoxicity assessment in gastric mucosa. *Digestion* 47 (Suppl 1): 31–34

55 Eidt S, Lorenzen J, Ortmann M (1996) Depth of infiltration of primary gastric B-cell lymphomas-correlation with proliferation, apoptosis and expression of p53 and bcl-2. *Pathol Res Pract* 192: 925–930

56 Wu MS, Shun CT, Wang HP, Sheu JC, Lee WJ, Wang TH, Lin JT (1997) Genetic alterations in gastric cancer: relation to histological subtypes, tumor stage and *Helicobacter pylori* infection. *Gastroenterology* 112: 1457–1465

57 Farinati F, Della Libera G, Cardin R, Molari A, Plebani M, Rugge M, Di Mario F, Naccarato R (1996) Gastric antioxidant, nitrites and mucosal lipoperoxidation in chronic gastritis and *Helicobacter pylori* infection. *J Clin Gastroenterol* 22: 275–281

58 Fuchs CS, Mayer RJ (1995) Gastric carcinoma. *N Engl J Med* 333: 32–41

59 Mowat C, Carswell A, McColl KEL (1998) Omeprazole lowers gastric juice ascorbic acid and elevates gastric juice nitrite concentrations. *Gastroenterology* 114: A236

60 Verdu E, Viani F, Armstrong D, Fraser R, Siegrist HH, Pignatelli B, Idström J-P, Cederberg C, Blum AL, Fried M (1994) Effect of omeprazole on intragastric bacterial counts, nitrates, nitrites and N-nitroso compounds. *Gut* 35: 455–460

61 Thorens J, Froehlich F, Schwitzer W, Saraga E, Bille J, Gyr K, Duroux P, Nicolet M, Pignatelli B, Blum AL (1996) Bacterial overgrowth during treatment with omeprazole compared with cimetidine: a prospective randomised double blind study. *Gut* 39: 54–59

62 Pignatelli B, Malaveille C, Rogatko A, Hautefeuille A, Thuillier P, Muñoz N et al (1993) Mutagens, N-nitroso compounds and their precursors in gastric juice from patients with and without precancerous lesions of the stomach. *Eur J Cancer* 29A: 2031–2039

63 Moss SF, Calam J, Agarwal B, Wang S, Holt PR (1996) Induction of gastric epithelial apoptosis by *Helicobacter pylori*. *Gut* 38: 498–501

64 Jackson LM, Wu K, Mahida YR, Jenkins D, Donnelly MT, Hawkey CJ (1998) COX-1 expression in human gastric mucosa infected with *Helicobacter pylori*: constitutive or induced? *Gastroenterology* 114: A160

65 Carlsson R, Bate C, Dent J, Frison L, Gnarpe H, Hallerbäck B, Unge P, Lundell L (1998) Does *H. pylori* infection influence the response to treatment with acid inhibition in patients with gastroesophageal reflux disease? In: R Carlsson: *Gastroesophageal reflux disease: a study of pathophysiology, clinical diagnosis and management*. University of Göteborg, 61–72

66 Holtmann G, Cain CR, Malfertheiner P (1998) The impact of *H. pylori* on healing of reflux esophagitis during treatment with pantoprazole. *Gastroenterology* 114: A151

67 Yeomans ND, Tulassay Z, Juhasz L, Racz I, Howard JM, Van Rensburg CJ, Swannell AJ, Hawkey CJ (1998) A comparison of omeprazole with ranitidine for ulcers associated with nonsteroidal antiinflammatory drugs. *N Engl J Med* 338: 719–726

68 Stok DL, Williams JG (1991) Alkaline reflux oesophagitis. *Gut* 32: 1090–1092

69 Hudson N, Balsitis M, Filipowicz F, Hawkey CJ (1993) Effect of *Helicobacter pylori* colonisation on gastric mucosal eicosanoid synthesis in patients taking non-steroidal anti-inflammatory drugs. *Gut* 34: 748–751

Proton Pump Inhibitors
ed. by L. Olbe

Comparison of different proton pump inhibitors

Karl-Uwe Petersen

Oberdorfstr. 22, D-52072 Aachen, Germany

Introduction

As proton pump inhibitors (PPIs) have revolutionized treatment of acid-related diseases, alone, or in drug combinations for eradication of *Helicobacter pylori*, it does not come as a surprise that the first representative of the class, omeprazole, has been joined by a number of similar agents including lansoprazole, pantoprazole and, as the latest entry, rabeprazole. It is the purpose of this overview to delineate differences and similarities and put them into the perspective of clinical relevance. Some of these aspects are covered in broader detail in other chapters of this book.

By and large, the events leading to inhibition of the H^+,K^+-ATPase by the various PPIs can be described in identical terms: After intestinal absorption, the drugs are distributed by the bloodstream and gain diffusional access to the canalicular system of the parietal cell. In this acid compartment, they are trapped and acid-activated to form short-lived sulfenamides ready to bind to sulfhydryl groups of the H^+,K^+-ATPase. Elimination depends on hepatic metabolism, followed by renal and faecal excretion. Along this way, a number of differences between the various PPIs can be identified.

Bioavailability

Magnitude

While absorption of PPIs is fast and extensive, bioavailability is limited by first-pass metabolism to different extents (Tab. 1), being highest for lansoprazole and pantoprazole.

It is a common mistake to confuse such data with the outcome of bioequivalence studies which, comparing various preparations of the same compound, are designed to allow predictions of relative therapeutic performances. By contrast, the class of PPIs embraces individual agents. Their recommended doses have been selected in individual dose-ranging studies identifying the dose with the largest effect [1–6]. In such studies, lower bioavailabilities are compensated for by higher doses, so that, finally, bioavailability has no bearing on the clinical performance.

Table 1. Pharmacokinetic properties of proton pump inhibitors at standard dosages

	Omeprazole (20 mg)	Lansoprazole (30 mg)	Pantoprazole (40 mg)
Bioavailability (%)	64 [13]	85 [71]	77 [12]
C_{max} (μmol/l)	0.2 [13]	2.85 [19]	7.0–8.6 [30] 6.2 [22]
t_{max} (h)	1–3 [12]	1.5–2.2 [21, 32]	1.9–2.5 [72]
AUC (μmol × h/l)	1.5 [13] 0.6–3.5 [12]	6.8 [19] 7.3 [32]	5.2–13.0 [12] 13.0, 9.0 [72] 10.5 [22]
Protein binding (%)	95 [12]	97 [12]	98 [12]
Volume of distribution (l/kg)	0.34 [12]	0.39–0.45 [71, 73]	0.16 [30]
Excretion pathways (renal/faecal) (%)	80/20 [74]	20/80 [32]	80/20 [30]
Clearance (l/h)	60 [19]	11–17 [19]	9 [19]
$t_{1/2}$ (h)	0.7 [74][a]	1.4–1.5 [1, 19]	1.0–1.5 [30]
$t_{1/2}$ (liver failure) (h)	3 [75]	6–7 [32]	7–9 [30]

Where available, values collected during multiple dosing are indicated. The multitude of pharmacokinetic studies in conjunction with high levels of interindividual variation account for some discrepancies in the values found in the published literature; for calculations in the figures, AUC values of 2.0 (omeprazole), 7.0 (lansoprazole) and 11.0 (pantoprazole) were considered representative.

[a] Single dose.

C_{max}, peak plasma concentration; t_{max}, time to reach to C_{max}; AUC, area under the concentration time curve.

Time dependence

As a further difference, it takes several days for omeprazole to reach its steady-state bioavailability [5]. Corresponding data for lansoprazole and pantoprazole are not available, although unchanged values of C_{max} and area under the time concentration curve (AUC) indicate the absence of relevant increases after the first dose [7, 8]. At face value, this discrepancy would suggest that the latter drugs reach maximum acid inhibitory efficacy with the first dose and, by this, are apt to provide faster pain relief. Hence, it may be surprising that omeprazole as well as lansoprazole and pantoprazole take several days to reach steady-state inhibition of acid secretion [9–11]. For instance, 40 mg of pantoprazole reduced acid output by 51 and 85% after the first and seventh dose, respectively [11]. This type of behavior, however, is predictable from the way the parietal cell organizes its supply with active H^+, K^+-ATPase molecules [12]: unless acid secretion is maximally stimulated, a substantial portion of the pump molecules are stored in the cytosol, so that the first PPI dose, regardless of its magnitude, will miss a sizable fraction of pumps. These pumps, together with newly synthesized molecules, will later be recruited into the canalicular membrane to be hit by the next dose. This cycle will repeat until a steady state is reached. Thus efficiency of the first dose is limited by the kinetics of the proton pump rather than drug bioavailability.

Dose linearity

As opposed to lansoprazole and pantoprazole, hepatic metabolism seems to saturate at higher dosages of omeprazole (40 mg) [13]. Although dose linearity is a desirable feature, its advantages may be elusive since PPIs show considerable interindividual variation in bioavailability [14, 15].

Interfering factors

There are some differences in the effect of food on oral bioavailability. Generally, a foregoing breakfast causes some delay in appearance of the drugs in plasma. Bioavailability (AUC) of omeprazole remains unchanged [13], whereas that of lansoprazole is markedly reduced [16, 17]. No alteration of bioavailability was found with rabeprazole [18] and in the majority of cases with pantoprazole. However, 5 of 24 volunteers displayed no measurable plasma concentrations for a period of 8 h after oral intake [8]. Tentatively, this finding may be ascribed to pharmaceutical rather than drug-specific properties. Although an effect of food was not obtained in a further study with lansoprazole, application before breakfast is emphasized with this PPI [19].

As opposed to omeprazole and pantoprazole, concurrent intake of antacids evoked a slight reduction in bioavailability of lansoprazole [20]. The problem posed is only minor, inasmuch as PPI treatment will largely suspend the need for use of antacids.

Distribution

PPIs are mainly distributed to the extracellular fluid, as suggested by their low apparent volume of distribution (Tab. 1). In animal studies, all PPIs crossed the placenta. Excretion into breast milk was minor with omeprazole and pantoprazole, whereas lansoprazole achieved milk levels comparable to plasma concentration [21]. As a general precaution, the use of PPIs during pregnancy and lactation is advised against. If strong acid inhibition is considered essential, omeprazole, mainly because of the accumulated experience, would be the most suitable drug.

Acid trapping

Trapping in the acid compartment of the parietal cell is essentially governed by the pK_a value of the respective pyridine groups. Those of omeprazole (4.13), lansoprazole (4.01) and pantoprazole (3.96) are very close to each other, all of them predicting an ≈ 1000-fold accumulation at a canalicular pH value of 1. Rabeprazole, with an estimated pK_a of 4.9 [12], will achieve an almost 10-fold higher accumulation. This suggests that the maximally effective dose may be rather low. Again, as the pump kinetics define the ceiling of maximal acid inhibition, this does not indicate a higher clinical efficiency.

Acid activation

PPIs are prodrugs that require an acid environment to be converted into the active compound. Accumulation in the canalicular system of the parietal cell at a pH value of 1 or below provides the optimal surroundings for activation. At cytosolic pH, transformation rates are too slow to allow the build-up of any effective concentration of the active sulfenamide.

Acid stability

PPIs differ in their acid stabilities and hence in activation rates at a given pH value. As shown by Kromer et al. [22], *in vitro*, it takes about 2.8 h to achieve a 50% activation of pantoprazole at a pH of 5; the respective values with omeprazole and lansoprazole are ~ 1, with rabeprazole ~ 0.12 h. A lower pH stability will result in more sulfenamide molecules formed at sites other than the canalicular space.

Quantitative estimate of extragastric acid activation

Risk assessment requires a quantitative estimate of extragastric acid activation of the PPI. Modulated by bioavailability, application of standard doses will deliver different molar loads, that of omeprazole being the lowest (Fig. 1). Due to discrepant rates of elimination (Tab. 1), plasma concentrations of the various PPIs are maintained for different periods of time, and systemic exposure (AUC) will differ accordingly (Fig. 1). Using the AUC values indicated in Table 1 and taking protein binding into account, systemic exposure to free omeprazole and either lansoprazole or pantoprazole amounts to 0.1 and 0.2 µmol × h/l, respectively (Fig. 2). Lysosomal exposure will be very similar since the relations between lysosomal pH (~ 4.7–5) [23, 24] and the pK_a values of the inhibitors (4–5) preclude

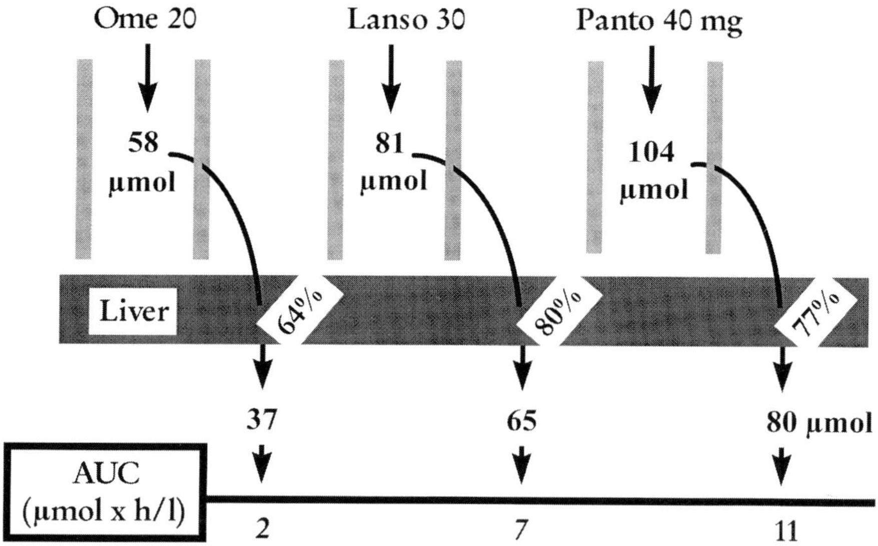

Figure 1. Effective loads of PPIs used at standard dosages. Molar loads depend on dose and bioavailability and, according to elimination rates, translate into different values of AUC. Ome, omeprazole; lanso, lansoprazole; panto, pantoprazole.

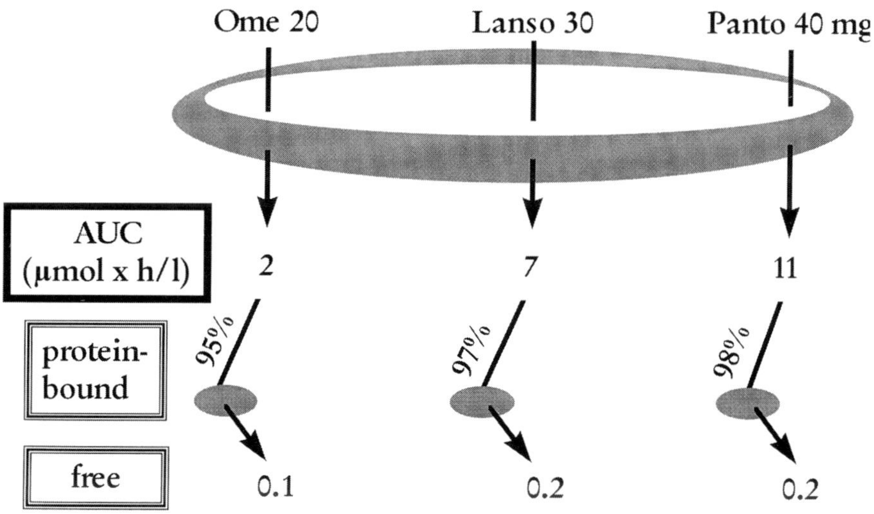

Figure 2. Protein-bound and free fractions of AUC associated with PPIs used at standard dosages (ome, omeprazole; lanso, lansoprazole; panto, pantoprazole).

any sizable accumulation. Published acid stability diagrams [12, 25] indicate that the fraction of omeprazole activated at lysosomal pH may exceed that of pantoprazole by a factor of 2.0 to 2.5. In absolute figures, this means virtually identical exposure to the respective active sulfenamides. Thus acid stability does not lend itself to differentiation of PPIs by safety characteristics.

Pertinent experimental data

Beil et al. [26] reported that omeprazole and pantoprazole at 300 µmol/l were unable to affect activities of a number of lysosomal enzymes *in vitro*. These concentrations are in large excess of the respective C_{max} values (Tab. 1). As C_{max} values refer to total rather than free drug concentrations, the safety margin is even wider.

Both omeprazole and pantoprazole react with vacuolar H^+ATPase, as inferable from their abilities to inhibit acidification in purified kidney lysosomes [27]. However, they did so with low potencies, concentrations needed for half-maximal inhibition (IC_{50}) being 75 and 195 µmol/l, respectively. Protection of the enzyme by 10 µmol/l glutathione suggested an extralysosomal action (at the neutral pH of the incubation medium), rather than an effect secondary to intralysosomal activation.

Sites of binding to the H^+,K^+-ATPase

As detailed elsewhere in this book, there are distinct differences in PPI reactions with the H^+,K^+-ATPase. Circumstantial and direct evidence indicates that binding to cysteine 813 is essentially linked to the inhibitory effect, with no functional consequences of binding to additional sites [28].

Rates of inhibition of H^+,K^+-ATPase

PPIs differ in the rates at which they suppress enzymic activity and acid transport, rabeprazole being the fastest and pantoprazole the slowest inhibitor. For full inhibition of ATP hydrolysis, rabeprazole took 5 min, omeprazole and lansoprazole 30 min, whereas pantoprazole had achieved a 50% reduction after a 45-min incubation [28]. These differences mainly reflect the divergent rates of acid activation.

In theory, these data suggest that PPI at equipotent dosages will reach identical levels of pump inihibition, as the number of available pumps sets the ceiling for efficiency, but may do so at different speeds. Such differences will be highest after the first dose; on repeated dosing, they will taper off as the number of pumps to be inhibited decreases and finally reaches steady state. Of course, effects on acid output *in vivo* will be modulated by individual pharmacokinetic and pharmaceutical properties of the respective drugs. It remains to be seen how far such effects translate into a quantifiable benefit in the clinical setting.

Elimination

There is no PPI excretion in the form of native drugs. The pharmacokinetics of omeprazole are unchanged in patients with renal impairment [29]. The same may be concluded for lansoprazole and pantoprazole [30–32]. Minor prolongation of elimination half-lives in the elderly may be explained in terms of age-dependent decreases in liver volume and liver blood flow [20].

At standard dosages, plasma elimination of omeprazole is fastest. Excretion occurs, to different proportions, by renal and faecal routes (Tab. 1). Omeprazole metabolism seems to be saturable, so that 40-mg doses of omeprazole and pantoprazole are excreted at the same rates (1.25 h) [22].

With hepatic metabolism as the predominant mechanism of PPI elimination, it is no surprise that liver failure gives rise to sizable prolongations of plasma elimination half-lives, which explain low-grade accumulation of lansoprazole and, more so, pantoprazole (Tab. 1). As pointed out below for slow metabolizers, this is no point of concern, given the wide safety margin of PPIs.

Metabolism

The PPIs are completely metabolized and excreted by renal and facal pathways (Tab. 1). Of the cytochrome P-450 (CYP) isoforms involved, CYP 2C19 (*S*-mephenytoin hydroxylase) is the most important, followed by CYP 3A4 [20, 33] (Fig. 3), whose role becomes more significant in people with reduced or absent expression of CYP 2C19 [34]. CYP3A4 seems to be more involved in formation of primary lansoprazole metabolites; however, subsequent processing is dominated by CYP 2C19 [35].

In some cases, the actions of CYP enzymes are complemented by additional hepatic (pantoprazole: phase II metabolism) or extrahepatic reactions (rabeprazole: chemical transformation yielding a thioether metabolite [33]). Nonetheless, the central role of 2C19 is underlined by this isoenzyme defining poor metabolizers of omeprazole [36], lansoprazole [37], pantoprazole [38, 39] and rabeprazole [40]. About fivefold elevations of AUC values are found in such cases [20]; increases with rabeprazole may be somewhat smaller [40]. Due to the large safety margin of PPIs, there is no need for dosage adjustments (which would require phenotyping). However, in long-term treatment (as in gastro-esophageal reflux disease (GERD)) the

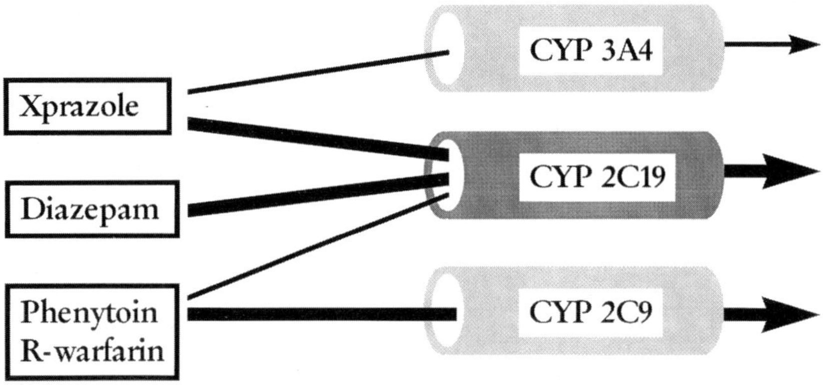

Figure 3. Relative contributions of CYP isoforms to the metabolism of PPIs (Xprazole) and marker substrates of CYP 2C9 and 2C19 (CYP, cytochrome P-450).

recommended strategy is to titrate dosages down to the lowest level that still affords symptomatic relief; using this approach, slow metabolizers will accept lower dosages.

Interactions with the CYP system

Considerable attention has been given to possible drug interactions with the class of substituted benzimidazoles. Two major aspects have unfolded: competition for the metabolising CYP enzymes and induction of certain CYP isoforms.

Omeprazole and CYP 2C19

The CYP isoform most involved in PPI bioconversion is CYP 2C19 [20, 33]. This enzyme makes minor contributions to the metabolism of a relatively small number of xenobiotics (e.g., phenytoin, tolbutamide and the less effective warfarin enantiomer, *R*-warfarin), and is essential to that of an even lesser number including diazepam (Fig. 3).

Omeprazole's interaction potential with drugs that are only partly under control of CYP 2C19 (Fig. 3) is negligible. At a dose of 40 mg, the drug was found to produce a 10% reduction of the AUC of tolbutamide, an effect considered to be of no clinical significance [20]. Effects on phenytoin pharmacokinetics were lacking at a dose of 20 mg and inconsistent at 40 mg of omeprazole [41]. Even so, monitoring of plasma concentration is recommendable, with and without cotreatment with other drugs. This is because the elimination half-life of phenytoin is *per se* highly variable and further complicated by the drug inhibiting its own metabolism [42].

Of warfarin, only the less effective *R* enantiomer was affected by 20 mg of omeprazole (12% increase in plasma concentration), and changes in coagulation time were trivial or absent [41], data that do not justify a general caveat against the use of omeprazole in combination with anti-coagulants. This notion is strengthened by a recent report indicating a lack of interaction between 40 mg of omeprazole and acenocoumarol [43].

Omeprazole 20 mg has been shown to decrease the clearance of diazepam by 27% [44], an effect doubled at 40 mg [45]. These effects must be weighed against the background of a high variability in diazepam clearance, with plasma elimation half-lives ranging from to 20 to 99 h [46]. Modulating factors are old age, compromised liver function and deficient expression of CYP 2C19 [47]. The clinical significance of the omeprazole-diazepam interaction has not been established [48]; it even appears doubtful in the light of published experience with the more powerful inhibitor [44], cimetidine [49, 50].

Usually, diazepam is dosed according to individual susceptibility, and the possibility of high plasma levels reached in poor metabolizers is not thought to constitute a need for drug monitoring. Hence not much relevance can be attributed to the action of 20 mg of omeprazole. For general reasons, the use of benzodiazepines that are not subject to phase I metabolism (e.g., oxazepam) is advisable in the elderly and those with severely impaired hepatic function [47]. The same may hold for the use of high-dose omeprazole.

Omeprazole and CYP 3A4

CYP 3A4 is of minor relevance to bioconversion of PPIs (cf. Fig. 3). This is in agreement with the lacking potential of omeprazole to interact with CYP 3A4 substrates such as corticosteroids, lidocaine and quinidine [20]. Also, carbamazepine metabolism is controlled in major part by CYP 3A4 [51]. On these grounds, a report on omeprazole increasing the AUC of carbamazepine (single dose of 400 mg) in healthy volunteers [52] is difficult to interpret. The interaction could not be confirmed in patients on continuous treatment with carbamazepine [53]. These discrepancies could be related to time-dependent changes in carbamazepine elimination, which, by inducing CYP 3A4 [54], accelerates its own metabolism. Autoinduction roughly halves plasma concentrations of the anticonvulsant within 3 to 6 weeks [55]. Thus inception and discontinuation of omeprazole during carbamazepine treatment seems to pose no problem. During initiation of carbamazepine dosing, drug monitoring is generally recommended, regardless of ongoing therapy with other drugs [55].

A mutual increase in AUC has been found with coadministration of omeprazole and clarithromycin [56], an interaction that might prove advantageous in eradication of *H. pylori*. No such effects have been reported with lansoprazole and pantoprazole. On closer scrutiny, competition for the metabolising enzyme(s) is a less convincing explanation for the omeprazole-clarithromycin interaction. This is because the latter agent is mainly metabolized by CYP 3A4 [57], whose role in omeprazole metabolism is minor. Clearly, more in-depth work is needed to confirm and understand these synergistic effects.

Pantoprazole

A low propensity of pantoprazole to interact with the metabolism of other drugs has largely been ascribed to pronounced phase II metabolism [12]. Minute changes seen in tests of possible interactions with phenytoin and *R*-warfarin went in the expected direction [20], but were, even if significant, of no clinical relevance. Unfortunately, doses exceeding the standard dose of 40 mg have not been studied (e.g., with warfarin, phenytoin and carbamazepine [58]), although higher dosages, for instance 2 × 40 mg in eradication of *H. pylori*, are in clinical use as well.

Lansoprazole

Information on possible drug interactions with lansoprazole is incomplete [59]. Some pertinent drugs have been studied only at standard dosage (prednisone [60]), not at all (carbamazepine), or data were published only in descriptive terms (warfarin [61]). However, compounds representative of most CYP isoforms have been studied with negative results [20, 60], with the notable exception of 2D6 (not investigated).

Induction of CYP 1A isoforms

CYP 1A1 and 1A2 are engaged in bioconversion of a limited number of drugs, including caffeine and theophylline [20]. Both omeprazole and lansoprazole are able to induce these isoforms *in vitro* [62, 63]. Such induction seems to be transient, as reported for omeprazole *in vitro* [63]. As to pantoprazole, a less pronounced induction has been reported in rat liver microsomes [64], while only elevated CYP1A1 messenger RNA (mRNA) levels were observed in a human hepatoma cell line [65].

In vivo, induction by omeprazole translated into acceleration of caffeine demethylation by 40 mg of omeprazole [66]. However, as analyzed elsewhere [41], quantitative changes (an ~ 13% increase in exhalation of $^{13}CO_2$) were trivial. Omeprazole doses up to 80 mg failed to influence theophylline elimination kinetics [20]. A dose of 20 mg left the metabolism of phenacetin unchanged [67]. By contrast, both 30 and 60 mg of lansoprazole produced measurable decreases (13%) in the AUC of theophylline [68, 69].

Negative results with pantoprazole in this area are less than conclusive, since the interaction potential with theophylline has only been studied at a pantoprazole dose of 30 mg applied by 2-min injections [58], so that the period of liver exposure was lower than in the clinical setting. Even so, a nonsignificant decrease in elimination half-life by 10% was noted. Lansoprazole hastening of theophylline elimination appears inconsiderable from a practical point of view. More important are concerns over possible links between cancerogenesis and inducibility of 1A isoforms. The ambiguities of this issue have been mooted previously. In the present context, it may suffice to emphasize that the 1A induction by PPIs is trivial in magnitude, probably transient and may even have positive aspects [41].

Rabeprazole

Information on rabeprazole is still limited. Similar to the other PPIs, its potential to interact with other drugs and its ability to induce CYP 1A isoenzymes seem to be low [65, 70].

Tolerability

There are no consistent differences between the various PPIs in terms of tolerability.

Outlook

PPIs share quite a number of properties, and discriminating features are rather subtle. Even where easily identifiable, they may interest more from theoretical than practical points of view. Their high efficacies and wide margins of safety make them first-line drugs in the treatment of acid-related diseases, even after the advent of *H. pylori*-related therapy.

References

1 Berlin I, Molinier P, Duchier A, Cournot A, Durrel J, Dellatolas F, Duchier J (1992) Dose-ranging study of lansoprazole, a new proton pump inhibitor, in patients with high gastric acid secretion. *Eur J Clin Pharmacol* 43: 117–119
2 Earnest DL, Dorsch E, Jones J, Jennings DE, Greski-Rose PA (1998) A placebo-controlled dose-ranging study of lansoprazole in the management of reflux esophagitis. *Am J Gastroenterol* 93: 238–243
3 Londong W (1994) Effect of pantoprazole on 24-h intragastric pH and serum gastrin in humans. *Aliment Pharmacol Ther* 8 (Suppl 1): 39–46

4 Müller P, Simon B, Khalil H, Luhmann R, Leucht U, Schneider A (1992) Dose-range finding study with the proton pump inhibitor pantoprazole in acute duodenal ulcer patients. *Z Gastroenterol* 30: 771–775
5 Wilde MI, McTavish D (1994) Omeprazole. An update of its pharmacology and therapeutic use in acid-related disorders. *Drugs* 48: 91–132
6 Zeitoun P (1989) Comparison of omeprazole with ranitidine in the treatment of reflux oesophagitis. *Scand J Gastroenterol* Suppl 166: 83–87
7 Tolman KG, Sanders SW, Buchi KN, Karol MD, Jennings DE, Ringham GL (1997) The effects of oral doses of lansoprazole and omeprazole on gastric pH. *J Clin Gastroenterol* 24: 65–70
8. Benet LZ, Zech K (1994) Pharmacokinetics – a relevant factor for the choice of a drug? *Aliment Pharmacol Ther* 8 (Suppl 1): 25–32
9 Lind T, Cederberg C, Ekenved G, Haglund U, Olbe L (1983) Effect of omeprazole – a gastric proton pump inhibitor – on pentagastrin stimulated acid secretion in man. *Gut* 24: 270–276
10 Müller P, Dammann HG, Leucht U, Simon B (1989) Human gastric acid secretion following repeated doses of AG-1749. *Aliment Pharmacol Ther* 3: 193–198
11 Simon B, Müller P, Marinis E, Luhmann R, Huber R, Hartmann R, Wurst W (1990) Effect of repeated oral administration of BY 1023/SK & F 96022 – a new substituted benzimidazole derivative – on pentagastrin-stimulated gastric acid secretion and pharmacokinetics in man. *Aliment Pharmacol Ther* 4: 373–379
12 Huber R, Kohl B, Sachs G, Senn-Bilfinger J, Simon WA, Sturm E (1995) The continuing development of proton pump inhibitors with particular reference to pantoprazole. *Aliment Pharmacol Ther* 9: 363–378
13 Andersson T, Andren K, Cederberg C, Heggelund A, Lundborg P, Röhss K (1990) Bioavailability of omeprazole as enteric coated (EC) granules in conjunction with food on the first and seventh days of treatment. *Drug Invest* 2: 184–188
14 Hatlebakk JG, Berstad A (1996) Pharmacokinetic optimisation in the treatment of gastro-oesophageal reflux disease. *Clin Pharmacokinet* 31: 386–406
15 Pue MA, Laroche J, Meineke I, de Mey C (1993) Pharmacokinetics of pantoprazole following single intravenous and oral administration to healthy male subjects. *Eur J Clin Pharmacol* 44: 575–578
16 Bergstrand R, Grind M, Nyberg G, Olofsson B (1995) Decreased oral bioavailability of lansoprazole in healthy volunteers when given with a standardised breakfast. *Clin Drug Invest* 9: 67–71
17 Delhotal-Landes B, Cournot A, Vermerie N, Dellatolas F, Benoit M, Flouvat B (1991) The effect of food and antacids on lansoprazole absorption and disposition. *Eur J Drug Metab Pharmacokinet* 3 (Spec Issue): 315–320
18 Yasuda S, Ohnishi A, Ogawa T, Tomono Y, Hasegawa J, Nakai H, Shimamura Y, Morishita N (1994) Pharmacokinetic properties of E3810, a new proton pump inhibitor, in healthy male volunteers. *Int J Clin Pharmacol Ther* 32: 466–473
19 Zimmermann AE, Katona BH (1997) Lansoprazole: a comprehensive review. *Pharmacotherapy* 17: 308–326
20 Andersson T (1996) Pharmacokinetics, metabolism and interactions of acid pump inhibitors. Focus on omeprazole, lansoprazole and pantoprazole. *Clin Pharmacokinet* 31: 9–28
21 Barradell LB, Faulds D, McTavish D (1992) Lansoprazole. A review of its pharmacodynamic and pharmacokinetic properties and its therapeutic efficacy in acid-related disorders. *Drugs* 44: 225–250
22 Kromer W, Krüger U, Huber R, Hartmann M, Steinijans VW (1998) Differences in pH-dependent activation rates of substituted benzimidazoles and biological in vitro correlates. *Pharmacology* 56: 57–70
23 Myers BM, Tietz PS, Tarara JE, LaRusso NF (1995) Dynamic measurements of the acute and chronic effects of lysosomotropic agents on hepatocyte lysosomal pH using flow cytometry. *Hepatology* 22: 1519–1526
24 Heilmann P, Beisker W, Miaskowski U, Camner P, Kreyling WG (1992) Intraphagolysosomal pH in canine and rat alveolar macrophages: flow cytometric measurements. *Environ Health Perspect* 97: 115–120
25 Kromer W (1995) Similarities and differences in the properties of substituted benzimidazoles: a comparison between pantoprazole and related compounds. *Digestion* 56: 443–454

26 Beil W, Staar U, Sewing KF (1992) Pantoprazole: a novel H^+/K^+-ATPase inhibitor with an improved pH stability. *Eur J Pharmacol* 218: 265–271
27 Simon WA, Keeling DJ, Laing SM, Fallowfield C, Taylor AG (1990) By 1023/SK & F 96022: biochemistry of a novel (H^+, K^+)-ATPase inhibitor. *Biochem Pharmacol* 39: 1799–1806
28 Besancon M, Simon A, Sachs G, Shin JM (1997) Sites of reaction of the gastric H, K-ATPase with extracytoplasmic thiol reagents. *J Biol Chem* 272: 22438–22446
29 Naesdal J, Andersson T, Bodemar G, Larsson R, Regardh CG, Skanberg I, Walan A (1986) Pharmacokinetics of ^{14}C-omeprazole in patients with impaired renal function. *Clin Pharmacol Ther* 40: 344–351
30 Fitton A, Wiseman L, Pantoprazole (1996) A review of its pharmacological properties and therapeutic use in acid-related disorders. *Drugs* 51: 460–482
31 Karol MD, Machinist JM, Cavanaugh JM (1997) Lansoprazole pharmacokinetics in subjects with various degrees of kidney function. *Clin Pharmacol Ther* 61: 450–458
32 Spencer CM, Faulds D (1994) Lansoprazole. A reappraisal of its pharmacodynamic and pharmacokinetic properties, and its therapeutic efficacy in acid-related disorders. *Drugs* 48: 404–430
33 VandenBranden M, Ring BJ, Binkley SN, Wrighton SA (1996) Interaction of human liver cytochromes P450 in vitro with LY307640, a gastric proton pump inhibitor. *Pharmacogenetics* 6: 81–91
34 Böttiger Y, Tybring G, Gotharson E, Bertilsson L (1997) Inhibition of the sulfoxidation of omeprazole by ketoconazole in poor and extensive metabolizers of S-mephenytoin. *Clin Pharmacol Ther* 62: 384–391
35 Katsuki H, Nakamura C, Arimori K, Fujiyama S, Nakano M (1997) Genetic polymorphism of CYP2C19 and lansoprazole pharmacokinetics in Japanese subjects. *Eur J Clin Pharmacol* 52: 391–396
36 Sohn DR, Kobayashi K, Chiba K, Lee KH, Shin SG, Ishizaki T (1992) Disposition kinetics and metabolism of omeprazole in extensive and poor metabolizers of S-mephenytoin 4′-hydroxylation recruited from an Oriental population. *J Pharmacol Exp Ther* 262: 1195–1202
37 Sohn DR, Kwon JT, Kim HK, Ishizaki T (1997) Metabolic disposition of lansoprazole in relation to the S-mephenytoin 4′-hydroxylation phenotype status. *Clin Pharmacol Ther* 61: 574–582
38 Schulz HU, Hartmann M, Steinijans VW, Huber R, Luhrmann B, Bliesath H, Wurst W (1996) Lack of influence of pantoprazole on the disposition kinetics of theophylline in man. *Int J Clin Pharmacol Ther* 34 (Suppl): S51–S57
39 Tanaka M, Ohkubo T, Otani K, Suzuki A, Kaneko S, Sugawara K, Ryokawa Y, Hakusui H, Yamamori S, Ishizaki T (1997) Metabolic disposition of pantoprazole, a proton pump inhibitor, in relation to S-mephenytoin 4′-hydroxylation phenotype and genotype. *Clin Pharmacol Ther* 62: 619–628
40 Yasuda S, Horai Y, Tomono Y, Nakai H, Yamato C, Manabe K, Kobayashi K, Chiba K, Ishizaki T (1995) Comparison of the kinetic disposition and metabolism of E3810, a new proton pump inhibitor, and omeprazole in relation to S-mephenytoin 4′-hydroxylation status. *Clin Pharmacol Ther* 58: 143–154
41 Petersen KU (1995) Review article: omeprazole and the cytochrome P450 system. *Aliment Pharmacol Ther* 9: 1–9
42 Reynolds, JEF (ed) (1996) *Martindale. The extra pharmacopoeia*. Royal Pharmaceutical Society, London, 384
43 de Hoon JN, Thijssen HH, Beysens AJ, Van Bortel LM (1997) No effect of short-term omeprazole intake on acenocoumarol pharmacokinetics and pharmacodynamics. *Br J Clin Pharmacol* 44: 399–401
44 Andersson T, Andren K, Cederberg C, Edvardsson G, Heggelund A, Lundborg P (1990) Effects of omeprazole and cimetidine on plasma diazepam levels. *Eur J Clin Pharmacol* 39: 51–54
45 Gugler R, Jensen JC (1985) Omeprazole inhibits oxidative drug metabolism. Studies with diazepam and phenytoin *in vivo* and 7-ethoxycoumarin *in vitro*. *Gastroenenterology* 89: 1235–1241
46 Jack DB (1992) *Handbook of pharmacokinetic data*. Macmillan, New York

47 Baldessarini (1996) Drugs and the treatment of psychiatric disorders. In: JG Hardman, LE Limbird (eds): *Goodman & Gilman's The pharmacological basis of therapeutics*. McGraw-Hill, New York, 424
48 Reynolds, JEF (ed) (1996) *Martindale. The extra pharmacopoeia*. Royal Pharmaceutical Society, London, 702
49 Gough PA, Curry SH, Araujo OE, Robinson JD, Dallman JJ (1982) Influence of cimetidine on oral diazepam elimination with measurement of subsequent cognitive change. *Br J Clin Pharmacol* 14: 739–742
50 Greenblatt DJ, Abernethy DR, Morse DS, Harmatz JS, Shader RI (1984) Clinical importance of the interaction of diazepam and cimetidine. *N Engl J Med* 310: 1639–1643
51 Kerr BM, Thummel KE, Wurden CJ, Klein SM, Kroetz DL, Gonzalez FJ, Levy RH (1994) Human liver carbamazepine metabolism. Role of CYP3A4 and CYP2C8 in 10,11-epoxide formation. *Biochem Pharmacol* 47: 1969–1979
52 Naidu MUR, Shobha JC, Dixit VK, Kumar A, Kumar TR, Sekhar KR, Sekhar EC (1994) Effect of multiple dose omeprazole on the pharmacokinetics of carbamazepine. *Drug Invest* 7: 8–12
53 Böttiger Y, Bertilsson L (1995) No effect on plasma carbamazepine concentration with concomitant omeprazole treatment. *Clin Drug Invest* 9: 180–181
54 Bertilsson L, Tybring G, Widen J, Chang M, Tomson T (1997) Carbamazepine treatment induces the CYP3A4 catalysed sulphoxidation of omeprazole, but has no or less effect on hydroxylation via CYP2C19. *Br J Clin Pharmacol* 44: 186–189
55 Pippenger CE (1987) Clinically significant carbamazepine drug interactions: an overview. *Epilepsia* 28 (Suppl 3): S71–S76
56 Gustavson LE, Kaiser JF, Edmonds AL, Locke CS, DeBartolo ML, Schneck DW (1995) Effect of omeprazole on concentrations of clarithromycin in plasma and gastric tissue at steady state. *Antimicrob Agents Chemother* 39: 2078–2083
57 Rodrigues AD, Roberts EM, Mulford DJ, Yao Y, Ouellet D (1997) Oxidative metabolism of clarithromycin in the presence of human liver microsomes. Major role for the cytochrome P4503A (CYP3A) subfamily. *Drug Metab Dispos* 25: 623–630
58 Steinijans VW, Huber R, Hartmann M, Zech K, Bliesath H, Wurst W, Radtke HW (1996) Lansoprazole of pantoprazole drug interactions in man: an updated review. *Int J Clin Pharmacol Ther* 34 (Suppl 1): S31–S50
59 Zech K, Steinijans VW, Huber R, Kolassa N, Radtke HW (1996) Pharmacokinetics and drug interactions – relevant factors for the choice of a drug. *Int J Clin Pharmacol Ther* 34 (Suppl): S3–S6
60 Cavanaugh JH, Karol MD (1996) Lack of pharmacokinetic interaction after administration of lansoprazole or omeprazole with prednisone. *J Clin Pharmacol* 36: 1064–1071
61 Cavanaugh JH, Winters EP, Cohen A, Locke CS (1991) Lack of effect of lansoprazole on steady-state warfarin metabolism. *Gastroenterology* 100 (Suppl): A40
62 Curi-Pedrosa R, Daujat M, Pichard L, Ourlin JC, Clair P, Gervot L, Lesca P, Domergue J, Joyeux H, Fourtanier G et al (1994) Omeprazole and lansoprazole are mixed inducers of CYP1A and CYP3A in human hepatocytes in primary culture. *J Pharmacol Exp Ther* 269: 384–392
63 Daujat M, Charrasse S, Fabre I, Lesca P, Jounaidi Y, Larroque C, Poellinger L, Maurel P (1996) Induction of CYP1A1 gene by benzimidazole derivatives during Caco-2 cell differentiation. Evidence for an acryl-hydrocarbon receptor-mediated mechanism. *Eur J Biochem* 237: 642–652
64 Masubuchi N, Hakusui H, Okazaki O (1997) Effects of pantoprazole on xenobiotic metabolizing enzymes in rat liver microsomes: a comparison with other proton pump inhibitors. *Drug Metab Dispos* 25: 584–589
65 Krusekopf S, Kleeberg U, Hildebrandt AG, Ruckpaul K (1997) Effects of benzimidazole derivatives on cytochrome P450 1A1 expression in a human hepatoma cell line. *Xenobiotica* 27: 1–9
66 Rost KL, Brösicke H, Brockmöller J, Scheffler M, Helge H, Roots I (1992) Increase of cytochrome P450IA2 activity by omeprazole: evidence by the 13C-[N-3-methyl]-caffeine breath test in poor and extensive metabolizers of S-mephenytoin. *Clin Pharmacol Ther* 52: 170–180

67 Xiaodong S, Gatti G, Bartoli A, Cipolla G, Crema F, Perucca E (1994) Omeprazole does not enhance the metabolism of phenacetin, a marker of CYP1A2 activity, in healthy volunteers. *Ther Drug Monit* 16: 248–250

68 Granneman GR, Karol MD, Locke CS, Cavanaugh JH (1995) Pharmacokinetic interaction between lansoprazole and theophylline. *Ther Drug Monit* 17: 460–464

69 Kokufu T, Ihara N, Sugioka N, Koyama H, Ohta T, Mori S, Nakajima K (1995) Effects of lansoprazole on pharmacokinetics and metabolism of theophylline. *Eur J Clin Pharmacol* 48: 391–395

70 Prakash A, Faulds D (1998) Rabeprazole. *Drugs* 55: 261–267

71 Delhotal-Landes B, Flouvat B, Duchier J, Molinie P, Dellatolas F, Lemaire M (1993) Pharmacokinetics of lansoprazole in patients with renal or liver disease of varying severity. *Eur J Clin Pharmacol* 45: 367–371

72 Huber R, Hartmann M, Bliesath H, Luhmann R, Steinijans VW, Zech K (1996) Pharmacokinetics of pantoprazole in man. *Int J Clin Pharmacol Ther* 34: S7–S16

73 Gerloff J, Mignot A, Barth H, Heintze K (1996) Pharmacokinetics and absolute bioavailability of lansoprazole. *Eur J Clin Pharmacol* 50: 293–297

74 Regardh CG, Andersson T, Lagerstrom PO, Lundborg P, Skanberg I (1990) The pharmacokinetics of omeprazole in humans – a study of single intravenous and oral doses. *Ther Drug Monit* 12: 163–172

75 Andersson T, Olsson R, Regardh CG, Skanberg I (1993) Pharmacokinetics of [^{14}C]omeprazole in patients with liver cirrhosis. *Clin Pharmacokinet* 24: 71–78

Pharmaceutical considerations

Proton Pump Inhibitors
ed. by L. Olbe

Pharmaceutical considerations

Åke G. Pilbrant

Pharmaceutical R & D, ASTRA Hässle AB, S-431 83 Mölndal, Sweden

Introduction

Since the launch of the first proton pump inhibitor (PPI), omeprazole, in 1988 there has been ever increasing interest in this new chemical class of drugs. Now, 10 years later, there are four compounds on the market, which all share common features (Fig. 1, Tab. 1). The PPIs are substituted benzimidazoles which inhibit gastric acid secretion by blocking H^+K^+-ATPase [1]. They are amphiphilic compounds, that is they are both acids and bases. The pyridine nitrogen is protonised with a pK_a of around 4. The positively charged ion is rapidly rearranged to a highly reactive sulphenamide which *in vivo* binds covalently to and inhibits the proton pump, the H^+K^+-ATPase within the parietal cell [2, 3]. The only place in the body where the pH is low enough to cause this rearrangement is the secretory cannaliculi of the

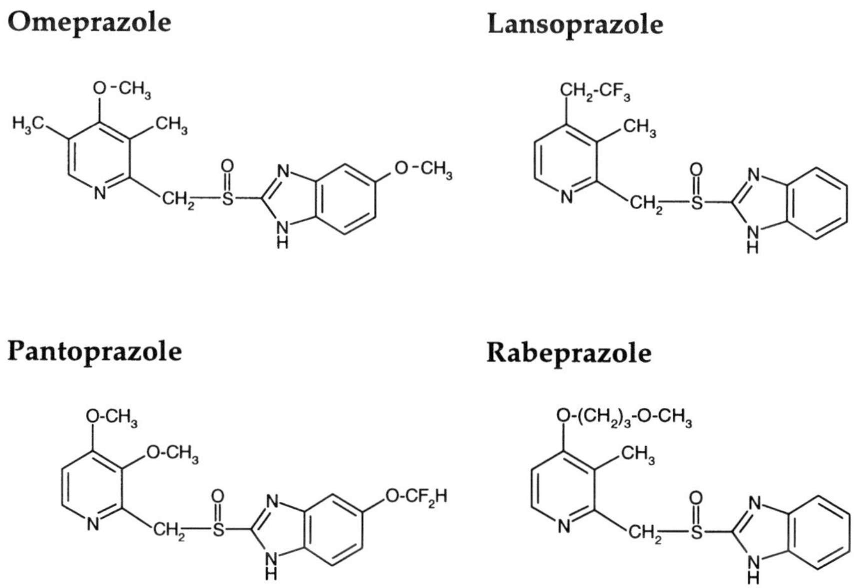

Figure 1. Commercially available PPIs.

Table 1. Physico-chemical data of PPIs

	Omeprazole	Lansoprazole	Pantoprazole	Rabeprazole
pK_a 37 °C	3.98, 8.7 [16]	3.89, 8.7 [16]	3.77, 8.2 [16]	5.0, 8.8[a]
pK_a 25 °C	4.0, 8.8 [6]	4.1, 8.8 [30]	4.0 [31]	4.9 [31]
Half-life of degradation in water solution, 37 °C				
at pH 2	105 s [16]	85 s [16]	195 s [16]	
at pH 7	23 h [16]	13 h [16]	39 h [16]	80 min[b]
Water solubility, mg/ml	0.15 [16]	0.06 [5]		

[a] Calculated according to Brändström et al [4].
[b] Astra Hässle AB. Data on file.

stimulated parietal cells. *In vitro* the rearrangement to the reactive sulphenamide can take place when the PPI comes in contact with anything reacting acidic whether in solution or in the solid state. The sulphenamide will then react further and cause degradation of the PPI to a number of usually heavily coloured degradation products [4]. This reactivity together with a rather low water solubility and an inherent instability makes the pharmaceutical formulation of the PPIs a real challenge. The difficulties are mirrored by a great number of patents and patent applications covering different aspects of pharmaceutical products and processes.

Physicochemical properties

The PPIs can be protonised in two steps. First, a proton binds to the pyridine nitrogen with a pK_a of around 4. At very low pH values another proton can bind to the benzimidazole nitrogen. This pK_a value is difficult to determine because of the rapid degradation of the PPIs at low pH values. In alkaline solutions the benzimidazole hydrogen can leave with a pK_a of around 9, forming a negatively charged ion.

The water solubility of the neutral compounds is rather low, less than 0.1 %. The charged ions have better water solubility, and the PPIs are freely soluble in sodium hydroxide solutions.

The stability of the PPIs in water solution is highly dependent on pH. The positively charged ion present in solution at low pH values degrades rapidly. The half-life of degradation of the PPIs in dilute solutions at pH 2 is in the range of a few minutes. The uncharged compounds in water solution degrade with a half-life of tenths of hours, while the negatively charged ionic species are fairly stable in solution; the half-life of degradation is close to a year. The kinetics and mechanisms of reaction of omeprazole have been thoroughly studied by Brändström et al. [4]. A pH/stability profile for lansoprazole has been published [5].

The solid-state stability of the PPIs is rather good. The pure chemical compounds can be stored for longer periods of time at room temperature, although its is preferable to store them at refrigerator temperature or in deep freeze. Contact with acidic reacting substances as well as low amounts of residual solvents induces degradation [6]. The stability of PPIs in pharmaceutical formulations can be improved by admixing alkaline reacting compounds [7–8]. Alkaline anionic salts of PPIs, for example potassium, sodium, calcium and magnesium salts, have much better storage stability than the neutral compounds [9].

Characteristics influencing dosage form design

After oral administration of easily bioavailable pharmaceutical formulations, the PPIs are rapidly and completely absorbed, with peak blood concentrations obtained within 10 to 20 min [6, 10]. They are rapidly eliminated from the body, with plasma half-lives of about 1 h.

The susceptibility for degradation in acid media, such as the contents of the stomach, precludes the use of conventional oral dosage forms. From the low water solubility coupled with the rapid absorption follows that there exists a potential for dissolution rate-limited absorption.

Since the PPIs bind covalently to the proton pump, the effect on gastric acid secretion is long lasting and depends on the total amount of the PPI absorbed and is not proportional to the blood concentration of the PPI at any particular time. This also means that the rate of absorption is not critical for the long-term effect – only the total amount absorbed.

Oral dosage forms

Formulation principles

There are two main options for getting around the risk of acid-catalysed degradation of the PPI in the stomach after oral administration.

1. To secure a neutral/alkaline gastric pH by coadministration of pH buffering substances. This was done in early human pharmacological studies with omeprazole [6] but can hardly be applied to a marketable pharmaceutical formulation for longer use.
2. To ensure that the active drug is not released in the stomach by using an enteric coating which dissolves only in solutions with a pH of 5.5 or higher, such as is the case in the small intestine.

An enteric-coating can be applied on whole tablets or onto individual pellets/particles/granules which then are dispensed into gelatin capsules or mixed with tablet excipients and compressed into tablets.

Astra, the pioneer of the PPI area, invented a pharmaceutical formulation of omeprazole: individually enteric-coated pellets dispensed in hard gelatin capsules [7]. Lansoprazole is presented in a similar capsule formulation [8], wheras pantoprazole [11] and rabeprazole [12] are formulated as single-unit enteric-coated tablets. In some markets Astra has recently also introduced a tablet containing a multitude of small, individually enteric-coated pellets [13].

Gastric emptying of enteric-coated dosage forms

Single-unit enteric-coated dosage forms must be swallowed whole, and they do not dissolve in the stomach. It is well known that insoluble enteric-coated tablets of a size >3–5 mm in diameter may reside in the stomach during quite some time if they are administered together with food [14], whereas a multiple dose unit of small enteric-coated pellets will show a much less variable gastric emptying time [15]. This may affect the time required to obtain a response on gastric acid secretion after the first dose. The effect on gastric acid secretion after a single dose of a PPI is long lasting, and during continuous dosing it is of less importance when – during a dosage interval – the absorption actually takes place. The pharmacodynamic effects at steady state after administration of enteric-coated whole tablets or capsules containing enteric-coated pellets will not differ [16].

Pharmacopoeial requirements

Pharmacopoeial requirements on enteric-coated articles include testing of the function of the enteric coating *in vitro*. The test article is placed in 0.1 M hydrochloric acid at 37°C for 2 h. The amount of drug released to the medium should be less than 10% – that is testing the integrity of the enteric coating. The pH of the medium is then shifted to pH 6.8, and the release of the drug to this medium should reach a certain minimum value within a specified time – a test to show that the enteric coating dissolves at a pH resembling that of the small intestine. Since the PPIs degrade rapidly in acid solution to a cascade of degradation products, the first part of the test, the acid stage, cannot be applied as such. It is possible to perform the testing in two separate steps. First, a number of enteric-coated units are individually exposed to acid for 2 h, the tablets or pellets are collected and dissolved in alkaline solution, and the amount of drug remaining intact after acid exposure is determined. Another set of enteric-coated units are then first exposed to acid during 2 h, the pH of the medium is shifted to pH 6.8 and the amount of drug released to the medium after a specified time is determined. However, because of the rapid degradation of the PPIs in acid solution, it is sufficient to perform only the second part of the test. The same information about the function of the enteric coating is gained.

Dissolution rate-limited absorption

Although the PPIs are rapidly absorbed from a solution, their low solubility in water coupled with the susceptibility of degradation in solutions of acid to near-neutral pH-values indicate that the rate of dissolution from a dosage form can limit the rate and extent of bioavailability [6].

Influence of food

Absorption from a controlled-release dosage form has a greater potential of being influenced by concomitant food intake than that from an immediate release formulation. Absorption from enteric-coated dosage forms, which dissolve first in the small intestine, are of course influenced by gastric emptying. In this respect enteric-coated tablets, due to their size, show a greater variability than small, individually enteric-coated multiple-unit formulations. The presence of food can also interfere with the dissolution and absorption of the active drug. When single oral doses of pantoprazole sodium sesquihydrate enteric-coated tablets were given to 19 healthy subjects prior to a high caloric breakfast, the area under the plasma concentration vs time curve (AUC) and the maximum plasma concentration (C_{max}) were the same as when the tablets were given in the fasting state [17]. The gastric emptying of the tablets given together with food were much more variable, resulting in an increased variability in time [t_{max}) to reach C_{max}. This delay in gastric emptying is of no clinical importance during continuous dosing, although it may delay the effect on gastric acid secretion after the first dose of a treatment. The influence of food on the absorption of omeprazole from a multiple-unit enteric-coated pellet formulation (Losec® capsules) was studied in 12 healthy subjects. In two periods of 7 days the capsules were given either before or after breakfast. When the capsules were given after the meal, the time for appearance of omeprazole in blood plasma seemed to be prolonged, but the total amount absorbed was not affected [18]. Different results were found for lansoprazole capsules, with C_{max} reduced about 50% and AUC reduced about 27% when the capsules were given together with a standard meal [19]. In another study in 12 healthy male subjects single doses of lansoprazole 30 mg capsules containing enteric-coated pellets were administered with or without breakfast. When co-administered with breakfast, t_{max} was doubled, and the AUC and C_{max} were decreased by approximately 50% [20].

Influence of antacids

In the clinical situation, where treatment with a PPI is indicated, antacids are often used for symptom relief. Antacids increase the pH of the stomach contents to pH values where the enteric coating of PPI dosage forms is soluble. Antacids usually have a short-term effect on gastric pH. If a PPI dosage form is taken together with antacids, there is a risk that the enteric coating will dissolve or partly dissolve while the dosage form still remains in the stomach. If the gastric pH returns to normal, the remaining PPI will rapidly degrade. It has been shown for omeprazole [21, 22] and pantoprazole [23] that this is not the case. The bioavailability of these two drugs is not influenced by concomitant administration of antacids. For lansoprazole capsules, however, the bioavailability was slightly decreased when the capsules were given together with antacids [19, 24]. When antacids were administered 1 h before the lansoprazole capsules, there was no influence on lansoprazole bioavailability [19].

Dispersion of enteric-coated dosage forms in liquids

For the PPIs, which degrade rapidly in acidic media, it is essential that the enteric coating functions. It is also important that the dosage forms be swallowed intact. They cannot be crushed or chewed. For patients having difficulties swallowing tablets or capsules, for example patients with erosive reflux oesophagitis, this can be a real challenge. Dosage forms containing small individually enteric-coated units can be dispersed, preferably in an acid-reacting fruit juice, before intake [25]. If the enteric-coated units are small enough, it is also possible to feed a dispersion through a nasogastric tube. For enteric-coated whole tablets there is no such opportunity.

Storage stability

Given the physicochemical characteristics of the PPIs, it is difficult to develop dosage forms with good long-term stability with regard to chemical stability as well as biopharmaceutical properties. The pharmaceutical products must be capable of being stored and handled at elevated temperatures and at high relative humidity. Functional and well-designed packages are important for good storage stability. According to current guidelines, a pharmaceutical product which can be stored at 40°C/75% relative humidity during 6 months without changes in its physicochemical characteristics can be assigned a shelf-life of 3 years. The market acceptance of the PPIs and especially omeprazole has created great interest, and a vast number of omeprazole products of different origin are available. All of these do not live up to the quality of the Astra brand-name products. A number of omeprazole products available in different countries were tested regarding their storage stability at 40°C/75% relative humidity [26, 27]. After storage for 6 months less than 20% of the products had acceptable quality with regard to potency, content of degradation products, discoloration and *in vitro* dissolution rate. The use of some of these products will certainly lead to suboptimal treatment results.

Parenteral dosage forms

The stability characteristics of the PPIs precludes the development of ready-to-use solutions for parenteral administration. In alkaline water solutions, where the PPIs are present mainly in anionic form, the stability (and solubility) is sufficient for the preparation of a solution which can be filtered sterile, dispensed aseptically into sterile injection vials and freeze-dried. For stability and solubility reasons the pH of the concentrated dispensing solution needs to be above pH 11. If the lyophilised substance is reconstituted with a small amount of water, the solution will have a high pH which might be given by slow intravenous injection; but this is accompanied by a high risk of causing pain at the injection site or even thrombophlebitis. It is recommended to dissolve the lyophilised substance in 50 to 100 ml of saline or 5% dextrose for infusion. The dilute solution in saline will have a pH of about 10 and can be given as a short-term infusion over 20 to 30 min without problems. Omeprazole (Losec®) is available both as a lyophilised substance for infusion (for reconstitution in 100 ml of saline or 5% dextrose for infusion) and as a lyophilised substance for intravenous injection. For the latter a solvent ampoule (water/polyethylene glycol) containing pH-buffering substances is provided. The pH of the injection solution, 10 ml containing 40 mg of omeprazole, is adjusted to pH 9. This solution can be given as an intravenous injection over at least 2.5 minutes. Lansoprazole [28] and pantoprazole [27] have also been formulated as lyophilised substances for extemporaneous reconstitution. These products are available only in a few countries.

The reconstituted solutions are stable for short periods of time. The lyophilised substances should only be reconstituted in the recommended solutions. The PPIs cannot be added to other infusion solutions. Parenteral nutritional solutions have too low a pH, causing rapid degradation of the active drug. Other solutions for infusion contain different metal ions which will precipitate the PPI out of solution.

Formulations for other routes of administration

Many other routes of administration for the PPIs have been discussed, for example rectal, transdermal, nasal and so on. However, the chemical structure of the PPIs is such that the active substances might cause allergic contact skin reactions. This property of the PPIs prohibits the development of pharmaceutical preparations for most routes other than oral and parenteral.

References

1 Fellenius E, Berglindh T, Sachs G, Olbe L, Elander B, Wallmark B (1981) Substituted benzimidazoles inhibit gastric acid secretion by blocking (H^+K^+)ATPase. *Nature* 290: 159–161

2 Wallmark B, Brändström A, Larsson H (1984) Evidence for acid-induced transformation of omeprazole into an active inhibitor of (H^+K^+)-ATPase within the parietal cell. *Biochem Biophys Acta* 778: 549–558

3 Lindberg P, Nordberg P, Alminger T, Brändström A, Wallmark B (1986) The mechanism of action of the gastric acid secretion inhibitor omeprazole. *J Med Chem* 29: 1327–1329

4 Brändström A, Lindberg P, Bergman N-Å, Alminger T, Ankner K, Junggren U, Lamm B, Norberg P, Erickson M, Grundevik I et al (1989) Chemical reactions of omeprazole and omeprazole analogues. *Acta Chem Scand* 43: 536–611

5 Tabata T, Makino T, Kashihara T, Hirai S, Kitamori N, Toguchi H (1992) Stabilization of a new antiulcer drug (lansoprazole) in the solid dosage forms. *Drug Dev Ind Pharm* 18: 1437–1447

6 Pilbrant Å, Cederberg C (1985) Development of an oral formulation of omeprazole. *Scand J Gastroenter* 20 (Suppl 108): 113–120

7 Lövgren KI, Pilbrant ÅG, Yasumura M, Morigaki S, Oda M, Ohishi N (1988) New pharmaceutical preparation for oral use. *US Patent* 4,786,505

8 Makino T, Tabata T, Hirai S (1991) Stabilized pharmaceutical composition and its production. *US Patent* 5,045,321

9 Brändström AE (1987) Omeprazole salts. *Eur Patent* EP-B1-0124495

10 Regårdh C-G, Gabrielsson M, Hoffman K-J, Löfberg I, Skånberg I (1985) Pharmacokinetics and metabolism of omeprazole in animals and man – an overview. *Scand J Gastroenterol* 20 (Suppl 108): 79–94

11 Dietrich R, Ney H (1992) Pantoprazol enthaltende orale Darreichungsformen. *Eur Pat Appl* 0 519 365 A1

12 Saeki Y, Koyama N, Aoki S (1989) Peroral preparation of an acid-unstable compound. *Eur Pat Appl* 0 342 522 A1

13 Bergstrand PJA, Lövgren KI (1996) Multiple unit pharmaceutical preparations containing proton pump inhibitor. PCT *Int Appl* 96 01624

14 Blythe RH, Grass G, Mac Donnell DR (1959) The formulation and evaluation of enteric coated aspirin tablets. *Am J Pharmacol* 131: 206–216

15 Bogentoft C, Carlsson I, Ekenved G, Magnusson A (1978) Influence of food on the absorption of acetylsalicylic acid from enteric-coated dosage forms. *Eur J Clin Pharmacol* 14: 351–355

16 Pilbrant Å (1993) Formulation of proton pump inhibitors. In: *Current status on targeted drug delivery to the gastrointestinal tract.* Capsugel Symposia series. Capsugel Library, Bornem, 35–42

17 Huber R, Hartmann M, Bliesath H, Lühmann R, Steinijans VW, Zech K (1996) Pharmacokinetics of pantoprazole in man. *Int J Clin Pharmacol Ther* 34 (Suppl 1): S7–S16

18 Andersson T, Andrén K, Cederberg C, Heggelund A, Lundborg P, Röhss K (1990) Bioavailability of omeprazole as enteric coated granules in conjunction with food on the first and seventh days of treatment. *Drug Invest* 2: 184–188

19 Delhotal-Landes B, Cournot A, Vermerien N, Dellatolas F, Benoit M, Flouvat B (1991) The effect of food and antacids on lansoprazole absorption and disposition. *Eur J Drug Metabol Pharmacokin* 16: 315–320

20 Bergstrand R, Grind M, Nyberg G, Olofsson B (1995) Decreased oral bioavailability of lansoprazole in healthy volunteers when given with a standardized breakfast. *Clin Drug Invest* 9: 67–71

21 Howden CW, Reid JL (1988) The effect of antacids and metoclopramide on omeprazole absorption and disposition. *Brit J Clin Pharmacol* 25: 779–781

22 Tuynman HARE, Festen HPM, Röhss K, Meuwissen SGM (1987) Lack of effect of antacids on plasma concentrations of omeprazole given as enteric-coated granules. *Br J Clin Pharmacol* 24: 833–835

23 Hartmann M, Bliesath H, Huber R, Koch H, Steinijans VW, Wurst W (1994) Simultaneous intake of antacids has no influence on the pharmacokinetcs of the gastric H^+K^+-ATPase inhibitor pantoprazole. *Gut* 35 (Suppl 4): A76

24 Gerloff J, Barth H, Mignot A, Fuchs W, Heintze K (1993) Does the proton pump inhibitor lansoprazole interact with antacids? *Naunyn Schmiedebergs Arch Pharmacol* 347 (Suppl): R31
25 Chun AHC, Eason CJ, Shi HH, Cavanaugh JH (1995) Lansoprazole: an alternative method of administration of a capsule dosage formulation. *Clin Ther* 17: 441–447
26 Davidson AG, McCallum A (1996) A survey of the stability of omeprazole products from 13 countries. *Drug Dev Ind Pharm* 22: 1173–1185
27 Karlsson A, Lindqvist J, Lövgren K, Rosén L, Tivert A-M (1996) An investigation of the pharmaceutical quality of non-Astra authorised omeprazole products – a comparative study. *Int Pharm J* 10: 210–213
28 Takechi N, Hamaguchi N (1995) Injectable solutions containing anti-ulcer benzimidazoles and amides. *Eur Pat Appl* 0 649 655 A1
29 Dietrich R (1996) Method of producing a pantoprazole lyophilisate. *PCT Pat Appl* WO 96/17607
30 Kristi A, Vrecer F (1996) Investigation of the acido-basic and partition properties of the proton pump inhibitor lansoprazole. *Eur J Pharm Sci* 4 (Suppl): S117
31 Huber R, Kohl B, Sachs G, Senn-Bilfinger J, Simon WA, Sturm E (1995) Review article: the continuing development of proton pump inhibitors with particular reference to pantoprazole. *Aliment Pharmacol Ther* 9: 363–378

Clinical experience with proton pump inhibitors

Proton Pump Inhibitors
ed. by L. Olbe

Helicobacter pylori infection and peptic ulcer disease

Peter Malfertheiner

Klinik für Gastroenterologie, Hepatologie und Infektiologie, Universitätsklinik Magdeburg, Leipziger Str. 44, D-39120 Magdeburg, Germany

Introduction

At the stage when peptic ulcers appeared to become clinically controlled by more and more potent acid inhibitory agents, the traditional concept of ulcer pathogenesis was turned upside down by the discovery of a microorganism specialized to infect the human gastric mucosa. *Helicobacter pylori* infection is now recognized as the predisposing key factor and has assigned to the gastric acid a contributory though important role in gastric and duodenal ulcerogenesis. The discovery of this bacterium has reopened the chapters of gastric physiology and pathophysiology and has substantially modified the clinical management of peptic ulcer disease by offering the anti-*H. pylori* therapy as the definitive cure for the great majority of patients suffering from gastric and duodenal ulcers. The new classification of peptic ulcers attains to a clear distinction of *H. pylori*-positive ulcers or ulcers of other and less frequent etiologies (Tab. 1), thereby addressing the proper management for each entity. Management now consists of antibiotics in addition to acid-suppressive agents.

It has been a long scientific "odyssey" from the first descriptions of spiral organisms in the stomach of mammals and humans in the past century [1–3], to the more recent dogma of the human stomach as a sterile organ [4] not conducive to the survival of bacteria, to the detection and isolation of *H. pylori* by Warren and Marshall [5, 6]. The lessons from the discovery of *H. pylori* go beyond the new conception of ulcer pathogenesis

Table 1. Classification of peptic ulcers in stomach and duodenum

H. pylori infection-positive
Drug (i.e, NSAIDs)-induced
H. pylori + NSAIDs
Acid hypersecretion (i.e., Zollinger-Ellison)
Anastomosis ulcer
Tumors (i.e., cancer, lymphoma)
Other rare specific causes (i.e., Morbus Crohn, eosinophilic gastroduodenitis)

and the "revolutionized" management of peptic ulcer disease. They remind us that reading the older medical literature can be a tremendous source of knowledge and vision, and that dogmata such as that concerning the normoacidic sterile stomach can prevent progress. Finally, scientific interactions in the field of *H. pylori* infection point to the beneficial effect of closely interacting medical disciplines, in this case pathology, gastroenterology and microbiology.

It is a happy accident that the introduction *H. pylori* therapy and the introduction of the first proton pump inhibitor (PPI) omeprazole coincided. Instead of the expected battle of two controversial approaches to curing peptic ulcer disease – either *H. pylori* eradication with antibiotics or potent acid suppression by PPIs – they merged in a single strategy for healing ulcers.

H. pylori and ulcer pathogenesis

The chain of scientific facts leading to the evidence that *H. pylori* is the key pathogen in peptic ulcer disease comprises both epidemiological data and a complex puzzle of inflammatory events in the gastric and duodenal mucosa with repercussions in gastric physiology. The most convincing element in this chain of causality is still the clinical documentation of permanent ulcer cure which follows successful *H. pylori* eradication [7; for review see refs 8 and 9]. Epidemiological studies have uniformely attributed a fourfold increased risk of developing an ulcer to *H. pylori* infected vs noninfected persons, and this risk is estimated to be 25 times higher if the degree of inflammatory activity is high and antrum predominant [10, 11]. Approximately 90% of patients with duodenal ulcer and 70% with gastric ulcer carry *H. pylori* infection [8, 9].

The difference in prevalence of *H. pylori* among duodenal and gastric ulcers is due to the higher frequency of non-steroidal anti-inflammatory drugs (NSAIDs), the other well established etiological agents frequently involved in gastric ulcers (Tab. 1). The other side of the coin is that only about 10% of *H. pylori*-infected subjects in Western industrialized countries will eventually develop an ulcer, with others developing symptoms or much more rarely, neoplastic gastric pathologies. Approximately 80% of *H. pylori*-infected patients will experience prolonged chronic gastric inflammation without any further progression to relevant clinical disease. The obvious complexity of *H. pylori* as an ulcerogenic condition clearly suggests that additional factors are required to complete the pathogenetic cascade towards ulcer formation.

The pathogenetic pathway

In the pathogenetic cascade leading to peptic ulcer the following aspects need to be addressed briefly (Fig. 1): i) pattern and phenotype of gastritis; ii) alterations in the homeostasis of gastric hormones and acid secretion; iii) gastric metaplasia in the duodenum as a prerequisite for *H. pylori* colonization; iv) the interaction of *H. pylori* with the mucosal barrier; v) "ulcerogenic" strains; vi) genetic factors; vii) therapeutic proof of causality.

Pattern and phenotype of gastritis

Generally *H. pylori* colonizes the gastric epithelium from the prepyloric antrum to the cardia, and the outcomes of *H. pylori* infection are significantly influenced by the topographical predominance of the chronic inflammation. The characteristic pattern of gastritis in patients with duodenal ulcer (DU) is the antrum-predominant distribution of *H. pylori* with a high density of the bacteria and a high degree of inflammatory activity in this location [10, 12–14]. Following eradication therapy, gastric mucosal alterations are usually fully reversible in DU [15–17].

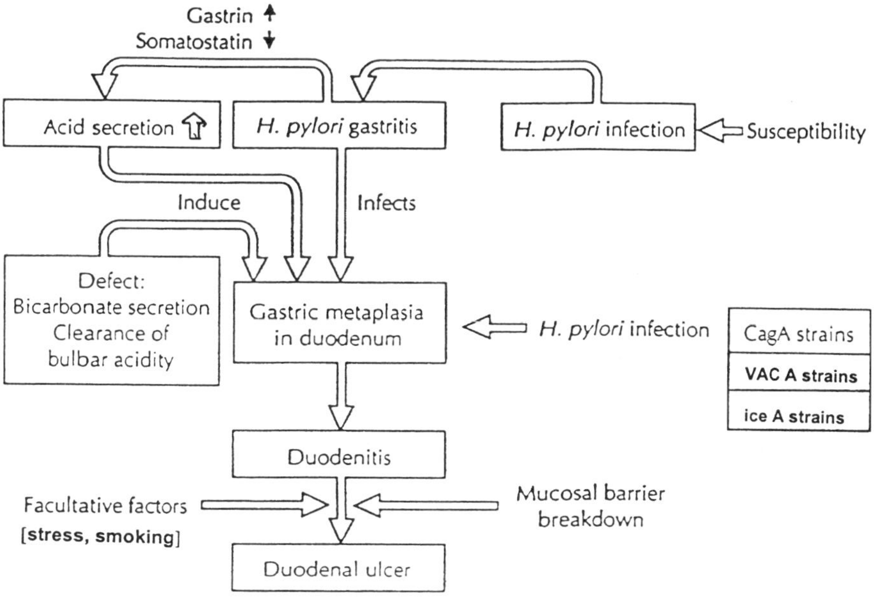

Figure 1. Pathogenetic cascade of *H. pylori* infection and duodenal ulcer formation (adapted and modified from ref. 31).

In gastric ulcer (GU), the topographic expression of chronic gastritis is such that the body mucosa and antral mucosa are equally affected. Unlike DU, acid secretion is decreased in patients with GU, because of the more severe involvement of the body mucosa. Acid-inhibitory drugs, in particular PPIs always lead to changes in the pattern of gastritis, with a reduction of bacteria and inflammatory activity in the antrum and an increase of both these conditions in the body [15–17].

Alterations in the homeostasis of gastric hormones and acid secretion

Antrum predominant chronic *H. pylori* infection is accompanied by an increase in both basal and stimulated gastric acid output, the effect being most pronounced in patients with DU [18–20]. The link between *H. pylori* infection and acid hypersecretion appears to be hormonal in nature and driven by hypergastrinemia (Fig. 2). The hypergastrinemia is consequent

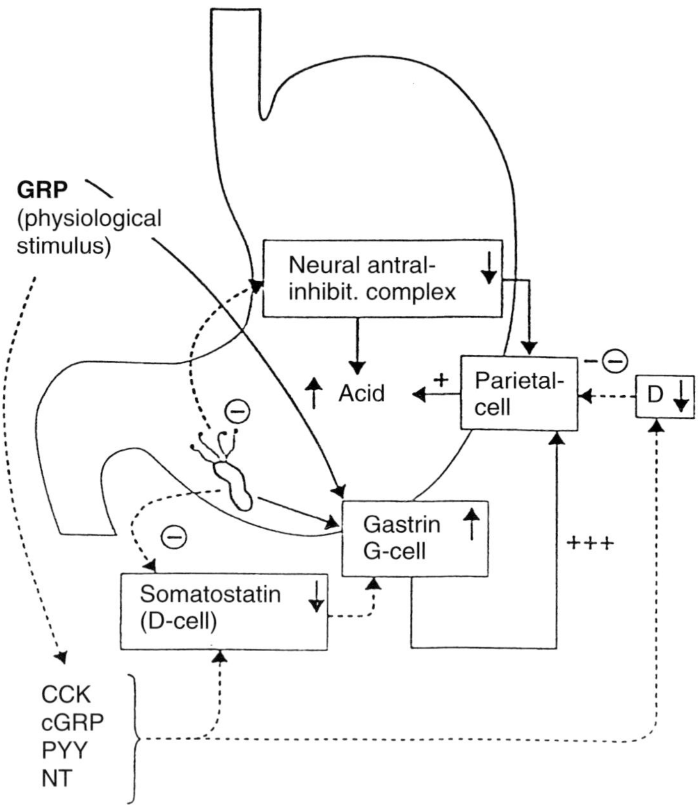

Figure 2. Physiological perturbations in antrum predominant gastritis that ultimately lead to increased gastric acid secretion mediated by hypergastrinemia and by the “knockout” of neutral inhibitory pathways controlling the parietal cell.

to the reduction in gastric somatostatin synthesis and release, which normally exerts an inhibitory control on gastrin release [21, 22].

More recent work has shown that, in addition to gastric hormones, neural pathways are also influenced by *H. pylori* infection (Fig. 2), with functional disruption of antral-fundic neural connections [23]. The impairment of the inhibitory neural control of gastrin and acid secretion elicited by a test meal in patients with *H. pylori*-positive DU [22] was recently demonstrated [24]. These abnormal responses, which in association with increased gastric emptying induce a higher duodenal acid load, are all reversed following *H. pylori* eradication [24]. Eradication of *H. pylori* infection rapidly reverses the accompanying hypergastrinemia and is associated with normalization of antral somatostatin levels, wheras it may be several months before acid hypersecretion returns to normal [19, 22, 25, 26]. Hypergastrinemia not only stimulates gastric acid secretion but in addition exerts a trophic effect on the parietal cell mass, and this may explain the sustained acid secretion following *H. plyori* eradication.

Gastric metaplasia in the duodenum is a prerequisite for H. pylori *colonization*

Gastric acid hypersecretion and more specifically the acid overload in the duodenum lead to the development of gastric metaplasia in the duodenal bulb [8, 27, 28]. The presence of gastric metaplasia in the duodenum increases the risk of duodenal ulcer 6-fold, whereas subsequent colonization of duodenal gastric metaplasia by *H. pylori* increases the risk 50-fold [29]. Because *H. pylori* colonization is specific and exclusive for gastric epithelial cells, gastric metaplasia in the epithelium of the duodenal bulb is crucial and essential for the organisms to colonize the duodenum [30]. Most likely this happens by migration from the antrum.

As in the stomach, chronic inflammation follows colonization of islands of duodenal gastric metaplasia by *H. pylori* and the inflamed duodenal mucosa becomes increasingly vulnerable to peptic acid attack and exposed to subsequent ulceration [31] (Fig. 1). Although *H. pylori* infection can be eradicated successfully, gastric metaplasia may persist or regress only partially [28, 32]. There is no continued increased risk for further duodenal ulcer relapse once *H. pylori* is eradicated.

Interaction of H. pylori *with the mucosal barrier*

Colonization of the gastric mucosa by *H. pylori* evokes a local inflammatory response, which results in mucosal injury of varying degrees [33]. The acute inflammatory response seems to be initiated by the release of epithelium-derived cytokines, predominantly interleukin-8 (IL-8) [34, 35]. Together with bacterial products such as lipopolysaccarides (endotoxins) and heat-shock proteins, cytokines orchestrate the acute inflammatory response, promoting the influx of neutrophils and macrophages into the gastric mucosa [34, 36], which subsequently release lysosomal enzymes, leukotrienes and oxygen-free radicals [34, 36]. The next step in the inflammatory cascade is the activation of T and B lymphocytes by bacterial antigens with the release of further proinflammatory cytokines, including IL-1, IL-2, IL-6 and tumour necrosis factor-α (TNF-α), as well as generation of specific immunglobulin (Ig)A and IgG antibodies directed against *H. pylori* [37, 38]. All these factors contribute to mucosal damage by promoting the release of factors with ulcerogenic potential such as platelet activating factor (PAF) and components of the complement pathway [38, 39].

"Ulcerogenic" strains

Pathogenetic properties (virulence factors) vary among strains. *H. pylori* isolated from patients with peptic ulcer disease appear to be more virulent, with some evidence that they exert a stronger adhesive property and produce greater amounts of enzymes with toxic potential [8]. Among them urease and phospholipases A_2 and C are of particular interest. *H. pylori* strains from ulcer patients produce higher amounts of urease, and this enzyme catalyzes production of ammonia, which in high concentration followed by formation of complexes such as NH_4Cl is toxic [40]. Phospholipases A and C disrupt a defensive element of the mucosal barrier, that is the surfactant composed of a phospholipid-rich layer responsible for maintaining the mucosal hydrophobicity involved in maintaining the integrity of the gastric epithelium [41, 42]. The released phospholipids appear to be ingested by *H. pylori* [43]. Several other bacterial products are released in close proximity to the epithelial cells, exerting a direct harmful effect [44].

Infection with certain *H. pylori* genotypes is linked to more severe morbidity. The most important genotypes are vac A- and cag A-positive, present in almost all patients with peptic ulceration. The *H. pylori*-derived vacuolating cytotoxin (vac A), an 87-kDa protein, causes vacuolar degeneration in cultured gastric cell preparations and gastric ulceration in experimental animals [44]. Although present in all *H. pylori* strains, the vac A gene, depending on its allelic form, is expressed in only 60%, lending strong support to the hypothesis of strain-dependent virulence. The cytotoxin-associated gene A (cag A), which is restricted to cytotoxin-producing strains of *H. pylori*, encodes for an ~120–160-kDa immunodominant protein that is now recognized as a marker of greater virulence, leading to an enhanced local inflammatory response [45–48].

Among *H. pylori*-infected individuals, bacterial strains expressing cag A protein are closely associated with peptic ulcer (present in 92% of cases) and, to a lesser extent, with chronic gastritis (~60% in Western populations) [49, 50]. Cytotoxin vac A and cag A gene products are frequently coexpressed, thus offering the possibility that cag A seropositivity may serve as a marker of disease. The cag A gene is now recognized to be part of large cag pathogenicity island which embraces other genes such as pic A and pic B [51]. These and a series of other genes have been characterized, and their function is to enhance mucosal inflammation through induction of cytokines [51]. A novel additional gene has been discovered recently and defined as ice A (induced by contact with epithelium) which has also to be incorporated among markers associated with peptic ulcer disease [52].

Genetic factors

In studies of twins, a genetic predisposition to acquire *H. pylori* has been shown with an increased affinity in monozygotes vs dizygotes [53]. Concerning peptic ulcer disease earlier studies showed, blood group O to have an associated higher risk [54]. More recently, increased *H. pylori* adhesion to gastric mucosa was shown in patients carrying Lewis b antigens, which are expressed on blood and gastric epithelial cells [55].

The pathogenetic importance of these findings are controversial, as the presence of these antigens is believed by some to contribute to an increase in mucosal damage through increased adhesion, whereas others suggest that binding of *H. pylori* to these antigenes would help to eliminate *H. pylori* during the shedding of the surface gastric epithelial cells attached by the bacteria. Several other adhesion-promoting factors have since been reported, but no conclusions can be drawn regarding their specific role in the ulcerogenic pathway. A Japanese working group contributed a new finding to this issue of genetics by reporting that subjects with human lymphocyte antigen (HLA) type DQA 1301 have an increased prevalence of ulcer disease [56].

The therapeutic proof of causality

The list of therapy studies is long, and all studies unequivocally report that *H. pylori* eradication leads to cure of gastric as well as duodenal ulcer [7–9]. The effect is lasting, as shown in long-term follow-up studies [57]. In addition, healing of the ulcer lesions is accelerated if antibiotics are added to acid-secretory inhibitors [58]. Finally, complications of peptic ulcer disease can also be kept from relapsing following *H. pylori* eradication, and this is superior to acid-inhibitory therapy alone (Tab. 2) [59–64]. All these facts taken together led in 1994 to the NIH consensus statement that antibiotic treatment in addition to antisecretory therapy is required in all patients with *H. pylori*-positive peptic ulcers [65].

Table 2. Ulcer bleeding relapses dependent on *H. pylori* status (follow up 6–24 months)

Author	Year	Bleeding relapse (%)	
		H. pylori-positive	*H. pylori*-negative
Graham	1993	29	0
Labenz	1994	37	0
Jaspersen	1995	29	0
Riemann	1995	12[a]	0
Rokkas	1995	31	0
Santander	1996	12[a]	0

[a] Patients under ranitidin.

Clinical experience with PPI

Numerous treatment regimes have been investigated for eradication of *H. pylori* infection, and initially these were performed predominantly in patients with DU. Historically, the first substances in use were bismuth salts (bismuth subcitrate and bismuth subsalicylate) [66], followed by several antibiotics among the 5-nitroimidazoles, penicillins and chinolones.

Antibacterial monotherapy was ineffective in the eradication of *H. pylori*, since such regimes typically achieved cure rates of $<20\%$ after 2 to 4 weeks of therapy [67]. Use of monotherapy with antibiotics was eventually strongly discouraged due to the possible risk of development of antibacterial resistance [66]. The next step was the addition of a bismuth compound to metronidazole or amoxicillin that increased the overall eradication rate to approximately 50% [68]. This result was unacceptably low, and hence the use of such dual therapy (bismuth plus one antibiotic) was not pursued further. The problem of antibiotic resistance in cases with therapy failure became increasingly recognized with the use of these therapies; the use of amoxycillin was exceptional in this respect, as no introduction of resistance was reported. The standard approach to eradicating *H. pylori* became a 14-day course of bismuth-based triple therapy, comprising colloidal bismuth, a nitroimidazole (typically metronidazole) and either tetracycline or amoxicillin. Using this kind of regimen, the 1988 pivotal study by Rauws and Tytgat confirmed that no ulcer relapse occurred following successful *H. pylori* eradication [7].

Although *H. pylori* eradication rates of 80 to 90% were obtained in most clinical trials with bismuth triple therapies, the success of these regimes in community use was limited by poor tolerability [69], poor patient compliance because of the complex dosage regimens, and acquisition of resistance to nitroimidazoles [70–73]. However, these regimens clarified the requirements, pitfalls and challenges of *H. pylori* eradication therapies (Fig. 3). Furthermore, in patients with active ulcer disease, the addition of an antisecretory agent was often necessary to provide rapid symptom relief.

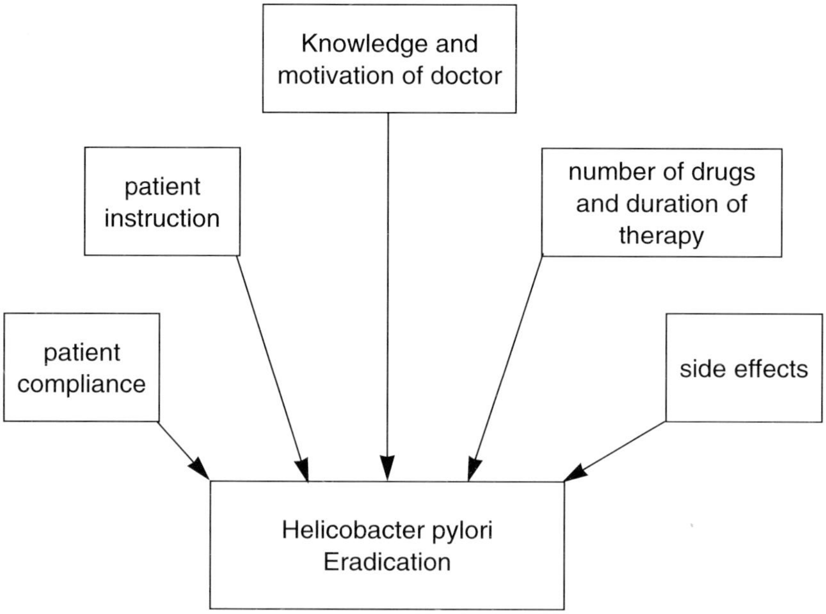

Figure 3. Requirements and influences on *H. pylori* eradication therapies in patients with peptic ulcer disease.

At the same time, omeprazole use started in many countries, providing a new dimension in healing peptic ulcers and speeding up symptom relief in these patients. A linear relationship between the degree of suppression of 24-h intragastric acidity and the rate of duodenal ulcer healing was demonstrated for antisecretory drugs [74], with the PPIs producing the most marked acid suppressant effect and the highest healing rates. The primary determinants of both duodenal and gastric ulcer healing include the degree and duration of suppression of intragastric acidity [75, 76]. Mathematical models proposed that if intragastric pH is maintained above 3 for 18–20 h per day, ulcer healing rates of 100% can be achieved within 4 weeks for duodenal ulcer [75] and within 8 weeks for gastric ulcer [76]. Similarly, an intragastric pH target threshold of 4 is predictive for healing in erosive esophagitis. While the optimal target pH for eradication of *H. pylori* remains to be established, it is likely that an intragastric pH in excess of 5 may be required.

The rationale for use of PPI in *H. pylori* therapy

Omeprazole as well as two other PPIs lansoprazole and pantoprazole, subsequently came into use, all possessing intrinsic activity against *H. pylori*, that is well documented *in vitro* [77–79]. With reduced acid secretion,

H. pylori colonization is suppressed, but the organism is rarely eradicated [80–85].

During omeprazole monotherapy, *H. pylori* organisms are cleared from the gastric antrum, but they grow and flourish in the corpus and fundus of the stomach [16, 17]. Thus to detect *H. pylori* in patients treated with PPIs, biopsies from both the gastric antrum and corpus should always be taken from 4 weeks after eradication therapy. The mechanism of PPI action against the bacterium have not been completely elucidated. As PPIs are known to inhibit growth of *H. pylori* even at neutral pH [80], specific mechanisms in addition to acid suppression must be assumed. Inhibition of alcohol dehydrogenase [81] and bacterial urease [77–79] have been demonstrated *in vitro*, and *in vivo* at high PPI doses. Omeprazole must, however, also dispose of a non-urease-dependent inhibitory mechanism since it works in the absence of urease and in a urease-deficient strain [89]. Inhibition of bacterial adenosine triphosphate (ATP)ase was supposed to be the target of bactericidal PPI action on *H. pylori* [77, 84, 90]. This putative mechanism has, however, been questioned and is addressed elsewhere in this book (see Sachs et al.; Blum and Martínek, this volume).

With regard to host factors, PPI may interfere with the mucosal inflammatory response, as *in vitro* data show inhibition of polymorphonuclear granulocyte chemotaxis [91].

Omeprazole and clarithromycin have been shown to reciprocally increase their concentration in the gastric mucosa [92], which is not the case with metronidazole and amoxycillin [93]. This partially may explain the optimal synergism of PPI and clarithromycin as observed in clinical trials.

The clinical experience

Omeprazole is clearly the most thoroughly investigated PPI in *H. pylori* eradication therapy. Its effectiveness in combination with antimicrobials has been proven in a series of well-designed studies. The use of pantoprazole and lansoprazole in *H. pylori* eradication therapy have subsequently also been well documented (Tab. 3).

The mode of action and rare adverse effects of the different PPIs are similar. Antibacterial therapy in combination with omeprazole was first described in 1989 by Unge and co-workers [80]. Their pilot study indicated that omeprazole and amoxicillin have a synergistic antibacterial effect, achieving an eradication rate two to three times higher than that of amoxicillin alone. The mechanism claimed to be involved is the better bioavailability of amoxicillin with omeprazole, but this was not confirmed [80, 88]. More likely, omeprazole prolongs the local stability of amoxicillin in the acidic milieu, rendering it less acidic and allowing a higher antibacterial concentration in a lower volume of gastric juice. The inconsistency of eradication rates with some trials reporting eradication rates equal to

Table 3. PPI-triple-therapies

Author (year)	Country	Therapy	Illness	No. of patients	Rates of eradications %
Lind (1996)	Europe and Can.	Ome 2 × 20 mg + Cla 2 × 250 mg + MET 2 × 400 mg	DU	111	95
		Ome 2 × 20 mg + Cla 2 × 500 mg + Amo 2 × 1000 mg		110	96
		Ome 2 × 20 mg + Cla 2 × 250 mg + Amo 2 × 1000 mg		111	84
		Ome 2 × 20 mg + Amo 2 × 1000 mg + MET 2 × 400 mg		119	79
Misiewicz (1996)	GB	Lan 2 × 30 mg + Cla 2 × 250 mg + MET 2 × 400 mg	DU + NUD	114	90
		Lan 2 × 30 mg + Cla 2 × 250 mg + Amo 2 × 1000 mg		116	90
		Lan 2 × 30 mg + Amo 2 × 1000 mg + MET 2 × 400 mg		120	72
		Ome 2 × 20 mg + Amo 2 × 1000 mg + MET 2 × 400 mg		115	82
Labenz 1997		Pan 2 × 40 mg + Cla 2 × 250 mg + Amo 2 × 1000 mg	DU	57	86

Main studies proving the efficacy of each of the marketed PPI based triple therapies. DU, duodenal ulcer; NUD, non-ulcer dyspepsia.

or greater than 80% [99] and others less than 60% [94–106] ended dual therapies as a first option. In dual therapies a duration of 10–14 days was found to be crucial, wheras shorter regimens were significantly less efficacious [98, 108]. The optimal daily dosage of omeprazole was twice (or three times) with doses varying from 20 to 80 mg. In three dose-finding studies a good correlation with increasing omeprazole dose and eradication rate was documented [101, 106, 107]. Three times omeprazole 40 mg and amoxicillin 750 mg achieved an eradication of >90%. However, in one trial, even the highest dose of omeprazole (160 mg/day) with amoxicillin yielded only an eradication rate of 69% [107].

The rate of adverse effects with PPI-based dual therapy ranged between 6 and 12%. Most patients experienced diarrhea and/or exanthema. Withdrawal rates were low, not exceeding 2%. Eradication rates obtained with PPI-amoxicillin regimen are negatively influenced by smoking [100, 108]. With clarithromycin being the most effective choice for anti-*H. pylori* monotherapy [109, 110] the dual therapy partnership with PPI was expected to achieve higher eradication rates. With this combination, *H. pylori* eradication rates ranged from 78 to 84% in a 2-week course of omeprazole plus clarithromycin [111–113]. The optimal dosage of omeprazole was 40 mg once or twice daily, and that of clarithromycin 500 mg two or three times daily. Adverse effects leading to discontinuation of therapy are rare, but a metallic taste resulting from high clarithromycin concentrations in the tongue may affect more than 50% of patients. Dual therapies using other PPIs such as lansoprazole have similarly reported eradication rates below 70% with either clarithromycin or amoxicillin [114, 115].

Following an interim period of PPI-based dual therapies with highly variable results, the breakthrough came in 1993. By adding a second antibacterial agent (tinidazole two times 500 mg) to omeprazole (20 mg used as single dose) and clarithromycin (250 mg two times per day), and by shortening the therapy course to 7 days, Bazzoli and co-workers created the recipe that eventually (following some modifications) turned out to be the optimal, new standard therapy for *H. pylori* cure [116]. The concept of adequate acid suppression combined with two synergistically acting antibiotics was the rationale for the selection of these drugs.

Several authors took up this concept and performed slight modifications of the original Bazzoli 7-day triple therapy, confirming unequivocally its high efficacy [117–121]. The short-course PPI-based triple regimens are generally well tolerated and achieve effective 24-h control of gastric acid secretion, which promotes rapid symptom resolution and ulcer healing with eradication rates ≥90%. In the largest trial conducted to date in the search of the optimal PPI antibiotic combinations, the MACH 1 study [122], a randomized, placebo-controlled, double-blind trial involving 787 patients with duodenal ulcer, *H. pylori* eradication was achieved in 96% of patients treated for 7 days with omeprazole (20 mg twice daily), amoxicillin (1 g twice daily) and high-dose clarithromycin (500 mg twice daily) and in 95% of those recieving omeprazole, metronidazole and low-dose clarithromycin (250 mg twice daily) [57]. These two regimens, equally potent, became the therapeutic gold standard and the reference therapy for all novel therapies. A subsequent study of 539 patients with DU (MACH 2) was set up to evaluate PPI triple therapy also in condition of metronidazole-resistant strains [123].

This issue has become increasingly more important, as *H. pylori* strains with metronidazole resistance vary between 20 and 70% around the world [124]. In the MACH 2 study 27% of strains were indeed found to be metronidazole resistant, but in spite of this 76% of patients with metronidazole-resistant, but in spite of this 76% of patients with metronidazole resistance were cured with the OMC regimen, whereas with OAC no interference was to be expected, and it worked effectively in 94% of metronidazole-resistant strains. That OMC is still effective in 76% of metronidazole-resistant strains, an effect that decreases to 43% with MC and without omeprazole, confirms the special not yet elucidated synergistic effect of omeprazole with the two antibiotics. Similar efficacy in metronidazole-resistant strains was shown with the combination lansoprazole, clarithromycin and metronidazole [126].

Clarithromycin resistance in most countries in the order of 1 to 12% prevalence is not yet a major issue, but causes more problems, as only 1 out of 2 patients with *H. pylori*-resistant strains would respond to the PPI triple therapy (OAC). Combinations of PPI with metronidazole (independent of the dose in the range from 800 to 1600 mg) and amoxicillin were consistantly 10% less effective than PPI-MC or PPI-AC [125]. Another important point emerging from all the studies is that clarithromycin with metronidazole as a partner in the PPI triple regimens requires only a dose of 2×250 mg, whereas in combination with amoxicillin regimens the required dose of clarithromycin is 2×500 mg.

Quadruple therapy, in which a PPI is added to the standard bismuth-based triple regimen, can achieve *H. pylori* eradication in 98% of patients [126], and may be warranted when prior eradication therapy has been unsuccessful or in patients with bacterial resistance to antibiotics [127]. A concept for selecting the optimal therapy following failure is proposed in Table 4.

In summary, the mechanisms underlying the synergistic action of the PPIs with antibiotics is still not fully understood. PPIs exert a direct antimicrobial effect *in vitro* against *H. pylori* and may also inhibit microbial urease activity, a crucial factor for *H. pylori* colonisation. *In vivo* by increasing intragastric pH PPIs may prevent inactivation of acid-labile antibiotics and proteolytic degradation of *H. pylori*-specific immunoglobulins, as well as enhance host immunity by providing a more favourable environment for leucocyte function. The lessons from clinical trials and clinical practice are that PPI-based triple therapies with either clarithromycin and amoxicillin or clarithromycin and 5-nitroimidazole unequivocally represent the best

Table 4. *H. pylori* therapies following failure

Result of resistance testing	Recommended therapy
MET-resistant CLA-sensitive	PPI-CLA-AMO (standard dose)
MET-resistant CLA-sensitive	PPI-CLA-AMO (standard dose)
MET-sensitive CLA-resistant	PPI-AMO-MET (standard dose)
MET-resistant CLA-resistant	PPI-BIS-MET or PPI-AMO (omeprazole 3 × 40 mg, amoxycillin 3 × 750 (or 1000) mg) 10–14 days

and world's most experienced therapy to date for curing *H. pylori* infection, this being the gold standard against which novel therapies must be measured.

References

1 Bizzozero G (1893) Über die schlauchförmigen Drüsen des Magendarmkanals und die Beziehung ihres Epithels zu dem Oberflächenepithel der Schleimhaut. *Arch mikr Anat* 82–152
2 Salomon H (1896) Über das Spirillum des Säugetiermagens und sein Verhalten zu den Belegzellen. *Centralbl f Bakt* 19: 433–442
3 Doenges JL (1939) Spirochetes in the gastric glands of *Macacus rhesus* and of man without related disease. *Arch Pathol* 27: 469–477
4 Palmer ED (1954) Investigation of the gastric mucosa spirochetes of the human. *Gastroenterology* 27: 218–220
5 Warren JR (1983) Unidentified curved bacili on gastric epithelium in active chronic gastritis. *Lancet* I: 1273–1275
6 Marshall BJ (1983) Unidentified curved bacili on gastric epithelium in active chronic gastritis. *Lancet* I: 1273–1275
7 Rauws EAJ, Tytgat GNJ (1990) Cure of duodenal ulcer associated with eradication of *Helicobacter pylori. Lancet* 335: 1233–1235
8 Malfertheiner P, Bode G (1993) *Helicobacter pylori* and the pathogenesis of duodenal ulcer disease. *Europ J Gastroenterol Hepatol* 5 (Suppl): 51–58
9 Tytgat GNJ, Lee A, Graham DJ, Dixon MF, Rokkas T (1993b) The role of infectious agents in peptic ulcer disease. *Gastroenterol Int* 6: 76–89
10 Sipponen P (1992) Natural history of gastritis and its relationship to peptic ulcer disease. *Digestion* 51 (Suppl 1): 70–75
11 Schubert TT, Bologna SD, Nensey Y et al. (1993) Ulcer risk factors: interactions between *Helicobacter pylori* infection, nonsteroidal use, and age. *Am J Med* 94: 413–418
12 Neri M, Susi D, Bovani I, Laerza F, Mezzeti A, Cuccurullo F (1994) Bacterial mucosal infiltration in *Helicobacter pylori*-associated gastritis: histological and clinical consequences. *Am J Gastroenterolog* 89: 1801–1805
13 Khulusi S, Mendall MA, Patel P, Levy J, Northfield TC (1994) Is there a quantifiable difference in *H. pylori* infection density between DU and non-DU patients? (Abstract) *Gastroenterology* 106: A106

14 Bayerdörffer E, Miehlke S, Lehn N, Manes GA, Sommer A, Höchter W, Hatz R, Stolte M (1993) Chronic type B gastritis as an important denominator of peptic ulcer healing. *Eur J Gastroenterol Hepatol* 5 (Suppl 3)
15 Graham DY (1994) *Helicobacter pylori*: consensus reached: peptic ulcer is on the way to becoming an historic disease. *Am J Gastroenterol* 89: 1137–1139
16 Stolte M, Bethke B (1990) Elimination of *H. pylori* under treatment with omeprazole. *Gastroenterology* 28: 271
17 Logan RPH, Walker MM, Misiewicz JJ et al (1995) Changes in the intragastric distribution of *Helicobacter pylori* during treatment with omeprazole. *Gut* 36: 12
18 Levi S, Beardshall K, Haddad G, Playford R, Gosh P, Calam J (1989) *Campylobacter pylori* and duodenal ulcers: the gastrin link. *Lancet* 1: 1167–1168
19 McColl KEL, El-Omar E (1994) Effect of *H. pylori* infection on gastrin and gastric acid secretion. In: RH Hunt, GNJ Tytgat (eds): *Helicobacter pylori*. Basic Mechanisms to Clinical Cure. Kluwer, Dordrecht, 245
20 Moss SF, Calam J (1993) Acid secretion and sensitivity to gastrin in patients with duodenal ulcer: effect of eradication of *Helicobacter pylori*. *Gut* 34: 888
21 Moss SF, Legon S, Bishop AE et al (1992) Effect of *Helicobacter pylori* on gastric somatostatin in duodenal ulcer disease. *Lancet* 340: 930
22 Odum I, Petersen HD, Andersen IB, Hansen BF, Rehfeld JF (1994) Gastrin and somatostatin in *Helicobacter pylori* infected antral mucosa. *Gut* 35: 615–618
23 Olbe L, Hamlet A, Dalenbäck J, Fändriks L (1996) A mechanism by which *Helicobacter pylori* infection of the antrum contributes to the development of duodenal ulcer. *Gastroenterology* 110: 1386–1394
24 Hamlet A, Olbe L (1996) The influence of *Helicobacter pylori* infection on postprandial duodenal acid load and duodenal bulb pH in humans. *Gastroenterology* 111: 391–400
25 McColl KEL, Fullarton GM, Chittajallu R, El Nujumi AM, Macdonald AMI, Dahill SW, Hilditch TE (1991) Plasma gastrin, daytime intragastric pH and nocturnal acid output before and at 1 and 7 months after eradication of *Helicobacter pylori* in duodenal ulcer patients. *Scand J Gastroenterol* 26: 339–346
26 El-Omar E, Penman I, Dorrian CA, Ardill JES, McColl KEL (1993) Eradicating *Helicobacter pylori* infection lowers gastrin mediated acid secretion by two thirds in patients with duodenal ulcer. *Gut* 34: 1060–1065
27 Kreiss C, Blum AL, Malfertheiner P (1995) Peptic ulcer pathogenesis. *Curr Opin Gastroenterol* 11 (Suppl 1): 25–31
28 Noah LA, Rolf TM, Bosma NB et al (1993) Gastric metaplasia and *Helicobacter pylori* infection. *Gut* 34: 1510
29 Carrick J, Lee A, Hazell S, Ralston M, Daskalopoulos G (1989) *Campylobacter pylori*, duodenal ulcer and gastric metaplasia: possible role of functional heterotopic tissue in ulcerogenesis. *Gut* 30: 790–797
30 Bode G, Malfertheiner P, Mader U, Stanescu A, Ditschuneit H (1991) Fine structure of active and healed duodenal ulcer. *Am J Gastroenterol* 86: 179–186
31 Malfertheiner P, Halter F (1994) Peptic ulcer pathogenesis. Year in *Helicobacter pylori*. *Curr Opin Gastroen* 30–34
32 Khulusi S, Badve S, Patel P, Lloyd R, Marrero JM, Finlayson C, Mendall M, A., Northfield TC (1996) Pathogenesis of gastric metaplasia of the human duodenum: role of *Helicobacter pylori*, gastric acid and ulceration. *Gastroenterology* 110: 452–458
33 Blaser MJ (1992) Hypothesis on the pathogenesis and natural history of *Helicobacter pylori*-induced inflammation. *Gastroenterology* 102: 720–727
34 Crabtree JE, Peichl P, Wyatt JL, Stachl U, Lindley IJ (1993) Gastric interleukin-8 and IgA IL-8 autoantibodies in *Helicobacter pylori* infection. *Scand J Immunol* 37: 65–70
35 Crowe SE, Alvarez L, Dytoc H, Hunt RH, Muller M, Sherman P et al (1995) Expression of interleukin 8 and CD54 by human gastric epithelium after *Helicobacter pylori* infection *in vitro*. *Gastroenterology* 108: 65–74
36 Dunn BE (1993) Pathogenic mechanisms of *Helicobacter pylori*. *Gastroenterology Clin North Am* 22: 43–57
37 Karttunen R (1991) Blood lymphocyte proliferation, cytokine secretion and appearance to T cells with activation surface markers in cultures with *Helicobacter pylori*. *Clin Exp Immunol* 83: 396–400

38 Hatz R, Bayerdörffer E, Lehn N, Enders G (1994) Immune response in *Helicobacter pylori* infection: implications for treatment of gastroduodenal disease. *Clin Immunother* 2: 295–306
39 Rosam AC, Wallace JL, Whittle BJR (1986) Potent ulcerogenic actions of platelet-activating factor on the stomach. *Nature* 319: 54–56
40 Smoot DT, Mobley HLT, Chippendale GR, Lewinson JF, Resau JH (1990) *Helicobacter pylori* urease activity is toxic to human gastric epithelial cells. *Infect Immun* 58: 1992–1994
41 Goggin PM, Marrero JM, Spychal RT, Jackson PA, Corbishley CM, Northfield TC (1992) Surface hydrophobicity of gastric mucosa in *Helicobacter pylori* infection: effect of clearance and eradication. *Gasterolology* 103: 1486–1490
42 Mauch F, Bode G, Ditschuneit H, Malfertheiner P (1993) Demonstration of a phospholipidrich zone in the human gastric epithelium damaged by *Helicobacter pylori*: *Gastroenterology* 105: 1698–1704
43 Hills BA (1993) Gastric mucosal barrier: evidence for *Helicobacter pylori* in gastric surfactant and deriving protection from it. *Gut* 38: 2071–2080
44 Figura N, Guglielmetti A, Rossolino A, Barberi A, Cusi G, Musmanno RA et al (1989) Cytotoxin production by *Campylobacter pylori* strains isolated from patients with peptic ulcers and from patients with chronic gastritis only. *J Clin Microbiol* 27: 225–226
45 Covacci A, Censini S, Bugnoli M, Petracca R, Burroni D, Macchina G et al (1993) Molecular characterisation of the 128-kDa immunodominant antigen of *Helicobacter pylori* associated with cytotoxicity and duodenal ulcer. *Proc Natl Acad Sci USA* 90: 5791–5795
46 Cover TL, Blaser MJ (1992) Purification and characterization of the vacuolating toxin from *Helicobacter pylori*. *J Biol Chem* 267: 10570–10575
47 Tummuru MK, Sharma SA, Blaser MJ (1995) *Helicobacter pylori* cag C, a homolog of the Bordetella pertussis toxin secretion protein, is required for induction of IL-8 in gastric epithelial cells. *Gastroenterology* A246
48 Peek RM, Miller GG, Tham KT, Perez-Perez GI, Zhao XM, Atherton JC et al (1995) Heightened cytokine expression and inflammatory response *in vivo* to cag A^+ *Helicobacter pylori* strains. *Lab Invest* 73: 760–770
49 Atherton JC (1997) The clinical relevance of strain types of *Helicobacter pylori*. *Gut* 40: 701–703
50 Blaser MJ (1995) Intrastrain differences in *Helicobacter pylori*: a key question in mucosal damage. *Ann Med* 27: 559–563
51 Censini S, Lange C, Xiang Z, Crabtree JE, Ghiara P, Borodovsky M, Rappuoli R, Covacci A (1996) cag a pathogenicity island of *Helicobacter pylori*, encodes type I-specific and disease-associated virulence factors. *Proc Natl Acad Sci USA* 93: 14648–14653
52 Van Doorn L-J, Figueiredo C, Sanna R, Plaisier A, Schneeberger P, De Boer W, Quint W (1998) Clinical relevance of the cag A, vac A and ice A status of *Helicobacter pylori*. *Gastroenterology* 115: 58–66
53 Malaty HM, Engstrand M, Pedersen NL, Graham DY (1994) *Helicobacter pylori* infection: genetic and environmental influences. *Ann Intern Med* 120: 982–986
54 Cowan WK (1973) Genetics of duodenal and gastric ulcer. *Clin Gastroenterol* 2: 539–546
55 Borén T, Falk P, Roth KA, Larson G, Normark S (1993) Attachment of *Helicobacter pylori* to human gastric epithelium mediated by blood group antigens. *Science* 262: 1892–1895
56 Azuma T, Konishi J, Tanaka Y, Hirai M, Ito S, Kato T, Kohli Y (1994) Contribution of HLA-DQA gene to host's response against *Helicobacter pylori*. *Lancet* 343: 542–543
57 Forbes GM, Glaser ME, Cullen DJE, Warren JR, Christiansen KJ, Marshall BJ et al (1994) Duodenal ulcer treated with *Helicobacter pylori* eradication: seven year follow-up. *Lancet* 343: 258–260
58 Huang JQ, Wilkinson JM, Hunt R H (1997) Antimicrobials accelerate healing of duodenal ulcer (DU) when given with proton pump inhibitors (PPI) or H_2-receptor antagonists (H2RA): A meta-analysis. *Gut* 41: A93
59 Graham DY, Hepps KS, Ramirez FC et al (1993) Treatment of *Helicobacter pylori* reduces the rate of rebleeding in peptic ulcer disease. *Scand J Gastroenterol* 28: 939–942
60 Labenz J, Börsch G (1994) Role of *Helicobacter pylori* eradication in the prevention of peptic ulcer bleeding relapse. *Digestion* 55: 19–23
61 Rokkas T, Karameris A, Mavrogeorgis A et al (1995) Eradication of *Helicobacter pylori* reduces the possibility of rebleeding in peptic ulcer disease. *Gastrointest Endosc* 41: 1–4

62 Jaspersen D, Koerner T, Schorr W et al (1995) *Helicobacter pylori* eradication reduces the rate of rebleeding in ulcer haemorrhage. *Gastrointest Endosc* 41: 5–7
63 Santander C, Gravalos RG, Cedenillay AG, Cantero J, Pajares JM (1996) Antimicrobial therapy for *Helicobacter pylori* infection vs long-term maintenance antisecretion treatment in the prevention of recurrent haemorrhage from peptide ulcer: prospective nonrandomized trail of 125 patients. *Am J Gastroenterol* 91: 1549–1552
64 Riemann JF, Schilling D, Schauwecker P, Wehlen G, Dorlars D, Kohler B, Maier M (1997) Cure with omeprazole plus amoxicillin vs long-term ranitidine therapy in *Helicobacter pylori*-associated peptic ulcer bleeding. *Gastrointest Endosc* 46: 299–304
65 NIH Consensus Conference (1994) *Helicobacter pylori* in peptic ulcer disease. NIH Consensus Development Panel on *Helicobacter pylori* in Peptic Ulcer Disease. *JAMA* 272(1): 65–69
66 Malfertheiner P, Nilius M Bismuth preparations. In: CS Goodwin, BW Worsley (eds): *Helicobacter pylori*: biology and clinical practice. CRC Press, Boca Raton. 1993:351–364
67 Hackelsberger A, Malfertheiner P (1996) A risk-Benefit assessment of drugs used in the eradication of *Helicobacter pylori* infection. *Drug Safety* 15(1): 30–52
68 Rauws EAJ, Langenberg W, Houthoff H J et al (1988) *Campylobacter pyloridis* associated chronic active antral gastritis: a prospective study of its prevalence and the effects of antibacterial and antiulcer treatment. *Gastroenterology* 94: 33–40
69 Malfertheiner P (1993) Compliance, adverse events and antibiotic resistance in *Helicobacter pylori* treatment. *Scand J Gastroenterol* 28 (Suppl 196): 34–37
70 Bianchi Porro G, Parente F, Lazzaroni M (1993) Short and long term outcome of *Helicobacter pylori* positive resistant duodenal ulcers treated with colloidal bismuth subcitrate plus antibiotics or sucralfate alone. *Gut* 34: 466–469
71 Axon ATR (1992) *Helicobacter pylori* therapy: effect on peptic ulcer disease. *J Gastroenterol Hepatol* 6: 131–137
72 Chiba N, Rao BV, Rademaker JW, Hunt RH (1992) Meta-analysis of the efficacy of antibiotic therapy in eradicating. *Helicobacter pylori*. *Am J Gastroenterol* 87: 1716–1727
73 Graham DY, Lew GM, Malaty HM et al (1992) Factors influencing the eradication of *Helicobacter pylori* with triple therapy. *Gastroenterology* 102: 493–496
74 Burget DW, Chiverton SG, Hunt RH (1990) Is there an optimal degree of acid suppresion for healing of duodenal ulcers? A model of the relationship between ulcer healing and acid suppression. *Gastroenterology* 99: 345–351
75 Jones DB, Howden CW, Burget DW et al (1987) Acid suppression in duodenal ulcer: a meta-analysis to define optimal dosing with antisecretory drugs. *Gut* 28: 1120–1127
76 Howden CW, Burget DW, Hunt RH (1994) Appropriate acid suppression for optimal healing of duodenal ulcer and gastro-oesophageal reflux disease. *Scand J Gastroenterol* 29(Suppl 201): 79–82
77 Nakao M, Malfertheiner P (1998) Growth inhibitory and bactericidal activities of lansoprazole compared with those of omeprazole and pantoprazole against *Helicobacter pylori*. *Helicobacter* 3(1): 21–27
78 Suerbaum S, Leying H, Klemm K et al (1991) Antibacterial activity of pantoprazole and omeprazole against *Helicobacter pylori*. *Eur J Clin Microbiol Infect Dis* 10: 92–93
79 Iwahi T, Satoh H, Nakao M et al (1991) Lansoprazole, a novel benzimidazole proton pump inhibitor and its related compounds have selective activity against *Helicobacter pylori*. *Antimicrob Agents Chemother* 35: 490–496
80 Unge P, Gad A, Gnarpe H et al (1989) Does omeprazole improve antimicrobial therapy directed towards gastric *Campylobacter pylori* in patients with antral gastritis? A pilot study. *Scand J Gastroenterol* 24(Suppl 167): 49–54
81 Hui WM, Lam SK, Ho J et al (1991) Effect of omeprazole on duodenal ulcer-associated antral gastritis and *Helicobacter pylori*. *Dig Dis Sci* 36: 577–582
82 Rauws EA, Langenberg W, Bosma A et al (1991) Lack of eradication of *Helicobacter pylori* after omeprazole (letter). *Lancet* 337: 1093
83 Weil J, Bell GD, Powell K et al (1991) Omeprazole and *Helicobacter pylori:* temporary suppression rather than true eradication. *Aliment Pharmacol Ther* 5: 309–313
84 Louw JA, Zak J, Jaskiewicz K et al (1992) Omeprazole may clear but not eradicate *H. pylori*. *Eur J Gastroenterol Hepatol* 4: 481–485
85 Sherman P, Shames B, Loo V et al (1992) Omeprazole therapy for *Helicobacter pylori* infection. *Scand J Gastroenterol* 27: 1018–1022

86 Bugnoli M, Bayeli PF, Rappuoli R et al (1993) Inhibition of *Helicobacter pylori* urease by omeprazole. *Eur J Gastroenterol Hepatol* 5: 683–685
87 Nagata K, Satoh H, Iwahi T et al (1993) Potent inhibitory action of gastric pump inhibitor lansoprazole against urease activity of *Helicobacter pylori*: unique action selective for *H. pylori* cells. *Antimicrob Agents Chemother* 37: 769–774
88 Axon ATR (1994) The role of acid inhibition in the treatment of *Helicobacter pylori* infection. *Scand J Gastroenterol* 29 (Supp 201): 16–23
89 McGowan CC, Cover TL, Blaser MJ (1994) The proton pump inhibitor omeprazole inhibits acid survival of *Helicobacter pylori* by a urease-independent mechanism. *Gastroenterology* 107: 1573–1578
90 Ge Z, Hiratsuka K, Taylor DE (1995) Nucleotide sequence and mutational analysis indicate that two *Helicobacter pylori* genes encode a P-type ATPase and a cation binding protein associated with copper transport. *Mol Microbiol* 15: 97–106
91 Wandall JH (1992) Effects of omeprazole on neutrophil chemotaxis, super oxide production, degranulation and translocation of cytochrome b-245. *Gut* 33: 617–621
92 Gustavson LF, Kaiser JF, Mukherjee DX et al (1994) Evaluation of pharmakokinetic drug interactions between clarithromycin and omeprazole (abstract). *Am J Gastroenterol* 89: 1373
93 Paulsen O, Höglund P, Walder M (1989) No effect of omeprazole-inducted hypoacidity on the bioavailability of amoxicillin or bacampicillin. *Scand J Infect Dis* 21: 219–223
94 Pommerien W, Braun M, Idström JP et al (1995) No interaction between omeprazole and amoxicillin during combination therapy in *Helicobacter pylori* positive healthy subjects (abstract). *Gastroenterology* 108: A194
95 Bayerdörffer E, Mannes GA, Sommer A et al (1992) High dose omeprazole treatment combined with amoxicillin eradicates *Helicobacer pylori. Eur J Gastroenterol Hepatol* 4: 697–702
96 Bayerdörffer E, Mannes GA, Sommer A et al (1993) Long-term follow-up after eradication of *Helicobacter pylori* with a combination of omeprazole and amoxicillin. *Scand J Gastroenterol* 28 (Suppl 169): 19–25
97 Bayerdörffer E, Miehlke S, Mannes GA et al (1995) Double-blind trial of omeprazole and amoxicillin to cure *Helicobacter pylori* infection in patients with duodenal ulcers. *Gastroenterology* 108: 1412–1417
98 Labenz J, Gyene E, Rühl GH et al (1993) Omeprazole plus amoxicillin: efficacy of various treatment regimes to eradicate *Helicobacter pylori. Am J Gastroenterol* 88: 491–495
99 Labenz J, Gyenes E, Rühl GH et al (1993) Amoxicillin plus omeprazole vs triple therapy for eradication of *Helicobacter pylori* in duodenal ulcer disease: a prospective, randomized, and controlled study. *Gut* 34: 1167–1170
100 Labenz J, Rühl GH, Bertrams J et al (1994) Medium and high dose omeprazole plus amoxicillin for eradication of *Helicobacter pylori* in duodenal ulcer disease. *Dig Dis Sci* 39: 1483–1487
101 Mannes GA, Bayerdörffer E, Hele C et al (1993) An increasing dose of omeprazole combined with amoxicillin increases the eradication rate of *Helicobacter pylori* (abstract). *Gastroenterology* 104 (Suppl): A140
102 Goh KL, Peh SC, Parasakthi N et al (1994) Omeprazole 40 mg combined with amoxicillin alone or with amoxicillin and metronidazole in the eradication of *Helicobacter pylori. Am J Gastroenterol* 89: 1789–1792
103 Collins R, Beattie S, O'Morain C (1993) High dose omeprazole plus amoxicillin in the treatment of acute duodenal ulcer. *Aliment Pharmacol Ther* 7: 313–315
104 McCarthy CJ, Collins R, Beattie S, Hamilton H, O'Morain C (1993) Short report: treatment of *Helicobacter pylori*-associated duodenal ulcer with omeprazole plus antibiotics. *Aliment Pharmacol Ther* 7: 463–466
105 Bell G, Powell K, Weil J et al (1991) Experience with omeprazole in combination with either amoxycillin or colloidal bismuth subcitrate in patients with metronidazole-resistant *Helicobacter pylori. Eur J Gastroenterol Hepatol* 3: 923–926
106 Miehlke S, Mannes GA, Lehn N, Hele C, Stolte M, Bayerdörffer E (1997) An increasing dose of omeprazole combined with amoxycillin cures *Helicobacter pylori* infection more effectively. *Aliment Pharmacol Ther* 11: 323–329

107 Pommerien W, Schultze V, Lembcke B et al (1995) Dose response of twice daily dosing of omeprazole combined with amoxicillin on *H. pylori* eradication in duodenal ulcer patients (abstract). *Gastroenterology* 108: A193
108 Labenz J, Leverkus F, Börsch G (1994) Omeprazole plus amoxicillin for cure of *Helicobacter pylori* infection: factors influencing the treatment success. *Scand J Gastroenterol* 29: 1070–1075
109 Graham DY, Operkun AR, Klein PD (1993) Clarithromycin for the eradication of *Helicobacter pylori*. *J Clin Gastroenterol* 16: 292–294
110 Peterson WL, Graham DY, Marshall B et al (1993) Clarithromycin as monotherapy for eradication of *Helicobacter pylori*: a randomized, double-blind trial. *Am J Gastroenterol* 88: 1860–1864
111 Logan RP, Gummett PA, Schaufelberger HD et al (1994) Eradication of *Helicobacter pylori* with clarithromycin and omeprazole. *Gut* 35: 323–326
112 O'Morain C, Dettmer A, Rambow A et al (1994) and the Clarithromycin European *H. pylori* Study Group: Dual therapy with clarithromycin and omeprazole for the treatment of active duodenal ulcers (abstract). *Am J Gastroenterol* 89: A1384
113 Labenz J, Stolte M, Domian C et al (1995) High dose omeprazole plus amoxicillin or clarithromycin cures *Helicobacter pylori* infection in duodenal ulcer disease. *Digestion* 56: 14–20
114 Harris AV, Gummett PA, Logan RP et al (1995) Eradication of *Helicobacter pylori* with lansoprazole and clarithromycin. *Aliment Pharmacol Ther* 9: 201–204
115 Cayla R, Zerbib F, de Mascarel A et al (1994) High dose of lansoprazole in combination with amoxycillin and clarithromycin twice daily for *H. pylori* eradication: results of a pilot study (abstract). *Am J Gastroenterol* 94: A1367
116 Bazzoli F, Zagari RM, Fossi S et al (1994) Short-term low-dose triple therapy for the eradication of *Helicobacter pylori*. *Eur J Gastroenterol Hepatol* 6: 773–777
117 Jaup BH, Norrby A (1995) Low-dose, short term triple therapy for cure of *Helicobacter pylori* infection and healing of peptic ulcers. *Am J Gasteroenterol* 90: 943–945
118 Labenz J, Stolte M, Rühl GH et al (1994) One week, low-dose triple therapy for the cure of *Helicobacter pylori* infection. *Eur J Gastroenterol Hepatol* 7: 9–11
119 Moayyedi P, Sahay P, Tompkins DS et al (1995) Efficacy and optimum dose of omeprazole in a new 1-week-triple therapy regimen to eradicate *Helicobacter pylori*. *Eur J Gastroenterol Hepatol* 7: 835–840
120 Adamek RJ, Szymanski C, Pfaffenbach B, et al (1995) Short term triple therapy with pantoprazole, clarithromycin and metronidazole for the healing of *Helicobacter pylori* infection. *Dtsch Med Wochenschr* 120: 358–360
121 Misiewicz JJ, Harris AW, Bardhan KD, Levi S, O'Morain C, Cooper BT, Kerr GD, Dixon MF, Langworthy H, Piper D et al (1997) One week triple therapy for *Helicobacter pylori*: a multicentre comparative study. *Gut* 41: 735–739
122 Lind T, Veldhuyzen van Zanten S, Unge P et al (1996) Eradication of *Helicobacter pylori* using one-week triple therapies combining omeprazole with two antimicrobials: the MACH 1 study. *Helicobacter* 1: 138–144
123 Lind T, Megraud F, Unge P, Bayerdörffer E, O'Morain C, Spiller R, Veldhuyzen van Zanten S, Dev Bardhan K, Hellblom M, Wrangstadh M et al (1997) The MACH 2 study – the role of omeprazole in eradication of *Helicobacter pylori* with one-week triple therapies – a randomised double-blind study; *submitted*
124 Megraud F (1994) *H. pylori* resistance to antibiotics. In: RH Hunt, GNJ Tytgat, *Helicobacter pylori* – basic mechanisms to clinical cure. Kluwer, Dordrecht, 570–583
125 Bayerdörffer E (1997) Is OAM giving satisfactory results? Astra Symposium Prague Proceedings; *in press*
126 De Boer W, Tytgat GNJ (1995) Only four days of quadruple therapy can effectively cure *Helicobacter pylori* infection. *Aliment Pharmacol Ther* 9: 633–638
127 The European *Helicobacter pylori* study group Current European concepts in the management of *Helicobacter pylori* infection. The Maastricht Consensus Report. *Gut* 41 (1): 8–13

Proton Pump Inhibitors
ed. by L. Olbe

Non-steroidal anti-inflammatory drug-associated ulcers

C.J. Hawkey

Department of Medicine, Division of Gastroenterology, University Hospital, Queen's Medical Centre, Nottingham NG7 2UH, UK

Introduction

The gastrointestinal side effects of nonsteroidal anti-inflammatory drugs, particularly with the development of ulcer bleeding and perforation, probably represent the most important iatrogenic problem in the developed world. Acute mucosal injury is almost universal after consumption of single doses of aspirin [1] and, although acute injury is a little slower to develop with nonaspirin non-steroidal anti-inflammatory drugs (NSAIDs), the prevalence of ulcers in patients taking NSAIDs or anti-inflammatory doses of aspirin has been shown to be around 20% [2]. In many cases these ulcers remain silent and cause no clinical harm, but a minority result in the ulcer complications of bleeding and perforation at a rate somewhere between 1 in 50 and 1 in 100 patient years [3]. As a result, it is likely that at least 1200 patients per annum in the United Kingdom die as a result of NSAID-associated ulcer complications [4]. Whilst it is important to stress that NSAIDs, particularly aspirin, have additional benefits in terms of protection against cardiovascular disease [5] and cancer [6] which almost certainly more than outweigh these risks, any strategy which could reduce NSAID-associated ulcer disease and complications is welcome.

Pathogenesis of NSAID-associated ulcer disease

Inhibition of prostaglandin synthesis is the shared property which defines nonsteroidal anti-inflammatory drugs. It leads to impairment of prostaglandin-dependent mucosal defence mechanisms, including gastric mucosal blood flow, and mucus and bicarbonate secretion [7]. As a consequence, superficial breaches of the epithelial barrier, which can be prevented by exogenous prostaglandins, develop [8].

Studies in laboratory animals and humans suggest that there is a second component of injury in which acid peptic attack deepens erosions resulting from compromised mucosal defence with development of deep erosions and ulcers [9, 10]. These studies also suggest that relatively powerful acid suppression, designed to achieve intragastric pH greater than 4 (at which level peptic activity diminishes) is necessary to prevent this phase of NSAID-associated gastric injury.

Rationale for prevention of gastroduodenal injury

Such considerations raise the possibility that NSAID-associated gastroduodenal injury can be prevented in humans in two main ways – by the use of prostaglandins or by profound acid suppression. Natural prostaglandins are too unstable *in vivo* to be useful agents, but the stable prostaglandin E1 analogue misoprostol has been developed and shown to prevent acute injury, endoscopic ulcers and hospitalisation with ulcer complications associated with NSAID use [11].

Acid suppression has many potential benefits. Aspirin and many of the nonaspirin NSAIDs are weak acids, so that at high pH a passive gastric absorption and trapping in the mucosa is reduced [12]. Furthermore, some NSAIDs break the gastric mucosal barrier, causing back diffusion and reduced intramucosal pH [13]. Acid is directly injurious to the mucosa and enhances the activity of pepsin [14].

In one pivotal study, Yeomans and his colleagues studied pylorus-ligated male Wistar rats. Indomethacin was given intraduodenally to avoid topical effects [9]. Endogenous gastric acid secretion was abolished by parental omeprazole. Exogenous acid was used to achieve a range of intragastric pHs. This study showed that extensive erosive changes developed in the presence of indomethacin when the pH was held below 4, but this was largely abolished once the intragastric pH of 4 was achieved.

Possible cytoprotective effects of omeprazole

Much less clear cut than its effects on acid are data suggesting that omeprazole may have acid-independent mucosally protective properties. In an early study Konturek and his colleagues presented data showing that omeprazole at a supposedly non-anti-secretory dose prevented aspirin- and ethanol-induced gastric lesions [15]. Even if acid had been suppressed, this is evidence in favour of a non-acid-mediated protective effect, since gastric acid suppression normally has no effect on on ethanol-induced gastric lesions. Similarly, Okabe and collegues reported that omeprazole 10 and 30 mg/kg given orally achieved relatively short-lived dose-dependent inhibition of hydrochloric acid/ethanol-induced lesions [16]. Since acid suppression alone does not protect against ethanol, they concluded a direct cytoprotective effect. Romano and colleagues took further the possibility that omeprazole was cytoprotective by investigating its ability to protect against sodium taurocholate-induced chromium-51 release from gastric epithelial cell monolayers maintained in culture [17]. This occurred without a change in pH, prostaglandin synthesis or the concentration of sulphasydrol compounds. Indomethacin did not reverse the protective effects of omeprazole.

There are several problems in interpreting these studies. First, other studies have failed to show a protective effect of omeprazole [18]. Second, not all studies have shown clearly that there was no effect on acid suppression. Third, a clearly defined mechanism for the proposed cytoprotective effects of omeprazole has not emerged. However, there have been some mechanistic studies of possible relevance. In humans, omeprazole and misoprostol but not cimitidine increased gastric mucosal blood flow and protected the mucosa against ethanol in a dose-dependent fashion [19]. Omeprazole has also been reported to enhance gastric mucus glycoprotein biosynthesis [20] though an underlying mechanism for this had not emerged, and other studies have shown a (possibly temporary and secondary) reduction in gastric mucus [21–27].

Synopsis

It seems most plausible that the ability of omeprazole to protect the gastroduodenal mucosa arises principally because of its effects on acid secretion. Its advantages in short- and long-term studies over H2 antagonists in protecting against NSAIDs can probably be explained on the basis of its greater potency of acid suppression. However, a number of other studies exist which are difficult to explain on this basis entirely. These data raise the possibility that omeprazole may have additional cytoprotective properties as well as its ability to inhibit acid secretion, which may be important in protecting the mucosa against nonsteroidal anti-inflammatory drugs, but there are too many contradiction in the data to conclude that this is definitely so.

Establishing the critical level of acid suppression

Short-term human studies

Daneshmend and colleagues studied 16 young healthy volunteers [10]. They received aspirin 900 mg bid with placebo, omeprazole 20 mg daily or omeprazole 40 mg bid for 7 days. At the end of this time subjects were intubated, and microscopic blood loss as an index of gastric mucosal injury was measured. On omeprazole 20 mg daily the intragastric pH rose from a range of 2.1 to 2.6 to 2.7 to 6.5, and 12 subjects had reductions in aspirin associated-microbleeding to levels similar to those seen with placebo (Fig. 1). On the higher dose of omeprazole the range of intragastric pH

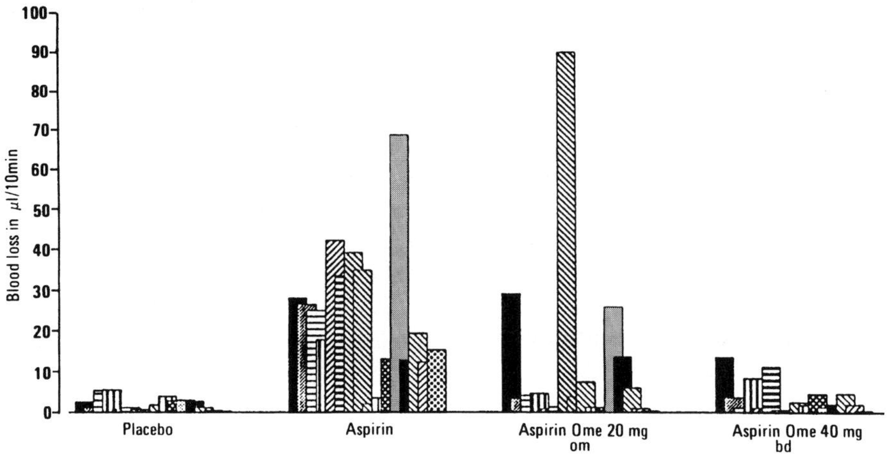

Figure 1. Individual rates of gastric mucosal blood loss in 16 normal adults on placebo, aspirin 900 mg mg bid, aspirin 900 mg bid plus omeprazole 20 mg each morning, and aspirin 900 mg bid plus omeprazole 40 mg bid. Reprinted by kind permission of the editor of *Gut*, 1990; 31: 514–517.

achieved was 5.6–6.9, and all subjects had microbleeding levels close to those seen in the absence of aspirin (Fig. 1).

Endoscopic studies also supported these data [25–27]. In one study, 15 healty subjects received either omeprazole 60 mg om or placebo for 4 days. One hour after the last intake of the drug, 1 g of aspirin was taken and endoscopy was carried out 2 h later. Fourteen out of 15 subjects showed more than one erosion if aspirin was taken with placebo, whilst none on omeprazole did ($p < 0.0001$).

In another study, omeprazole 40 mg daily reduced gastric mucosal injury associated with longer-term dosing of aspirin 650 mg qds for 2 weeks. In this study only 1 out of 20 subjects taking placebo had ≤5 erosions at the end of the study compared with 11 out of 20 on omeprazole ($p < 0.01$) [26].

In a third endoscopic study, 36 healthy volunteers were dosed with the lower doses of aspirin associated with cardiovascular protection (300 mg daily) for 14 days. In subjects receiving placebo the median injury score rose from 1 (baseline) to 10 at the end of 14 days. Subjects receiving 20 mg of omeprazole daily had a reduction in their median score to 1, that is comparable to baseline.

Human clinical studies

These considerations led to a clinical programme of research comparing omeprazole with placebo, ranitidine and misoprostol for prophylaxis, healing and maintenance of NSAID-associated ulcers and multiple erosions.

These were preceded by a trial of high-dose famotidine, which in many ways can be regarded as a surrogate for the effects of proton pump inhibitors.

Famotidine

The hypothesis that greater than normal levels of acid suppression were required to protect against NSAID-associated ulceration was initially tested in a study of famotidine at 2 doses, the normal clinical dose of 20 mg bid and a higher dose of 40 mg bid [28, 29]. These studies showed two important points. First, patients with an ulcer at initial endoscopy had a higher relapse rate than those without. Second, in both groups, famotidine 40 mg bid was effective in preventing both gastric and duodenal ulcers. Famotidine 20 mg bid was only effective at preventing duodenal ulcers.

Omeprazole vs misoprostol: The OMNIUM study [30]

Nine hundred and thirty-five NSAID users presenting with gastric or duodenal ulcer and/or ≥ 10 erosions in the stomach or in the duodenum were randomised to receive omeprazole 20 or 40 mg once daily in the morning or misoprostol 200 µg qds. They were treated for 4 or 8 weeks until there was no ulcer and fewer than five erosions at each site and no more than mild dyspeptic symptoms. Patients achieving this treatment success were re-randomised to maintenance treatment with omeprazole 20 mg, misoprostol 200 µg bid or placebo for up to 6 months. During this maintenance phase

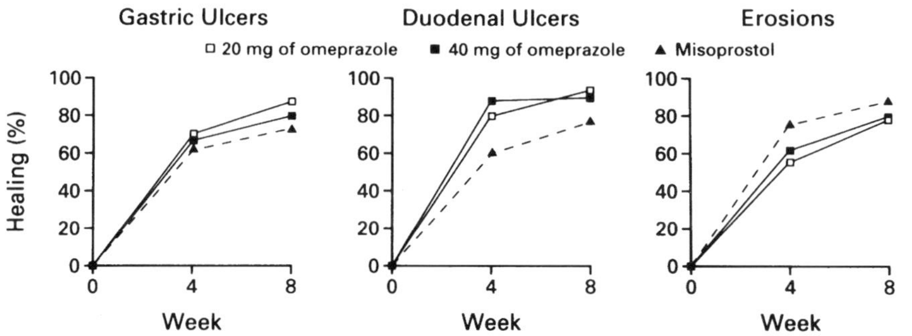

No. of Patients Healed/Total No.

20 mg of omeprazole	82/117	102/117	47/59	55/59	65/118	91/118
40 mg of omeprazole	88/132	105/132	57/65	58/65	67/109	86/109
Misoprostol	77/125	91/125	36/60	46/60	73/97	84/97

Figure 2. Cumulative rates of healing of gastric ulcers, duodenal ulcers and erosions at 4 and 8 weeks during treatment with 20 mg of omeprazole daily, 40 mg of omeprazole daily or 200 µg of misoprostol four times daily. Reprinted by kind permission of the editor of the *New England Journal of Medicine,* 1998; 338(11): 727–734.

they were endoscoped at 1, 3 and 6 months or when clinical need dictated. During both the healing and maintenance phase of the study, quality of life was assessed with the Nottingham Health Profile, the Psychological General Well-being Index, the Gastrointestinal Symptom Rating Scale and the Symptoms Related to Arthritis Scale.

Over 8 weeks duodenal ulcer healing was higher with omeprazole 20 and 40 mg than with misoprostol 200 µg qds (Fig. 2). Gastric ulcer healing was significantly higher with omeprazole 20 mg (but not 40 mg) compared with misoprostol. By contrast, misoprostol achieved faster healing in patients with multiple erosions in the stomach or duodenum only (Fig. 2). Dyspepsia and reflux symptoms improved significantly faster on omeprazole than misoprostol. Scores for abdominal pain, reflux and diarrhoea were better on omeprazole than misoprostol, as was the overall score for the gastrointestinal rating scale. The other quality-of-life scores showed no overall differences between the drugs.

During the maintenance phase the estimated proportion of patients remaining in remission by 6 months was 61% for patients taking omeprazole 20 mg daily (Fig. 3). This was significantly higher than with misoprostol 200 µg twice daily (48%, $p = 0.001$) or placebo (27%, $p < 0.001$). This was attributable to a smaller number of patients relapsing with duodenal ulcer on omeprazole (3% vs 10% misoprostol, 12% placebo). Fourteen percent of patients taking placebo, 7% taking misoprostol and 12% taking omeprazole had multiple erosions at relapse. Values for gastric ulcer were 32, 10 and 13%, respectively. The estimated proportion of patients remaining in remission on misoprostol was higher than on placebo. As in the healing phase, gastro intestinal symptom rating scale (GSRS) scores were better on omeprazole than misoprostol.

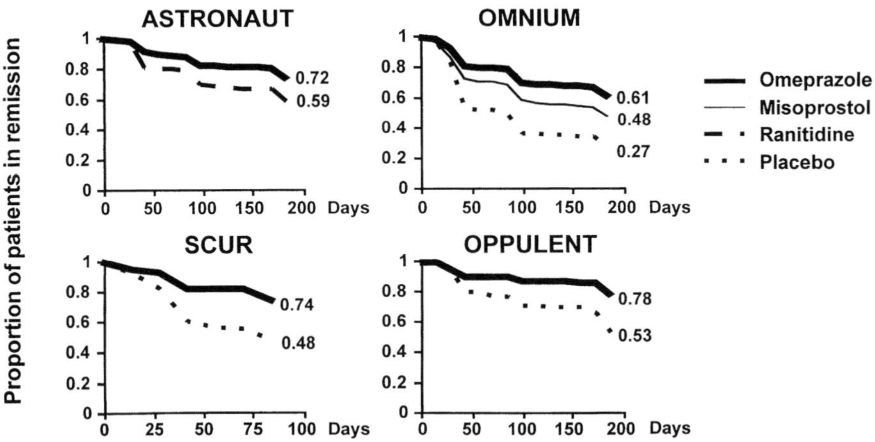

Figure 3. Maintenance of remission in four studies of omeprazole in NSAID users.

Omeprazole vs ranitidine: The ASTRONAUT study [31]
This study was conducted according to the same design as the OMNIUM study. Five hundred and forty-one patients on continuous NSAID therapy who presented with ulceration and/or more than 10 erosions (in either stomach or duodenum) were randomised to receive omeprazole 20 or 40 mg mane or ranitidine 150 mg bd as healing therapy over 4 or 8 weeks. The 432 patients achieving treatment success (as defined above) were re-randomised to receive omeprazole 20 mg or ranitidine 150 mg bd or 6 months.

Healing of gastric and duodenal ulcers and erosions was significantly higher with omeprazole than ranitidine (Fig. 4) (differences significant for omeprazole 20 mg vs ranitidine, for all endpoints and for omeprazole 40 mg vs ranitidine for gastric ulcer). Relief of overall upper gastrointestinal symptoms over the first 4 weeks was significantly greater in patients treated with omeprazole 20 mg than ranitidine.

During the maintenance phase significantly more patients remained in remission on omeprazole 20 mg than on ranitidine 150 mg bd (the estimated percentages in remission at the end of 6 months being 72% for omeprazole and 59% for ranitidine) (Fig. 3). Relapse with gastric ulcer, duodenal ulcer and erosions was more common with ranitidine treatment than with omeprazole.

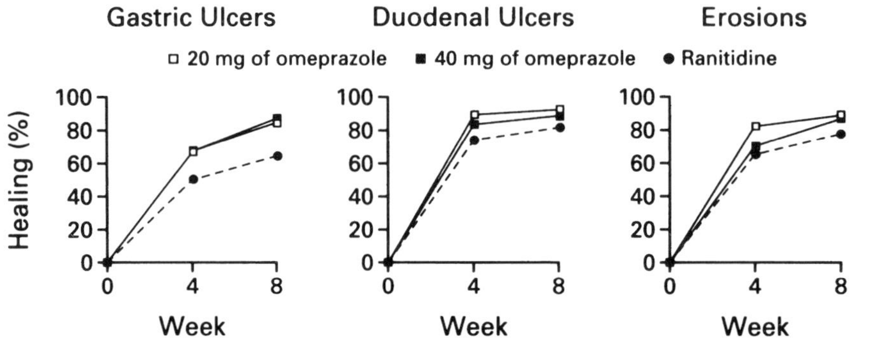

NO. OF PATIENTS HEALED/TOTAL

20 mg of omeprazole	47/70	59/70	32/36	33/36	50/61	54/61
40 mg of omeprazole	45/67	58/67	35/42	37/42	51/73	63/73
Ranitidine	35/70	45/70	31/42	34/42	37/57	44/57

Figure 4. Cumulative rates of healing of gastric ulcers, duodenal ulcers and erosions at 4 and 8 weeks during treatment with 20 mg of omeprazole daily, 40 mg of omeprazole daily or 150 mg of ranitidine given twice daily. Reproduced by kind permission of the editor of the *New England Journal of Medicine,* 1998; 338(11): 719–726.

Prognostic factors in the comparative studies

For both these studies *Helicobacter pylori* was a significant prognostic factor for healing and maintenance such that patients who were *H. pylori* positive healed faster and were more likely to remain in remission when treated with acid-suppressing drugs. The site and nature of the original lesion was a major determinant of the site and nature of the lesion at relapse. These data suggest that the value of maintenance treatment is in the prevention of ulceration of a pre-existing local mucosal defect, rather than the prevention of new lesions caused by *H. pylori*.

Primary and pragmatic prophylaxis studies

Because patients who do not present with ulcers may represent a different pathological process than those demonstrated to have ulcers, omeprazole was also assessed in two other studies. In one (the Scandinavian Ulcer Recurrence or SCUR study [32]) patients with a history of peptic ulcer or dyspepsia were randomised, without initial endoscopy, to receive omeprazole 20 mg once daily ($n = 86$) or placebo ($n = 91$) for up to 3 months. Omeprazole reduced the proportion of patients who experienced treatment failure from 50 to 24.7% (Fig. 3), much of this being due to a reduction in peptic ulcer from 16.7 to 4.7% and dyspeptic symptoms from 20.0 to 8.2%.

The OPPULENT study [33]
In this study, which was conducted in patients also participating in the OMNIUM study, patients whose initial endoscopy showed no peptic ulcer, 10 or fewer gastric erosions, 10 or fewer duodenal erosions and only mild dyspepsia were randomised to receive omeprazole 20 mg once daily ($n = 83$) or placebo ($n = 86$) and endoscoped routinely after 1, 3 and 6 months. In the study the estimated probability of remaining in remission for 6 months whilst receiving omeprazole was 0.78 compared with 0.53 placebo (Fig. 3), ($p = 0.004$). Much of this difference was due to a reduction in the number of patients developing peptic ulcer from 16.5% with placebo to 3.6% in patients receiving omeprazole.

Omeprazole-based H. pylori eradication regimes in the management of infected patients also taking NSAIDs
As a result of the OMNIUM and ASTRONAUT studies, the *Helicobacter* status of a large number of patients taking NSAIDs had been established. These and others entered a study in which patients with current or past known peptic ulcer and/or current moderate/severe dyspepsia who were *H. pylori* positive were randomised to receive omeprazole 20 mg bid, clarithromycin 500 mg bid, amoxycillin 1 g bid or omeprazole with placebo

antibiotics for 1 week [34]. They then received a further 3 or 7 weeks of omeprazole until their underlying lesions were healed. After this they were followed for up to 6 months, with endoscopy at 1, 3 and 6 monts, whilst receiving no maintenance treatment. In this study, which has yet to be reported in full, *H. pylori* eradication was found to make no difference to the overall outcome (estimated proportion remaining in remission 55 vs 51%. Interestingly, *H. pylori* eradication was associated with lower initial healing of peptic ulcers (particularly gastric ulcers).

Relationship between omeprazole, Helicobacter pylori and NSAIDs
In patients who were selected to enter the OMNIUM study who received placebo during the maintenance phase, *H. pylori* status had no influence. By contrast, in the SCUR study patients infected with *H. pylori* tended to do worse. Recently, *H. pylori* eradication (using a bismuth-based regime) has been reported to reduce the development of gastric ulcers over a period of 2 months in patients without a past history of peptic ulcer starting an NSAID (naproxen) for the first time. These apparently discrepant data can be harmonised if it is assumed that *H. pylori* is a harmful influence in patients who have not previously developed NSAID-associated mucosal injury. In such patients, who were by definition those who entered the OMNIUM study, local mucosal factors associated with prior ulceration appear to become preeminent determinants of relapse, and *H. pylori* status becomes irrelevant. Furthermore, in these patients, a positive *H. pylori* status is clearly associated with greater effectiveness for acid-suppressing drugs. Whether this is due to more profound depression of intragastric acidity in such patients or to additional levels of mucosal prostaglandins associated with *H. pylori* infection is not known.

References

1 Hawkey CJ, Hawthorne AB, Hudson N, Cole AT, Mahida YR, Daneshmend TK (1991) Separation of aspirin's impairment of haemostasis from mucosal injury in the human stomach. *Clin Sci* 81: 565–573
2 Hawkey CJ, Hudson N (1994) Mucosal injury caused by drugs, chemicals and stress. In: WS Haubrich, F Schaffner, JE Berk, WB Saunders (eds): *Bockus gastroenterology*, 5th edn. Saunders, vol 2, 656–699
3 Silverstein FE, Graham DY, Senior JR et al (1995) Misoprostol reduces serious gastrointestinal complications in patients with rheumatoid arthritis receiving non-steroidal anti-inflammatory drugs. A randomised, double blind, placebo controlled trial. *Ann Intern Med* 123: 241–249
4 Hawkey CJ (1990) Non-steroidal anti-inflammatory drugs and ulcers: facts and figures multiple, but do they add up? *Br Med J* 300: 278–284
5 Antiplatelet Trialists' Collaboration (1994) Collaborative overview of randomised trials of antiplatelet therapy-III: reduction of venous thrombosis and pulmonary embolism by antiplatelet prophylaxis among surgical and medical patients. *Brit Med J* 308: 235–246
6 Thun MJ, Namboodiri MM, Calle EE, Flanders WD, Heath CW Jr (1993) Aspirin use and risk of fatal cancer. *Cancer Res* 53: 1322–1327
7 Hawkey CJ, Rampton DS (1985) Prostaglandins and the gastrointestinal mucosa: are they important in its function, disease or treatment? *Gastroenterology* 89: 1161–1189

8 Whittle BJR (1981) Temporal relationship between cyclooxygenase inhibition as measured by prostacyclin biosynthesis and the gastrointestinal damage induced by indomethacin in the rat. *Gastroenterology* 80: 94–98
9 Elliott SL, Ferris RJ, Giraud AS, Cook GA, Skeljo MV, Yeomans ND (1996) Indomethacin damage to rat gastric mucosa is markedly dependent on luminal pH. *Clin Exper Pharmacol Physiol* 23: 432–434
10 Daneshmend TK, Stein AG, Bhaskar NK, Hawkey CJ (1990) Abolition by omeprazole of aspirin-induced gastric mucosal injury in man. *Gut* 31: 514–517
11 Walt RP (1992) Misoprostol for the treatment of peptic ulcer and anti-inflammatory drug-induced gastroduodenal ulceration. *New Engl J Med* 327: 1575–1580
12 Hogben CAM, Schanker LS, Tocco DJ, Brodie BB (1957) Absorption of drugs from the stomach II. *Hum J Pharmacol Exp Ther* 120: 540–545
13 Cvasta TE, Cooke AR (1972) The effect of several ulcerogenic drugs on the canine gastric barrier. *J Lab Clin Med* 79: 302–308
14 Samloff IM (1971) pepsinogens, pepsins and pepsin inhibitors. *Gastroenterology* 586–604
15 Konturek SJ, Brzozowski T, Radecki T (1983) Protective action of omeprazole, a benzimidazole derivative, on gastric mucosal damage by aspirin and ethanol in rats. *Digestion* 27 (3): 159–164
16 Okabe S, Miyake H, Awane Y (1986) Cytoprotective effects of NC-1300 and omeprazole on HCl ethanol-induced gastric lesions in rats. *Japanese J Pharmacol* 42 (1): 123–133
17 Romano M, Razandi M, Ivey KJ (1989) Protection of gastric epithelial cell monolayers from a human cell line by omeprazole *in vitro*. *Scand J Gastroenterol* 24 (5): 513–521
18 O'Brien PE, Frydman G, Holmes R, Malcontenti C, Phelan D (1990) Evaluation of putative cytoprotective of anti-ulcer drugs using quantitative histological techniques. *Dig Dis Sci* 35 (9): 1130–1139
19 Blandizzi C, Gherardi G, Marveggio C, Natale G, Carignani D, Del Tacca M (1995) Mechanisms of protection of omeprazole against experimental gastric mucosal damage in rats. *Digestion* 56 (3): 220–229
20 Ichikawa T, Ishihara K, Saigenji K, Hotta K (1991) Effects of omeprazole on gastric mucus glycoprotein biosynthesis. *Gastroenterologia Japonica* 26 (3): 390
21 Parodi MC, Cognein P, Fazzuoli L, Sacco T (1992) Effects of omeprazole on gastric mucus secretion, tissue prostaglandin synthesis, and acid inhibition in patients with duodenal ulcer: comparison with ranitidine treatment. *Current Therapeutic Research, Clinical Experimental* 52 (1): 13–23
22 Guslandi M, Franceschi M, Fanti L, Pellegrini A, Tittobello A (1992) Omeprazole-induced changes in gastric mucus secretion. *Methods Find Exp Clin Pharmacol* 13 (3): 219–223
23 Mizuguchi Y, Kawai T, Miwa K, Takei K, Mizumura Y, Sanada J, Niki S, Takeda K, Onoda K, Shinohara Y et al (1996) The effects of a proton pump inhibitor (omeprazole) on amounts of gastric mucus and gastric mucosal proliferation in rats. *J Tokyo Med Coll* 54 (5): 460–470
24 Ohara S, Murayama N, Kuwata H, Ishihara K, Hotta K (1988) Effects of omeprazole on rat gastric mucus glycoproteins with acetylsalicylic acid-induced gastric damage. *Arch Int Pharmacodynam Ther* 296: 92–201
25 Bigard MA, Isal JP (1988) Complete prevention by omeprazole of aspirin induced gastric lesions in healthy subjects. *Gut* 29: A712
26 Scheiman JM, Belcher EM, Loeffler KM, Elta GH (1994) Omeprazole ameliorates aspirin-induced gastroduodenal injury. *Dig Dis Sci* 39: 97–103
27 Simon B, Elsner H, Muller P (1995) Protective effects of omeprazole against low-dose acetylsalicyl acid. An endoscopic controlled double-blind study in healthy volunteers. *Arzneimittelforschung* 45 (6): 701–703
28 Taha AS, Hudson N, Hawkey CJ, Swannell AJ, Trye PN, Cottrell J, Mann SG, Simon TJ, Sturrock RD, Russell RI (1996) Famotidine for the prevention of gastric and duodenal ulcers caused by non-steroidal anti-inflammatory drugs. *New Engl J Med* 334: 1435–1439
29 Hudson N, Taha AS, Russell RI, Sturrock RG, Trye P, Cottrell J, Mann SG, Swannell AJ, Hawkey CJ (1997) Famotidine for healing and maintenance in non-steroidal anti-inflammatory drug-associated gastroduodenal ulceration. *Gastroenterology* 112 (6): 1817–1822
30 Hawkey CJ, Karrasch IA, Szczepanski L, Walker DG, Barkun A, Swannell AJ, Yeomans Nd (1998) Omeprazole compared with misoprostol for treating and preventing ulcers associated with nonsteroidal antiinflammatory drugs. *New Engl J Med* 338 (11): 727–734

31 Yeomans ND, Tulassay Z, Juhasz L, Racz I, Howard JM, van Rensburg CJ, Swannell AJ, Hawkey CJ (1998) A comparison of omeprazole and ranitidine for treating and preventing ulcers associated with nonsteroidal antiinflammatory drugs. *New Engl J Med* 338(11): 719–726
32 Ekström P, Carling L, Wetterhus S et al (1996) Prevention of peptic ulcer and dyspeptic symptoms with omeprazole in patients receiving continuous non-steroidal antiinflammatory drug therapy – A Nordic Multicentre Study. *Scand J Gastroenterol* 31: 753–758
33 Cullen D, Bardhan KD, Eisner M, Kogut M, Peacock RA, Thomson JM, Hawkey CJ (1998) Primary gastroduodenal prophylaxis with omeprazole for non-steroidal anti-inflammatory drug users. *Aliment Pharmacol Ther* 2: 135–140.
34 Hawkey CJ, Tulassay Z, Szczepanski L, van Rensburg CJ, Filipowicz-Sosnowska A, Lanas A, Wason CM, Peacock RA, Gillon KRW (1998) *Helicobacter pylori* eradication in patients taking non-steroidal, anti-inflammatory drugs: the HELP NSAIDS study. *Lancet* 352: 1016–1021.

Proton Pump Inhibitors
ed. by L. Olbe

Zollinger-Ellison syndrome

Robert T. Jensen

Digestive Diseases Branch, National Institute of Diabetes and Digestive and Kidney Diseases, National Institutes of Health, Bethesda, MD 20892-1804, USA

Introduction

The discovery of omeprazole and the subsequent development of other proton pump inhibitors (lansoprazole, pantoprazole) has had a profound effect on the management of Zollinger-Ellison syndrome (ZES) as well as other gastric hypersecretory states.These drugs have now become the drugs of choice for these conditions [1]. The focus of this chapter will be their impact on Zollinger-Ellison syndrome, because of all the gastric hypersecretory states this disease demonstrates the most profound gastric acid hypersecretion and has been the best studied. Although there are a few studies with lansoprazole and pantoprazole (Tab. 1), most of the detailed studies (Tab. 1) [2–13] have been performed using omeprazole, so these studies will be primarily emphasized in this chapter. To understand the impact of omeprazole on the treatment of ZES, it is essential to understand the treatment regimens that existed prior to its introduction in the early 1980s for treatment of ZES [2, 3, 14].

Pre-omeprazole treatment of gastric acid hypersecretion in patients with ZES

With the availability in the early 1970s of metiamide [14] followed by cimetidine, the first widely used histamine H_2-receptor antagonist in ZES [14], it became possible to control medically gastric acid hypersecretion for the first time in most patients with ZES. Numerous studies with cimetidine alone [15–19] or with an anticholinergic agent [12, 14, 19–23] – ranitidine – alone [17, 23–25] or with an anticholinergic agent [15, 23], and famotidine alone or with an anticholinergic agent [11, 14, 26] were subsequently published [14] (Tab. 1). Even though a number of these studies reported successful control of acid hypersecretion in all patients with ZES, a number of studies reported failure rates >40% (Tab. 1) [11, 14, 16, 18, 21, 24, 25]. An editorial [27] in 1984 concluded that the single most important determinant of treatment failure was the lack of adequate suppression of acid

Table 1. Comparison of the efficacy of H^+-K^+ ATPase inhibitors or histamine H_2-receptor antagonists in the long-term control of gastric acid hypersecretion in patients with ZES

Antisecretory drug	No. of patients	Mean duration of treatment (months)	Mean % failure	Year	Author [Ref.]
Histamine H_2-receptor antagonist					
Cimetidine	14	11	0	1978	Stadil [15]
	13	–	61	1979	Bonfils [16]
	17	26	65	1983	Deveney [18]
	13	28	0	1983	Jensen [19]
	13	27	0	1984	Collen [17]
Cimetidine + anticholinergic agent[a]	61	12	8	1978	McCarthy [20]
	20	33	50	1983	Stabile [21]
	18	29	6	1983	Malagelada [22]
	20	28	0	1983	Jensen [19]
	6	37	0	1986	Vinayek [23]
Ranitidine	15	18[b]	40	1982	Mignon [24]
	10	14	40	1983	Vezzadini [25]
	13	14	0	1984	Collen [17]
	14	18	0	1986	Vinayek [23]
Ranitidine + anticholinergic agent[a]	19	14	0	1984	Stadil [15]
	10	18	0	1986	Vinayek [23]
Famotidine + anticholinergic agent[a]	32	10	0	1985	Howard [26]
	13	(range 7–34)	61	1993	Corleto [11]
H^+-K^+ ATPase inhibitor					
Omeprazole	7	14	0	1984	Lamers [2]
	11	(range 1–9)[c]	0	1985	McArthur [3]
	11	15	2	1986	Delchier [4]
	9	(range 2–27)[c]	0	1986	Bardram [5]
	80	19	7.5[d]	1988	Lloyd-Davies [6]
	31	(range 0–18)[c]	3.2	1988	Hirschowitz [7]
	40	29[e]	0	1989	Maton [8]
	10	21	0	1989	Lehy [9]
	116	38	0	1993	Metz [10]
	8	20	0	1996	Corleto [11]
Lansoprazole	20	18	0	1993	Metz [33]
	21	31	0	1993	Jensen [36]
	9	–	0	1993	Mignon [37]
	26	28	4	1996	Hirschowitz [38]
Pantoprazole	10	12	0	1997	Rabebold [39]

[a] Isopropamide, propantheline or pirenzepine were used in a few patients.
[b] Approximate duration of treatment.
[c] Mean not determined, range given.
[d] Six patients underwent total gastrectomy and were listed as having had drug failures, although acid secretion was reported to have been controlled before surgery.
[e] Median dose reported.

secretion because of an inadequate dose of antisecretory agent, primarily owing to the failure to use a well-defined criterion of acid control.

A number of studies demonstrated that reduction of gastric acid hypersecretion to <10 mEq/h for the hour prior to the next dose of antisecretory medication would allow peptic ulcers to heal and prevent the further development of mucosal disease in the majority of patients with ZES [14, 20, 28]. Subsequent studies demonstrated that more stringent criteria were required in the small percentage of patients with previous Billroth II gastrectomies or with severe esophageal reflux disease [12, 14, 29, 30]. At present, except for these two latter groups of patients with ZES, the criterion of <10 mEq/h for the hour prior to the next drug dosage is almost universally used [14]. To achieve this degree of control of acid hypersecretion in patients with ZES with histamine H_2-receptor antagonists, not only were large doses required but anticholinergic agents frequently had to be added and frequent dosing was needed, with the result that almost all patients required drug at 4- to 6-h dosing [14, 17, 23, 31] (Fig. 1). When this criterion was used to treat gastric acid hypersecretion in patients with ZES, the failure rate was reduced to zero (Tab. 1) [14, 17, 19, 23]. The mean daily dose of cimetidine required to control gastric acid hypersecretion to these levels in patients with ZES at the National Institutes of Health (NIH) was 3.6 g/day for cimetidine, 1.2 g/day for ranitidine and 0.25 g/day for famotidine [14]. Side-effects with these high doses of histamine H_2-receptor antagonists were generally not a limiting factor [14]. Except for antiandrogen side-effects (impotence, gynecomastia) in males [14, 31] or occasional patients with drug interactions due to inhibition of the mixed-function oxidase system by high doses of cimetidine, side-effects did not limit their use. However, expense, the inconvenience of frequent dosing, the need for titration of the dosage in each patient because the dosage could not be predicted, side-effects due to anticholinergic agents added to potentiate the action of the histamine H_2-receptor antagonist, or the difficulty of completely controlling symptoms and healing the mucosa in patients with previously Billroth II resection [29], or moderate to severe esophageal reflux disease [30] were major limitations of the widespread successful use of histamine H_2-receptor antagonists in ZES [14]. Furthermore, expense, inconvenience, anticholinergic side-effects and a failure to adequately control symptoms in all patients affected patient compliance. Therefore, prior to the availability of omeprazole, medical therapy in all patients with ZES was only achieved in a few specialty centers with considerable expertise. Many specialty centers still had a high failure rate with these drugs (Tab. 1).

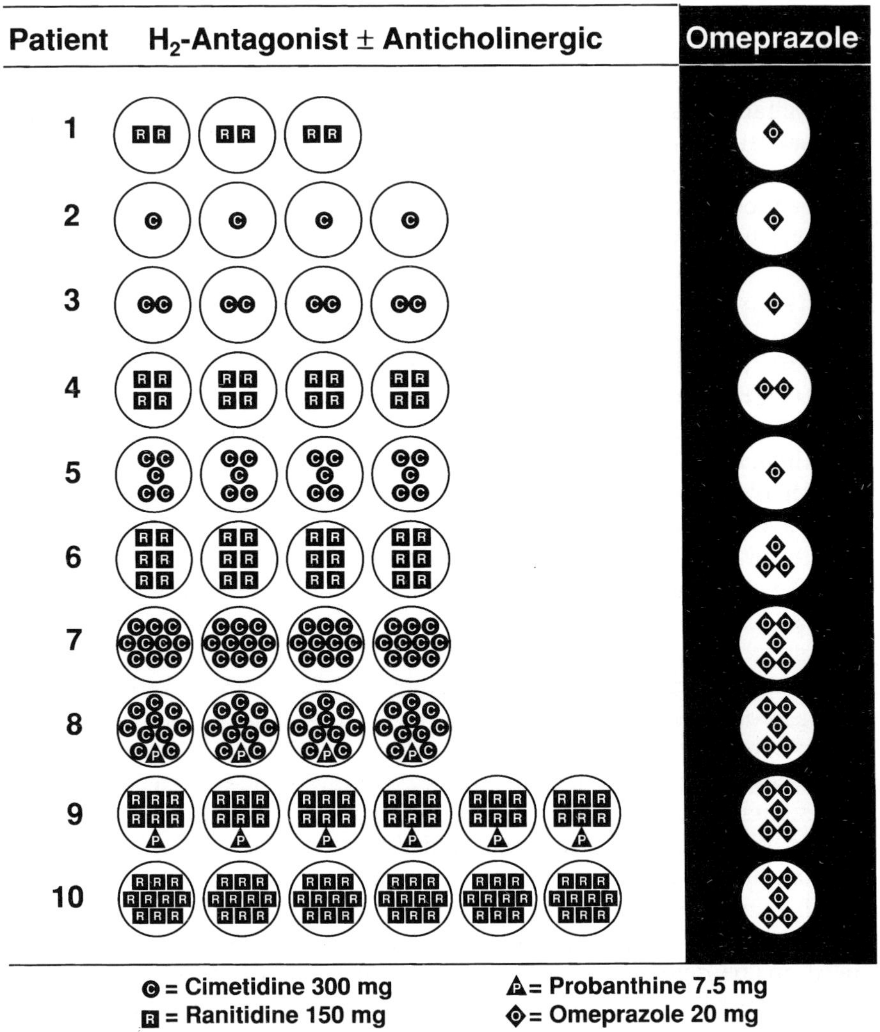

Figure 1. Comparative ability of histamine H_2-receptor antagonists (cimetidine, ranitidine alone or with an anticholinergic agent) or omeprazole to control gastric acid hypersecretion in the first 10 patients with ZES treated with omeprazole at the National Institutes of Health. Numbers refer to patient number. *Data on the left* show doses and frequency of histamine H_2-receptor antagonists. Each circle shows the number and type of histamine H_2-antagonist taken at each dosing. C, cimetidine (300 mg); R, ranitidine (150 mg); P, probanthine (15 mg). *Data on the right* show the number of omeprazole "O" (20 mg) tablets taken once per day required to control the acid secretion. Shown are the minimal doses of the antisecretory drug required to reduce acid secretion to < 10 mEq/h for the hour prior to next drug dosage. Figure was drawn by K. McArthur from data in ref. 3.

Omeprazole treatment in patients with ZES

The results of omeprazole treatment of ZES from 10 studies are summarized in Table 1 and include the results of the large, long-term NIH study involving 116 patients treated for up to 9 years [10]. Even with long-term treatment, omeprazole has controlled acid hypersecretion in most studies in all patients except for the rare patient (<0.5%) who cannot or will not regularly take oral medications.

The major advantage of omeprazole over the histamine H_2-receptor antagonists is its long duration of action (Fig. 2) [3, 11, 14, 32, 33]. Its long duration of action allows once-a-day dosing in 68 to 90% of patients with ZES [10, 14]. Figure 1 shows the dramatic efficacy of omeprazole in the first 10 patients treated with omeprazole starting in 1982 at the NIH. Many of these 10 patients had to take a large number of tablets of cimetidine or ranitidine either alone or with the anticholinergic agent probanthine every 4 to 6 h to control their acid hypersecretion prior to omeprazole (Fig. 1, left panel). With omeprazole, acid hypersecretion was controlled in all 10 patients with up to 100 mg/day (five tablets) of omeprazole taken once per day (Fig. 1, right panel). Data from studies that demonstrate the marked increased duration of action of omeprazole in patients with ZES, which allows once-a-day dosing, are summarized in Figure 2. In all of these studies except the one by Vinayek et al. [32], the minimal dose of histamine H_2-receptor antagonist or omeprazole that reduced gastric acid hypersecretion to control values was determinded i.e., <10 mEq/h, except in patients with moderate to severe gastroesophageal reflux disease or previous gastric acid-reducing surgery, where <5 mEq/h was used [12, 14, 29, 30]). Subsequently, the drug was stopped, and the increase in acid secretion was measured for up to 56 h (Fig. 2). The time from the last dose of drug for the acid secretion to reach one-half of the basal acid output ($BAO_{1/2}$) when no drug was present was calculated in each study. The total duration of action could not be determined in these studies because of the possible risk to the patients of prolonged periods without adequate control of the severe hypersecretion [14]; however, the time to reach the untreated $BAO_{1/2}$ after each drug was an excellent measure of their relative durations of action. With histamine H_2-receptor antagonists there was no significant difference between the duration to reach $BAO_{1/2}$ for cimetidine and ranitidine (10.7 vs 11.3 h, respectively) (Fig. 2); however, famotidine had a 30% longer duration of action of 14.1 ± 1.0 h [26] (Fig. 2). In contrast, omeprazole in two different studies [3, 32] (Fig. 2, left and right lower panels) had a duration of action greater than three-times longer ($BAO_{1/2}$ – 37 ± 3 and 34 ± 6 h) than the histamine H_2-receptor antagonists.

In most studies hypersecretion of gastric acid in patients with ZES is controlled with <80 mg of omeprazole per day; however, occasional patients require >200 mg/day [6, 10, 12–14]. In the recent NIH study [10] involving 116 patients treated for a mean of 38 ± 3 months (range 0.1–

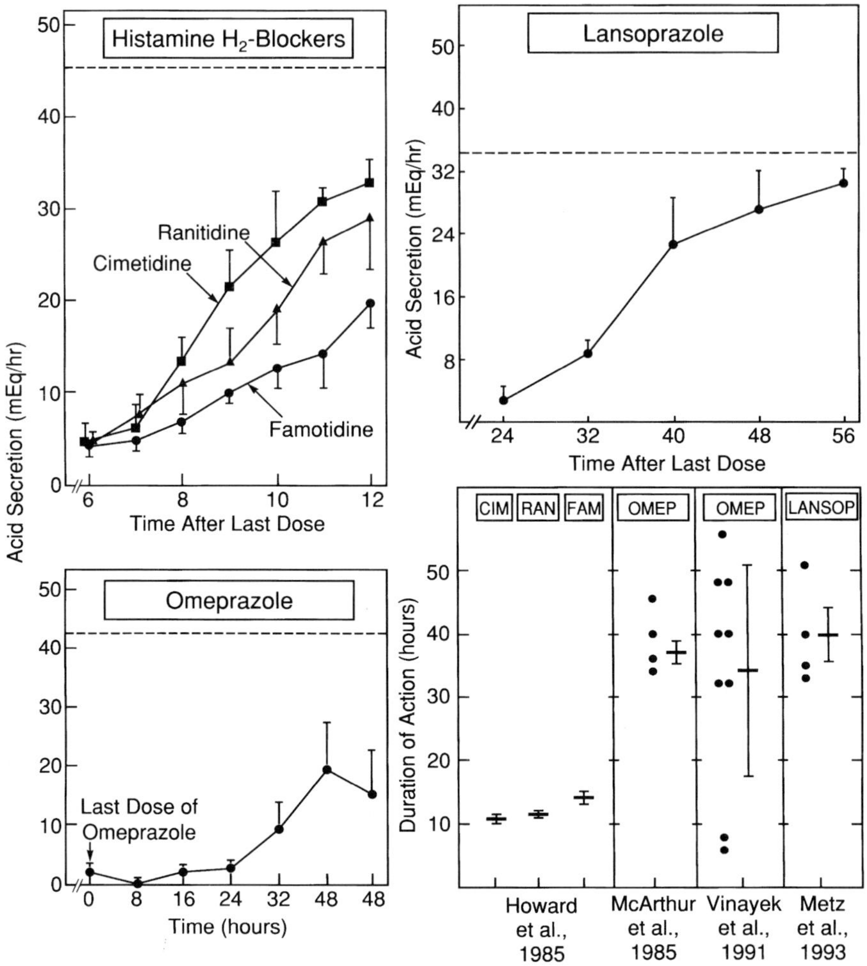

Figure 2. Duration of action of oral histamine H_2-receptor antagonists, omeprazole and lansoprazole, in patients with ZES. *Top left panel*: Duration of action of equipotent doses of famotidine, ranitidine and cimetidine in five patients with ZES. The minimum dose requirement for each drug to reduce gastric acid output to less than 10 mEq/h during the 6th hour after administration was determined in each patient. Thereafter, gastric acid output was measured from the beginning of the 6th hour to the end of the 12th hour in each patient with each of the three equipotent doses for famotidine, ranitidine, and cimetidine. The dotted line represents the mean BAO without any drug. *Top right panel*: Duration of action of lansoprazole was determined. The minimum lansoprazole dose to reduce acid to <10 mEq/h in the last hour before the next dose was determined. Data are from four patients. Acid secretion was measured 24 h after the last dose, then at every 8 h thereafter. *Bottom left panel*: Duration of action of omeprazole was determined. The minimum dose requirement for omeprazole to reduce gastric acid output to less than 10 mEq/h during the last hour before the next dose of drug was determined. Data are from five patients. Gastric acid output was measured every 8 h after the last dose of omeprazole. The dotted line represents the mean BAO for the five subjects being tested prior to receiving these drugs. Vertical bars represent 1 SEM. *Bottom right panel*: Time (hours) to reach $BAO_{1/2}$ are shown after stopping histamine H_2-antagonists [cimetidine (CIM), ranitidine (RAN) or famotidine (FAM)], after stopping omeprazole (OMEP) or lansoprazole (LANSOP).

9.5 years), 75% of patients had their acid secretion initially controlled with a once-per-day dosage, with 46% of patients requiring 60 mg taken once per day, 5% required 80 mg once per day and 24% required 100–120 mg once per day. In 25% of patients, twice-a-day dosing was required, with all patients initially well controlled on 60 mg twice per day [10]. None of the 116 patients required omeprazole dosing greater than twice per day, demonstrating that the need for dosing more frequently than twice per day is uncommon in patients with ZES [10, 14]. In an earlier NIH study [8] the median daily omeprazole dose was 100 mg/day, whereas in other studies the median dose was 60–80 mg/day [4, 6, 7, 9]. It had been proposed that this difference in drug dose might be due to a lesser percentage of patients receiving a split daily dose in the earlier NIH study. This conclusion was supported by another study at the NIH [8] that demonstrated that a number of patients with ZES who did not have satisfactory control of their acid hypersecretion with 120 mg of omeprazole taken once per day did have satisfactory control with a 60-mg dose taken twice a day [8]. Furthermore, in a number of patients acid hypersecretion was controlled with a twice-a-day dosing that, in total amount, was less than that required if taken as a single daily dose. These data demonstrate that if patients require higher doses of omeprazole (> 80 mg), more effective control of acid secretion can be obtained by dividing the dosage into a twice-a-day dose rather than continuing to increase the once-a-day dosing.

In long-term treatment studies with histamine H_2-receptor antagonists, patients averaged one dosage increase per year [12, 14]. In long-term treatment of ZES patients with omeprazole, the initial studies demonstrated that in one-third of the patients the initial omeprazole dosage could be decreased, in one-third of the patients it had to be increased and in one-third it remained stable [12]. These studies demonstrated that long-term tachyphylaxis does not occur. Recent studies [10, 11, 13, 34] demonstrate that the long-term maintenance doses of omeprazole reported in early studies [2–6, 8, 9] were too high and can be reduced to 20 mg daily or twice daily in 68% of all patients, and in 95% of patients with uncomplicated ZES i.e., without gastric acid-reducing surgery, multiple endocrine neoplasia-type I (MEN-I) or severe gastroesophageal disease. In one study [13] it was also possible to reduce the omeprazole dosage in 35% of patients with complicated ZES associated with previous gastric acid-reducing surgery, MEN-I or severe gastroesophageal reflux disease. It is not surprising that dose reduction was possible in a much smaller percentage of patients with complicated ZES. Previous studies demonstrated patients with ZES with

The OMEP data (McArthur [3]) are from data in *bottom left panel*; LANSOP data (Metz et al. [33]) are from data in *top right panel*; and histamine H_2-antagonist data are from the data in the *top left panel*. In the study by Vinayek [32], each patient received 80 mg of omeprazole orally, whereas in each of the other studies the minimal effective oral dose was used.

MEN-I and hyperparathyroidism were more resistant to gastric antisecretory drugs [13, 14] and patients with ZES with previous gastric acid-reducing surgery or severe gastroesophageal reflux disease required greater acid inhibition than patients without these conditions [13, 14, 29]. In a recent long-term NIH study [10] of 91 patients with ZES treated with omeprazole in which dose reduction was attempted for patients with well-controlled acid secretion and dose increases for patients in whom acid secretion was not well controlled, the mean daily omeprazole dosage was reduced from 62 ± 3 mg initially to 37 ± 3. In this study [10] 19% of patients required an upward dose adjustment, and 53% were able to undergo a dose reduction. After a mean follow-up of 38 ± 3 months (0.1 – 116 months) [10], the final omeprazole doses in 116 patients with ZES for the 78 patients (67%) taking a single daily dose were 20 mg (30% of total patients), 40 mg (7%), 60 mg (16%), 80 mg (7%), 100 mg (5%), and 120 mg (3%). Of the 116 patients in this study [10], 38% were taking a twice-daily omeprazole dose at the end of the study of 20 mg (10%), 40 mg (13%), 60 mg (10%) or 80 mg (1%).

Dose reduction during maintenance studies in patients with ZES was possible because of the recommended initial dosing schedule used in most studies. Because omeprazole is acid-labile and because of the need to rapidly control acid secretion in patients with ZES [3, 6, 13, 14, 34], it was recommended that patients with ZES be started on 60 mg omeprazole per day, the acid secretory rate determined 1 h before the next dose and, if the control was inadequate, the dose be increased until acid secretion was controlled (< 10 mEq/h) [6, 12, 14, 34]. Furthermore, even though omeprazole dosage in patients with ZES has been shown to correlate significantly with ranitidine dose and basal acid output [8, 10], the exact dosage cannot be predicted for a given patient; therefore initial dose titration is needed in each patient [10, 12, 35]. However, the efficacy of omeprazole increases over the first few days of its use [13, 34]. Therefore, the possibility of starting patients initially on low-dose omeprazole has been raised [13, 34]. This would be less expensive and would circumvent the need for later dose titration studies to decrease the omeprazole dosage. A recent study [34] examined this approach in 49 consecutive patients with ZES who were first treated with ranitidine for 2 weeks, and then a low dose of 20 mg of omeprazole was given on day 1 of the study. Gastric secretion was measured 1 h before the next omeprazole dose on day 2 and repeated on day 3 if acid secretion exceeded 10 mEq/h. In this study [34] 32% of patients failed to have their acid hypersecretion satisfactorily controlled owing to persistent symptoms or inadequate acid control. The BAO was the only clinical or laboratory feature that was significantly different between patients in which low-dose initial treatment was or was not successful with all patients with a BAO < 20 mEq/h having a successful outcome. It was concluded [34] because of the need to rapidly control gastric acid hypersecretion, owing to the high risk of developing complications from peptic ulcer disease in these patients, that patients should continue to be started on treatment with omeprazole 60 mg/day and the daily initial dose adjusted by acute titration as currently recommended. After the initial maintenance dose is established, attempts should be made to reduce the dose to 20 mg/day or twice per day. In only the minority of patients with ZES in whom the BAO is known to be <20 mEq/h (~20% of patients) should an initial low dose of omeprazole be used [34].

Use of other proton pump inhibitors in ZES

The use of either lansoprazole [33, 36–38] or pantoprazole [39] in patients with ZES is much more limited than omeprazole (Tab. 1). In four studies [33, 36–38] lansoprazole has been shown to be effective, and in one study [39] reported in preliminary form, pantoprazole has been reported to be effective in 10 patients with ZES (Tab. 1). In two NIH studies [33, 36] lansoprazole was found to have the same duration of action as omeprazole (Fig. 2), 69% of patients were controlled with a single daily dose, and the mean lansoprazole dose was similar to that reported with omeprazole. Furthermore, long-term maintenance dose reduction was possible in the majority of patients treated with lansoprazole, similar to that seen with omeprazole [36]. In a recent study [38] in which 26 patients with ZES were treated for a median time of 28 months (range 3–48 months), the initial mean dose was 66 ± 4 mg/day, and the drug remained effective long-term in all but one patient who developed a jejunal ulcer perforation. In this study [38] equi-effective doses of lansoprazole and omeprazole were compared in 13 patients. No correlation was found between doses of the two drugs; however, there was no difference in their mean doses (omeprazole – 48 mg/day, range 20–100, and lansoprazole – 53 mg/day, range 15–90 mg/day).

In the pantoprazole study [39] 10 patients were treated for 4 to 14 months (mean 12 months). Pantoprazole controlled symptoms in all patients and prevented development of mucosal disease with a single daily dose in 70% of patients. Some patients required daily doses up to 160 mg/day, particularly patients with high BAOs.

Safety and side-effects of long-term omeprazole treatment in patients with ZES

In the long-term NIH study involving 116 patients treated for up to 9.5 years [10], omeprazole caused no dose-related side-effects or idiosyncratic reactions in any patient, and no patient had to stop taking it because of an untoward effect. These results are similar to those of a number of other long-term treatment studies in patients with ZES [6, 8].

Potential concerns about the long-term use of omeprazole have been raised in respect to the possible consequences of increased hypergastrinemia (increased incidence of gastric carcinoid tumors) or due to long-term drug-induced hypo- or achlorhydria (malabsorption of vitamin B_{12}, iron or calcium) [40–50]. Rats, but not mice, given omeprazole for 2 years developed proliferation of the gastric enterochromaffin-like cells (ECL cells) and carcinoid tumors of the stomach [48, 50, 51]. Other causes of chronic hypergastrinemia such as long-term, high-dose ranitidine, fundectomy, partial corpectomy and long-term infusions of gastrin-17 also increase ECL cells [12, 50–54]. Furthermore, fundectomy and long-term, high-dose ranitidine can cause carcinoid tumors [12, 51–54]. Hypergastrinemic states in humans such as ZES or pernicious anemia are also associated with ECL cell hyperplasia and an increased risk of carcinoids [51, 55]. Numerous studies demonstrate that ECL cells are increased approximately twofold in ZES and that of the six types of endocrine cells in the stomach, only the ECL cells were increased [12, 56]. Recent analyses show the gastric carcinoid tumors that occur in patients with ZES occur almost entirely in the 20–25% of the patients who have MEN-I [9]. In two studies involving 200 patients and 48 patients [14, 57, 58], gastric carcinoids occurred in 13 and 30% of patients with ZES and MEN-I and in 0.6 and 0% of patients without MEN-I. Two recent studies report gastric carcinoids in patients with ZES and MEN-I have loss of heterozygosity on chromosome 11q13 in the region of the MEN-I gene [59, 60], demonstrating that ECL gastric carcinoids are an independent tumor type in MEN-I. In two studies with prolonged omeprazole treatment [9, 61] and one study with lansoprazole treatment [62] for up to 4 years in patients with ZES, there was no further increase in ECL cells. Therefore, at present there is no data to support the conclusion that long-term omeprazole treatment in patients with ZES and MEN-I increases the rate of development of carcinoids. In animal studies the evidence supports the conclusion that the ECL cell changes and carcinoids are the result of omeprazole-induced long-term hypergastrinemia [40, 51, 63]. In some studies [9, 33], but not others [6, 8, 38], treatment with omeprazole or lansoprazole of patients with ZES has caused further increases in serum gastrin levels. Furthermore, in two recent studies [43, 44] 36–43% of patients met at least one criterion of marked gastric acid hyposecretion while taking omeprazole long-term, and 31% of the patients had no acid during each of 3 years while taking omeprazole. These latter data demonstrate omeprazole-induced achlorhydria is relatively frequent in patients with ZES; therefore, physiological hypergastrinemia as well as tumor-induced hypergastrinemia could possibly occur together. The extent of ECL changes has been shown to correlate with the serum gastrin [51, 63, 64]; therefore, it is possible that long-term treatment with a proton pump inhibitor could contribute in ZES patients to more rapid ECL changes. Additional long-term studies involving more patients will be needed to resolve this issue completely.

A large number of studies support the conclusion that gastric acidity is important for the absorption of protein-bound vitamin B_{12} from food, non-heme iron in the diet and calcium [43–47]. Furthermore, a number of clinical conditions that cause hypo- or achlorhydria have been shown to cause anemia, decreased iron or vitamin B_{12} absorption or both, including vagotomy, atrophic gastritis and gastric resection [43–45]. Therefore, long-term treatment with potent acid suppressants such as the proton pump inhibitors could lead to malabsorption of one or both of these nutrients. Until recently, relatively few patients had been evaluated for the long-term effects of treatment with any proton pump inhibitor taken for any indication that provided data to address whether such chronic treatment could lead to malabsorption of these nutrients. In one study [46] in 34 patients with peptic diseases (primarily reflux disease) given treatment for up to 48 months, omeprazole did not cause any statistically significant decrease in iron body stores assessed by monitoring serum ferritin; however, after 4 years the mean serum vitamin B_{12} level was lower than at 2 years. Recently we have completed studies on patients with ZES who have been maintained long-term on omeprazole or other gastric antisecretory drugs to attempt to address their effects on body iron stores [43] or vitamin B_{12} [44].

In the study of the effect of long-term omeprazole treatment on body iron stores [43] 109 patients with ZES were studied. Eighty-two percent (89/109) patients were taking omeprazole and the remainder either histamine H_2-antagonists or no antisecretory drug following curative resection. The mean duration of omeprazole treatment was 6 years (range 1–12.5 years) and the total duration of any gastric acid antisecretory treatment was 10 years (range 1–21 years). Acid hyposecretion by at least one criterion was present in 45% of patients. There were no significant differences in serum ferritin levels, which are a measure of total body iron stores [65] in patients taking or not taking omeprazole, with or without drug-induced acid hyposecretion, with different durations of omeprazole treatment or with different total duration of antisecretory drug treatment [43]. These data support the conclusion that continuous treatment with omeprazole for 6 years or antisecretory drug treatment for 10 years did not decrease body iron stores or cause iron deficiency [43].

A similarly designed study [44] assessed the effect of long-term omeprazole treatment on serum vitamin B_{12} levels and serum folate levels. Of the 131 consecutive patients with ZES studied, 111 were taking omeprazole and 20 patients were taking histamine H_2-receptor antagonists. All patients had their acid hypersecretion controlled for at least 6 months prior to the study. Serum folate and vitamin B_{12} were assessed yearly. The mean duration of either omeprazole treatment (range 0.2–12 years), or treatment with histamine H_2-receptor antagonists (range 3–17 years) was 4.5 years. Vitamin B_{12} levels were significantly lower ($p = 0.03$) in patients taking omeprazole, but there was no difference in folate levels or in any hematological parameter in patients taking or not taking omeprazole. Serum vitamin B_{12} levels were significantly lower in patients with sustained acid hyposecretion or with complete achlorhydria ($p<0.0001$) compared with patients without hypo- or achlorhydria [44]. In 68 patients with two serum vitamin B_{12} levels at least 5 years apart, serum vitamin B_{12} levels decreased significantly (30%) ($p = 0.001$) only in patients rendered achlorhydric. Eight patients (6%) had vitamin B_{12} levels below the lower limit of normal, and the serum vitamin B_{12} levels prior to omeprazole treatment were normal in each of these patients [44]. These results show that long-term treatment with omeprazole can lead to significant decreases in serum vitamin B_{12} levels, but not serum folate levels. These results suggest that all patients with ZES treated long-term with proton pump inhibitors should have yearly serum vitamin B_{12} levels determined.

Use of intravenous omeprazole in patients with ZES

Many patients with ZES will require parenteral administration of a gastric antisecretory drug to control acid hypersecretion at some point in their treatment, whether because of surgery, chemotherapy or other inter-current illness [14, 66]. These patients are usually treated with intravenous gastric acid antisecretory medications during these periods while they are unable to take oral medication. The use of parenteral histamine H_2-receptor antagonists (cimetidine, ranitidine) [14, 35, 66] or omeprazole [67] to control gastric hypersecretion in patients with ZES during surgery has been particularly well studied. These studies demonstrate that histamine H_2-receptor antagonists are best administered by continuous infusion. However, because the dose requirement varies in individual patients (Fig. 3), prior to surgery all patients must be treated with continuous intravenous infusion of histamine H_2-receptor antagonist to determine the dose that controls the gastric acid hypersecretion. Relatively high doses of intravenous cimetidine or ranitidine are required by many patients (Fig. 3, top) [66]. The mean intravenous cimetidine dose required in one recent study was 2.9 mg/kg/h, but there was a wide range from 0.5 to 7 mg/kg/h. The minimal effective intravenous cimetidine dose correlated closely with the previous oral dose of cimetidine ($r = 0.96$, $p<0.001$), ranitidine or famotidine ($r = 0.95$, $p<0.001$). In this study patients were treated for up to 83 days with these intravenous cimetidine doses without side-effects or loss of efficacy. Another recent study [68] demonstrated that continuous intravenous infusion of ranitidine at 100% of the previously effective oral equivalent dose will effectively control acid output in 95% of patients with ZES, thus limiting the need for repeated dose adjustments and gastric output assessment in patients who require parenteral therapy. It must be stressed, however, that the adequacy of the administered dose should be checked by measuring acid output after a few hours to ensure that acid output is less than 10 mEq/h. It was recommended [14, 35, 66] that acid output be rechecked

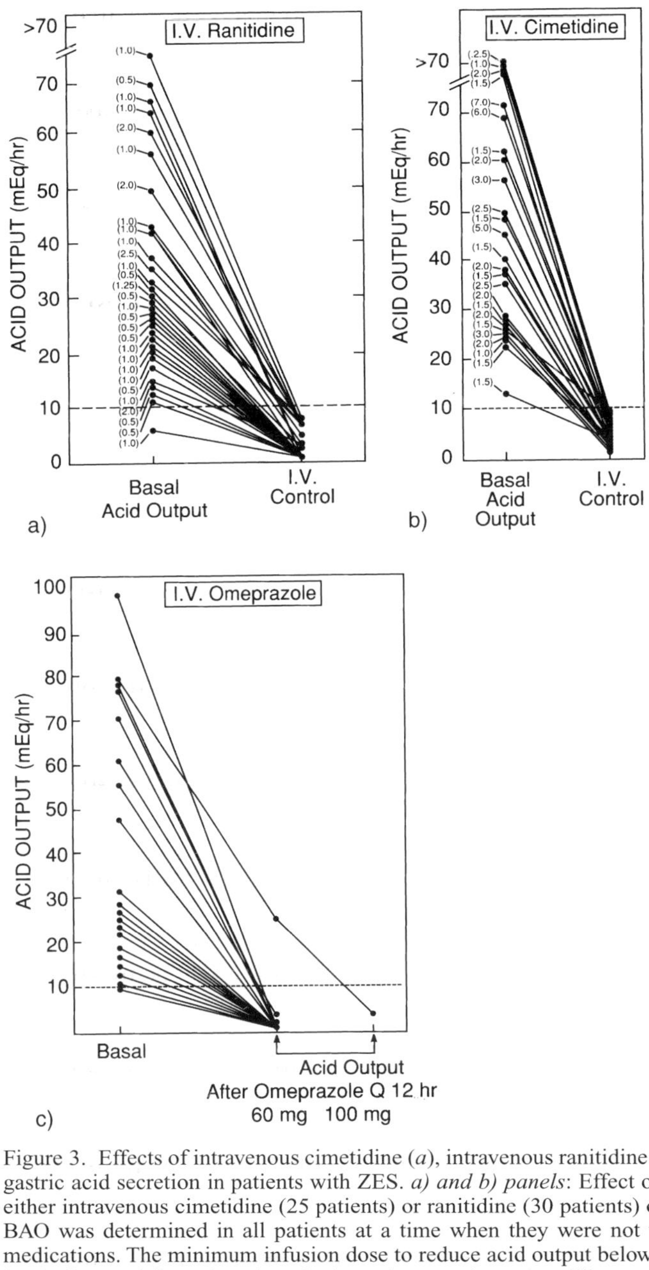

Figure 3. Effects of intravenous cimetidine (*a*), intravenous ranitidine (*b*) or omeprazole (*c*) on gastric acid secretion in patients with ZES. *a) and b) panels*: Effect of continuous infusion of either intravenous cimetidine (25 patients) or ranitidine (30 patients) on gastric acid secretion. BAO was determined in all patients at a time when they were not taking any antisecretory medications. The minimum infusion dose to reduce acid output below 10 mEq/h, the accepted level of control, in each patients is shown in parentheses in milligrams/kg/hour. *c)*: Effect of an intravenous bolus dose of omeprazole on gastric acid secretion during the last hour before the next dose of drug in 20 patients with ZES is shown. BAO was determined on a previous occasion in all patients at a time when they were taking no antisecretory medications. The *dotted line* represents an acid output of 10 mEq/h, the accepted level of control. Figure was drawn from data in studies by Saeed et al. [69] (cimetidine); Vinayek et al. [68] (ranitidine); and Vinayek et al. [67] (omeprazole).

in the early postoperative period because in some patients drug requirements increase after surgery. Intravenous omeprazole is not licensed in many countries, including the United States; however, a study performed at the NIH [67] demonstrates that parenteral omeprazole may be very useful in patients with ZES requiring parenteral gastric antisecretory agents such as at the time of surgery. In this study [67], 60 mg of omeprazole given by intermittent intravenous bolus every 12 h controlled acid secretion in 19 of 20 patients with ZES. One patient required 100 mg every 12 h (Fig. 3, bottom). No patient developed drug toxicity related to omeprazole even with treatment up to 15 days, and the drug remained effective [67]. An additional study [32] has examined the pharmacokinetics and pharmacodynamics of intravenous (i.v.) and oral omeprazole in patients with ZES. The mean elimination half-lives of i.v. and oral omeprazole were not different (2.3 ± 0.4 vs 2.4 ± 0.5 h) but were significantly ($p < 0.002$) longer than reported in normal subjects [32]. The mean durations of action of i.v. and oral omeprazole were not significantly different (34 ± 7.2 vs 35 ± 6.2 h) [32]. These data support the findings of the surgical i.v. omeprazole study [67], demonstrating that intermittent bolus injections of parenteral omeprazole should alleviate the need for continuous infusions of histamine H_2-receptor antagonists [32]. Because of the ease of administration and its potency, intermittent administration of intravenous omeprazole during surgery or during other periods of parenteral drug dosing would likely become the drug of choice, if it were available, for times requiring parenteral treatment of the acid hypersecretion in patients with ZES.

References

1 Jensen RT (1996) Gastrinoma. *Clin Gastroenterol* 10: 555–766

2 Lamers CBHW, Lind T, Moberg S, Jansen JBMJ, Olbe L (1984) Omeprazole in Zollinger-Ellison syndrome: effects of a single dose and of long term treatment in patients resistant to histamine H_2-receptor antagonists. *N Engl J Med* 310: 758–761

3 McArthur KE, Collen MJ, Maton PN, Cherner JA, Howard JM, Ciarleglio CA, Cornelius MJ, Jensen RT, Gardner JD (1985) Omeprazole: effective, convenient therapy for Zollinger-Ellison syndrome. *Gastroenterology* 88: 939–944

4 Delchier JC, Soule JC, Mignon M, Goldfain D, Cortot A, Travers B, Isal JP, Bader JP (1986) Effectiveness of omeprazole in seven patients with Zollinger-Ellison syndrome resistant to histamine H_2-receptor antagonists. *Dig Dis Sci* 31: 693–699

5 Bardram L, Stadil F (1986) Omeprazole in the Zollinger-Ellison syndrome. *Scand J Gastroenterol* 21: 374–378

6 Lloyd-Davies KA, Rutgersson K, Solvell L (1988) Omeprazole in the treatment of Zollinger-Ellison syndrome: a 4-year international study. *Aliment Pharmacol Ther* 2: 13–32

7 Hirschowitz BI, Denen J, Raufman J, LaMont B, Berman R, Humphries T (1988) A multicenter US study of omeprazole treatment of Zollinger-Ellison syndrome. *Gastroenterology* 94: A188 (abstract)

8 Maton PN, Vinayek R, Frucht H, McArthur KA, Miller LS, Saeed ZA, Gardner JD, Jensen RT (1989) Long-term efficacy and safety of omeprazole in patients with Zollinger-Ellison syndrome: a prospective study. *Gastroenterology* 97: 827–836

9 Lehy T, Mignon M, Cadiot G, Elouaer-Blanc L, Ruszniewski P, Lewin MJ, Bonfils S (1989) Gastric endocrine cell behavior in Zollinger-Ellison patients upon long-term potent antisecretory treatment. *Gastroenterology* 96: 1029–1040

10 Metz DC, Strader DB, Orbuch M, Koviach PD, Feigenbaum KM, Jensen RT (1993) Use of omeprazole in Zollinger-Ellison: a prospective nine-year study of efficacy and safety. *Aliment Pharmacol Ther* 7: 597–610
11 Corleto V, Annibale B, D'Ambra G, Saggioro A, Ferrua B, Cassetta MR, Della Fave G (1993) Efficacy of long-term therapy with low doses of omeprazole in the control of gastric acid secretion in Zollinger-Ellison syndrome patients. *Aliment Pharmacol Ther* 7: 167–173
12 Metz DC, Jensen RT (1995) Advances in gastric antisecretory therapy in Zollinger-Ellison syndrome. In: M Mignon, RT Jensen (eds): *Endocrine tumors of the pancreas: recent advances in research and management. Series: Frontiers of Gastrointestinal Research.* S. Karger, Basel, Switzerland, 240–257
13 Metz DC, Pisegna JR, Fishbeyn VA, Benya RV, Feigenbaum KM, Koviack PD, Jensen RT (1992) Currently used doses of omeprazole in Zollinger-Ellison syndrome are too high. *Gastroenterology* 103: 1498–1508
14 Jensen RT, Gardner JD (1993) Gastrinoma. In: VLW Go, EP DiMagno, JD Gardner, E Lebenthal, HA Reber, GA Scheele (eds): *The pancreas: biology, pathobiology and disease.* Raven Press, New York, 931–978
15 Stadil F, Stage JG (1978) Cimetidine and the Zollinger-Ellison (Z-E) syndrome. In: C Wastell, P Lance (eds): *Cimetidine, The Westminster Hospital Symposium.* London: Churchill Livingstone, 91–104
16 Bonfils S, Mignon M, Gratton J (1979) Cimetidine treatment of acute and chronic Zollinger-Ellison syndrome. *World J Surg* 3: 597–604
17 Collen MJ, Howard JM, McArthur KE, Raufman JP, Cornelius MJ, Ciarleglio CA, Gardner JD, Jensen RT (1984) Comparison of ranitidine and cimetidine in the treatment of gastric hypersecretion. *Ann Intern Med* 100: 52–58
18 Deveney CW, Stein S, Way LW (1983) Cimetidine in the treatment of Zollinger-Ellison syndrome. *Am J Surg* 146: 116–123
19 Jensen RT, Gardner JD, Raufman JP, Pandol SJ, Doppman JL, Collen MJ (1983) Zollinger-Ellison syndrome: current concepts and management. *Ann Intern Med* 98: 59–75
20 McCarthy DM (1978) Report on the United States experience with cimetidine in Zollinger-Ellison syndrome and other hypersecretory states. *Gastroenterology* 74: 453–458
21 Stabile BE, Ippoliti AF, Walsh JH, Passaro E Jr (1983) Failure of histamine H_2-receptor antagonist therapy in Zollinger-Ellison syndrome. *Am J Surg* 84(6): 1621–1623
22 Malagelada J, Edis AJ, Adson MA, Van Heerden JA, Go VLW (1983) Medical and surgical options in the management of patients with gastrinoma. *Gastroenterology* 84: 1524–1532
23 Vinayek R, Howard JM, Maton PN, Wank SA, Slaff JI, Gardner JD, Jensen RT (1986) Famotidine in the therapy of gastric hypersecretory states. *Am J Med* 81: 49–59
24 Mignon M, Vallot T, Hervoir P, Benfredo P, Bonfils S (1982) Ranitidine versus Cimetidine in the management of Zollinger-Ellison syndrome. In: AJ Riley, PR Salmon (eds): *Ranitidine, Proceedings of an International Symposium, World Congress of Gastroenterology, Stockholm*, Excerpta Medica, Amsterdam, 169–177
25 Vezzadini P, Bonora G, Tomassetti P, Pazzaglia M, Labo G (1983) Medical treatment of Zollinger-Ellison syndrome with ranitidine. *Int J Tiss Reac* 4: 339–343
26 Howard JM, Chremos AN, Collen MJ, McArthur KE, Cherner JA, Maton PN, Ciarleglio CA, Cornelius MJ, Gardner JD, Jensen RT (1985) Famotidine, a new, potent, long-acting histamine H_2-receptor antagonist: comparison with cimetidine and ranitidine in the treatment of Zollinger-Ellison syndrome. *Gastroenterology* 88: 1026–1033
27 Jensen RT (1984) Basis for failure of cimetidine in patients with Zollinger-Ellison syndrome. *Dig Dis Sci* 29: 363–366
28 Raufman JP, Collins SM, Pandol SJ, Korman LY, Collen MJ, Cornelius MJ, Feld MK, McCarthy DM, Gardner JD, Jensen RT (1983) Reliability of symptoms in assessing control of gastric acid secretion in patients with Zollinger-Ellison syndrome. *Gastroenterology* 84: 108–113
29 Maton PN, Frucht H, Vinayek R, Wank SA, Gardner JD, Jensen RT (1988) Medical management of patients with Zollinger-Ellison syndrome who have had previous gastric surgery: a prospective study. *Gastroenterology* 94: 294–299
30 Miller LS, Vinayek R, Frucht H, Gardner JD, Jensen RT, Maton PN (1990) Reflux esophagitis in patients with Zollinger-Ellison syndrome. *Gastroenterology* 98: 341–346

31 Jensen RT, Collen MJ, Allende HD, Pandol SJ, Raufman JP, Bissonnette BM, Duncan WC, Durgin PL, Gillin JC, Gardner JD (1983) Cimetidine-induced impotence and breast changes in patients with gastric hypersecretory states. *N Engl J Med* 308: 883–887
32 Vinayek R, Amantea MA, Maton PN, Frucht H, Gardner JD, Jensen RT (1991) Pharmacokinetics of oral and intravenous omeprazole in patients with the Zollinger-Ellison syndrome. *Gastroenterology* 101: 138–147
33 Metz DC, Pisegna JR, Ringham GL, Feigenbaum KM, Koviack PD, Maton PN, Gardner JD, Jensen RT (1993) Prospective study of efficacy and safety of lansoprazole in Zollinger-Ellison syndrome. *Dig Dis Sci* 38: 245–256
34 Termanini B, Gibril F, Stewart CA, Weber HC, Jensen RT (1996) A prospective study of the effectiveness of low dose omeprazole as initial therapy in Zollinger-Ellison syndrome. *Aliment Pharmacol Ther* 10: 61–71
35 Metz DC, Pisegna JR, Fishbeyn VA, Benya RV, Jensen RT (1993) Control of gastric acid hypersecretion in the management of patients with Zollinger-Ellison syndrome. *World J Surg* 17: 468–480
36 Jensen RT, Metz DC, Koviack PD, Feigenbaum KM (1993) Prospective study of the long-term efficacy and safety of lansoprazole in patients with Zollinger-Ellison syndrome. *Aliment Pharmacol Ther* 7 (Suppl 1): 41–50
37 Mignon M, Pospai D, Forestier S, Vatier J, Vallot T (1993) Treatment of patients with Zollinger-Ellison syndrome. *Clin Ther* 15: 22–31
38 Hirschowitz BI, Mohnen J, Shaw S (1996) Long-term treatment with lansoprazole for patients with Zollinger-Ellison syndrome. *Aliment Pharmacol Ther* 10: 507–522
39 Radebold K, Bornman PC, van Wyk MEC, Kaye P, Marks IN, Terblanche J (1997) Preliminary results of the proton-pump inhibitor pantoprazole in patients with Zollinger-Ellison syndrome. *Gastroenterology* 112: A37
40 Creutzfeldt W (1988) The achlorhydria-carcinoid sequence: role of gastrin. *Digestion* 39: 61–79
41 Wormsley KG (1988) Is chronic long-term inhibition of gastric secretion really dangerous. *Scand J Gastroenterol Suppl* 146: 166–174
42 Arnold R (1994) Safety of proton pump inhibitors – an overview. *Aliment Pharmacol Ther* 8: 65–70
43 Stewart CA, Termanini B, Sutliff VE, Serrano J, Yu F, Gibril F, Jensen RT (1998) Assessment of the risk of iron malabsorption in patients with Zollinger-Ellison syndrome treated with long-term gastric acid antisecretory therapy. *Aliment Pharmacol Ther* 12: 83–98
44 Termanini B, Gibril F, Sutliff VE III, Yu F, Venzon DJ, Jensen RT (1998) Effect of long-term gastric acid suppressive therapy on serum vitamin B_{12} levels in patients with Zollinger-Ellison syndrome. *Am J Med* 104: 422–430
45 Koop H (1992) Review article: metabolic consequences of long-term inhibition of acid secretion by omeprazole. *Aliment Pharmacol Ther* 6: 399–406
46 Koop H, Bachem MG (1992) Serum iron, ferritin and vitamin B_{12} during prolonged omeprazole therapy. *J Clin Gastroenterol* 14: 288–292
47 Dutta SK (1994) Editorial: vitamin B_{12} malabsorption and omeprazole therapy. *J Am Coll Nutr* 13: 544–545
48 Ekman L, Hansson E, Havu N, Carlsson E, Lundberg C (1985) Toxicological studies on omeprazole. *Scand J Gastroenterol* 20 (Suppl 108): 53–69
49 Marcuard SP, Albernaz L, Khazanie PG (1994) Omeprazole therapy causes malabsorption of cyanocobalamin (vitamin B_{12}). *Ann Intern Med* 120: 211–215
50 Havu N (1986) Enterochromaffin-like cell carcinoids of gastric mucosa in rats after life-long inhibition of gastric secretion. *Digestion* 35 (Suppl 1): 42–55
51 Hakanson R, Ekelund M, Sundler F (1984) Activation and proliferation of gastric endocrine cells. In: S Falkmer, R Hakanson, F Sundler (eds): *Evolution and tumor pathology of the neuroendocrine system*. Elsevier, Amsterdam, 371–398
52 Helander HF, Bordi C (1995) Morphology of gastric mucosa during prolonged hypergastrinemia. In: Mignon, RT Jensen (eds): *Endocrine tumors of the pancreas: recent advances in research and management. Series: Frontiers in Gastrointestinal Research*. S. Karger, Basel, Switzerland, 372–384
53 Mattsson H, Havu N, Brautigam J, Carlsson K, Lundell L, Carlsson E (1991) Partial gastric corpectomy results in hypergastrinemia and development of gastric enterochromaffinlike-cell carcinoids in the rat. *Gastroenterology* 100: 311–319

54 Havu N, Mattsson H, Ekman L, Carlsson E (1990) Enterochromaffin-like cell carcinoids in the rat gastric mucosa following long-term administration of ranitidine. *Digestion* 45: 189–195
55 Rindi G, Bordi C, Rappel S, La Rosa S, Stolte M, Solcia E (1996) Gastric carcinoids and neuroendocrine carcinomas: pathogenesis, pathology, and behavior. *World J Surg* 20: 168–172
56 D'Adda T, Corleto V, Pilato FP, Baggi MT, Robutti F, Delle Fave G, Bordi C (1990) Quantitative ultrastructure of endocrine cells of oxyntic mucosa in Zollinger-Ellison syndrome. Correspondence with light microscopic findings. *Gastroenterology* 99: 17–26
57 Lehy T, Cadiot G, Mignon M, Ruszniewski P, Bonfils S (1992) Influence of multiple endocrine neoplasia type 1 on gastric endocrine cells in patients with the Zollinger-Ellison syndrome. *Gut* 33: 1275–1279
58 Jensen RT (1993) Gastrinoma as a model for prolonged hypergastrinemia in man. In: JH Walsh (ed): *Gastrin*. Raven Press, New York, 373–393
59 Cadiot G, Vissuzaine C, Potet F, Mignon M (1995) Fundic argyrophil carcinoid tumor in a patient with sporadic-type Zollinger-Ellison syndrome. *Dig Dis Sci* 40: 1275–1278
60 Chandrasekharappa SC, Guru SC, Manickam P, Olufemi SE, Collins FS, Emmert-Buck MR, Debelenko LV, Zhuang Z, Lubensky IA, Liotta LA et al (1997) Positional cloning of the gene for multiple endocrine neoplasia-Type 1. *Science* 276: 404–407
61 Maton PN, Lack EE, Collen MJ, Cornelius MJ, David E, Gardner JD, Jensen RT (1990) The effect of Zollinger-Ellison syndrome and omeprazole therapy on gastric oxyntic endocrine cells. *Gastroenterology* 99: 943–950
62 Schenk BE, Festen HPM, Kuipers EJ, Klinkenberg-Knol EC, Meuwissen GM (1996) Effect of short- and long-term treatment with omeprazole on the absorption and serum levels of cobalamin. *Aliment Pharmacol Ther* 10: 541–545
63 Hakanson R, Sundler F (1986) Mechanisms for the development of gastric carcinoids. *Digestion* 35 (Suppl 1): 1–151
64 Lamberts R, Creutzfeldt W, Stockmann F, Jacubaschke U, Maas S, Brunner G (1988) Long-term omeprazole treatment in man: effects on gastric endocrine cell populations. *Digestion* 39: 126–135
65 Cook JD, Lipschitz DA, Miles LEM, Finch CA (1974) Serum ferritin as a measure of iron stores in normal subjects. *Am J Clin Nutr* 27: 681–687
66 London J, Frucht H, Doppman JL, Maton PN, Gardner JD, Jensen RT (1989) Zollinger-Ellison syndrome in the acute care setting. *J Intensive Care Med* 4: 272–283
67 Vinayek R, Frucht H, London JF, Miller LS, Stark HA, Norton JA, Cederberg C, Jensen RT, Gardner JD, Maton PN (1990) Intravenous omeprazole in patients with Zollinger-Ellison syndrome undergoing surgery. *Gastroenterology* 99: 10–16
68 Vinayek R, Hahne WF, Euler AR, Norton JA, Jensen RT (1993) Parenteral control of gastric hypersecretion in patients with Zollinger-Ellison syndrome. *Dig Dis Sci* 38: 1857–1865
69 Saeed ZA, Norton JA, Frank WO, Young MD, Maton PN, Gardner JD, Jensen RT (1989) Parenteral antisecretory drug therapy in patients with Zollinger-Ellison syndrome. *Gastroenterology* 96: 1393–1402

Proton Pump Inhibitors
ed. by L. Olbe

Gastro-oesophageal reflux disease

Lars Lundell[1] and John Dent[2]

[1] *Department of Surgery, Sahlgren's University Hospital, University of Gothenburg, Sweden*
[2] *Gastroenterology Unit, Royal Adelaide Hospital, University of Adelaide, South Australia*

Introduction

Gastro-oesophageal reflux disease (GORD) can be broadly defined as troublesome symptoms which occur as a consequence of the reflux of gastric juice with or without oesophageal mucosal damage. For nearly all patients with reflux disease, symptoms are the motivation for seeking diagnosis and/or therapy. Research shows that many clinicians do not appreciate how severely reflux symptoms affect a patient's quality of life [1–6]. Assessments of quality of life using standard instruments have demonstrated that patients with untreated reflux oesophagitis have marked impairment of their quality of life that is markedly influenced by anxiety about the source of the symptoms.

Over the last decade we have seen significant progress in assessment and treatment of GORD [7], and recently the nature and management of endoscopy-negative reflux disease have been substantially clarified. The proton pump inhibitors (PPIs) represent an enormous therapeutic advantage for reflux disease, to the extent that they have become the medical treatment of choice because of their superior efficacy in association with an excellent tolerability and safety profile. This efficacy of PPIs hinges on the superiority of these drugs to reduce food-stimulated acid secretion and consequently the pH of the refluxate. Even when a treatment option has been defined by a series of clinical trials, its use in clinical practice usually requires further refinement. This is particularly relevant when there are several options for management of the same disease as is the case of GORD. Important strategic questions relevant to the management of reflux disease still need to be further researched, but at the present state of knowledge the role of PPIs is central in the following clinical areas: to optimize the approach to diagnosis based on symptom analysis and the utility of the response to treatment in the diagnostic work-up, to achieve the most appropriate initial treatment allowing also a practical assessment of the outcome of ongoing drug therapy and then in the choice of long-term therapy, given the now well-documented chronicity of reflux disease.

Clinical evaluation and significance of reflux symptoms

Analysis of symptom pattern is vital for prompt and cost-effective diagnosis of reflux disease. In a substantial number of patients, evaluation of the nature of these sensations and the relationship of them to provocation of reflux, such as food ingestion and postural stress, allows a confident diagnosis without further assessment [8–12]. Endoscopy is not an effective alternative to symptom evaluation for several reasons, most important among them that two-thirds of people with troublesome reflux symptoms have no endoscopic oesophagitis [1, 13]. For reasons of practicality, cost and even diagnostic sensitivity, oesophageal pH monitoring cannot substitute for symptom evaluation [7]. Until this decade there was a substantial clinical emphasis on nighttime reflux and its associated symptoms, in contrast to what most patients report about the timing of their reflux symptoms [2, 3, 9]. It is now well established that GORD is primarily a disease of daytime, food-provoked oesophageal acid exposure. Contrary to widely held assumptions, nocturnal acid exposure is unusual in mild or moderate GORD and contributes significantly only to more severe forms of the disease [8].

Symptom frequency and intensity are the most important measures of the severity of GORD and will support a treatment aim of symptom relief. Patients enrolled in different clinical trials who had troublesome reflux symptoms but no endoscopic evidence of oesophagitis showed a similar distribution of severity of heartburn compared with patients with severe oesophagitis [13–20]. Consequently, oesophagitis and symptom severity should be taken as independent and equally important measures of severity of reflux disease and assessed separately. Trials with effective therapies have shown that symptom relief is an important measurable outcome variable which is reflected in normalisation of quality of life [20].

The clinical usefulness of a therapeutic test

Abolition of abnormal oesophageal acid exposure is a powerful predictor of successful treatment of reflux disease [17, 21, 22]. This information may assist in the management of individual patients in whom the cause of symptoms is unclear, and normalisation of acid exposure during therapy indicates successful treatment (Fig. 1). It should be noted that control of oesophageal acid exposure cannot always be achieved with standard doses of PPIs, as a minority of patients will require higher doses [23].

A therapeutic test with PPIs is a useful option for assistance with diagnosis provided that a careful symptom analysis suggests reflux disease. A therapeutic test can also be helpful for recognition of reflux-induced hoarseness and asthma and in patients with noncardiac chest pain [24–28]. These diseases have a high prevalence in the population, as does GORD

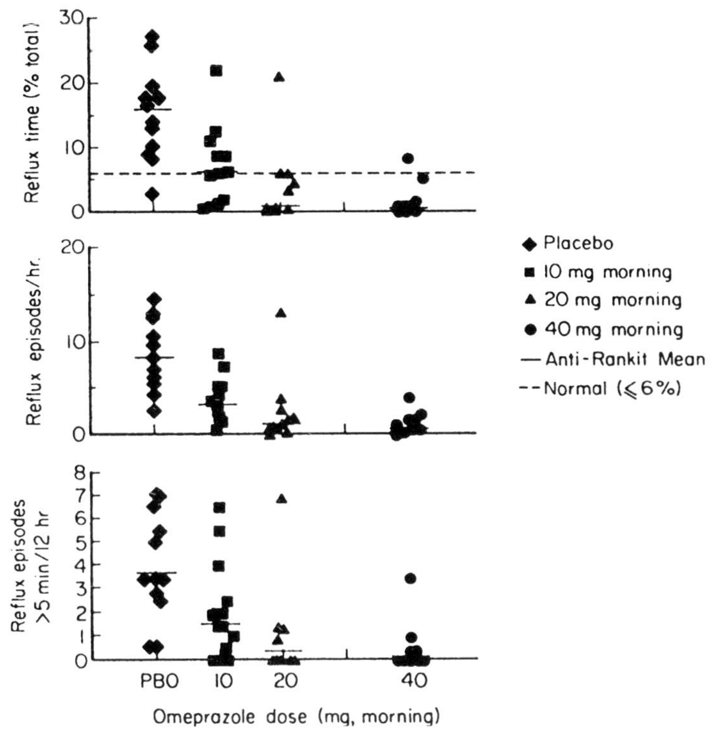

Figure 1. Oesophageal acid exposure as assessed by use of ambulatory 24-h pH monitoring before and during different doses of omeprazole [22].

[29], and they will co-exist in a proportion of patients whether they are linked or not. The effectiveness of a therapeutic test depends on the introduction of acid inhibition which is strong enough to abolish or almost completely prevent acid reflux and the continuation of treatment for a time period which is long enough to ascertain whether the symptoms have been resolved or at least substantially improved.

There are several reports on the role of a therapeutic test with PPIs in the treatment of GORD [30–33]. Empirical treatment with 80 mg daily of omeprazole was shown to be slightly more sensitive and cheaper than acid-perfusion testing and symptom-index pH monitoring in a group of patients with noncardiac chest symptoms of probable oesophageal origin. In one study, the diagnosis of endoscopy-negative reflux disease was evaluated by treatment with 40 mg of omeprazole for 1 week. The primary end point was the disappearance of symptoms, and a symptom reduction of >75% was considered a positive test result. The omeprazole therapeutic test was again shown to be slightly more sensitive than pH monitoring despite the fact that the dose of omeprazole used was probably not sufficiently high for optimal results in this setting. Another study [32] compared 24-h pH monitoring of

PPI therapy as a diagnostic test in patients with noncardiac chest symptoms potentially linked to GORD. In the group of patients treated with omeprazole 80 mg daily, all patients showed improvement in symptoms, and the majority showed abolition of acid reflux.

A further study [33] enrolled dyspeptic patients with heartburn, where the patients were randomly allocated to treatment with either 20 mg twice daily of omeprazole or placebo for 1 week. Symptom improvement was considered a positive therapeutic outcome, and the sensitivity of omeprazole administration was reported to be 71–81%, compared with 36–47% for placebo. It can therefore be concluded that the therapeutic test is a useful step in the evaluation of suspect reflux disease either before or after endoscopy and is an attractive substitute for pH monitoring in many patients.

There have been several studies on the effect of antireflux treatment with PPIs on asthma, usually comprising small samples of patients. Improved symptoms and/or lung functions have been observed in omeprazole-treated patients but in individual patients only, and it can thus be concluded that improvement of asthma by antisecretory treatment does occur but appears to be uncommon [34–38]. The situation concerning hoarseness and laryngitis is even less clear [39–40]. It can, however, be argued that in some patients with respiratory symptoms, in particular broncheal asthma, coexisting with symptomatic GORD, a therapeutic test with antireflux treatment seems advisable.

Studies suggest that a therapeutic test should consist of a PPI given preferably at least twice the natural dose for 1, possibly 2 weeks. In the case of investigation of the possibility that respiratory symptoms are caused by GORD, the period of treatment should probably be longer (2–4 weeks).

The short-term efficacy of PPIs

The general effectiveness of the PPIs for the treatment of GORD is now widely recognised and translated into clinical practice. PPIs have become the drug of choice for short-term treatment of well-defined reflux oesophagitis and are also increasingly popular options in the treatment of endoscopy-negative reflux disease. The first PPI, omeprazole, was originally shown to be highly effective in promoting healing of oesophagitis [41], and a historically interesting fact is that one of the present authors (J. D.) presented the first clinical results with omeprazole in severe peptic oesophagitis at the same meeting of the Australian Gastroenterological Society where Barry Marshall reported that the bacteria *Campylobacter pyloridis* might be the pathogenetic cause of peptic ulcer disease. Numerous studies subsequently documented the superiority of PPIs over H_2-receptor antagonists both with respect to healing of the oesophagitis and the relief of symptoms (Fig. 2). Clinical trials which have evaluated the dose response

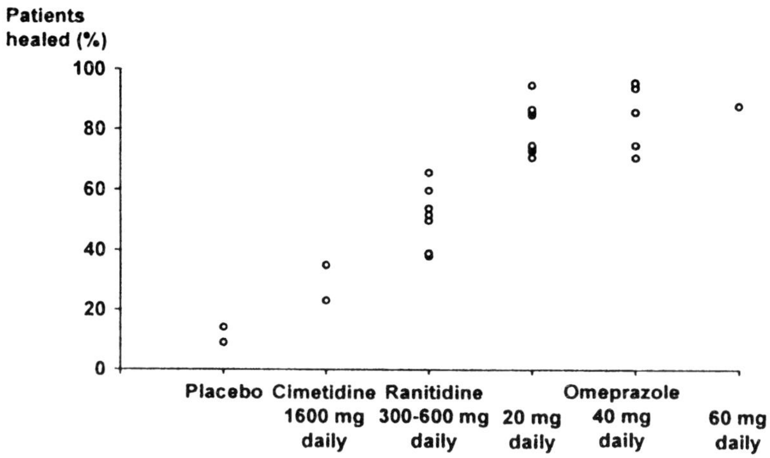

Figure 2. Endoscopic healing and symptom relief in patients with oesophagitis treated with either PPIs or H_2-receptor antagonists.

to omeprazole therapy have documented small increases or no significant differences in healing rates after 4 and 8 weeks between 20 and 40 mg daily of omeprazole [21, 41–53]. Patients needing a larger dose for healing have a reduced responsiveness to acid inhibition, as documented by insufficient reduction of oesophageal acid exposure during standard dose treatment [23]. The pretreatment severity of the oesophagitis is a primary prognostic factor for the subsequent mucosal healing and symptom relief of therapy. Other potentially important prognostic factors (such as smoking habits, body habitus, alcohol consumption etc.) have been considered to be relevant factors that influence reflux disease, but in a comprehensive analysis only the patient's age has been known to be an important prognostic factor for the outcome of PPI treatment, with PPI being more effective in older patients. This effect is most likely explained by an age-dependent difference in bioavailability.

When studies are evaluated which compare different PPIs, it is important to note whether equipotent doses are used [54, 55]. Gastric acidity studies during treatment have indicated that, for example, the efficacy of 20 mg of omeprazole daily compares with that of 30 mg of lansoprazole daily. In this particular aspect, this dose of lansoprazole was found inferior or equal to 40 mg of omeprazole. Lansoprazole may have a slightly higher bioavailability than omeprazole, which may explain some observations. Lansoprazole 30 mg was found to be slightly more effective in decreasing gastric acidity than 40 mg of pantoprazole when studied during the 1st and the 7th day of treatment [56–69]. When differences have been found in the levels of acid suppression produced by standard doses of different PPIs, these have been relatively small, and of unclear clinical significance.

All studies of the healing of oesophagitis during 4 to 8 weeks of PPI therapy have shown that symptom resolution is a good indicator of healing of oesophagitis. Data from diary cards confirmed the rapid symptomatic response with PPI therapy. The clinical implication is that there is no need for endoscopic control of healing of the oesophagitis provided that reflux-induced symptoms have resolved.

Endoscopy-negative reflux disease

Recent research in patients with endoscopy-negative reflux disease have shown chronicity and relapse when treatment is stopped and disability from symptoms with essentially the same pattern as are found in patients with reflux oesophagitis [3, 13, 16, 18]. Also, endoscopy-negative patients respond similarly to therapy. Data on therapeutic effects on endoscopy-negative GORD are only available for omeprazole in daily doses from 10 to 20 mg. In trials, absence of heartburn occurred significantly more often in patients treated with 20 mg daily of omeprazole than in those allocated to omeprazole 10 mg, ranitidine 150 mg bid and cisapride 10 mg given 4 times daily (Fig. 3) [13, 15–19, 34, 70, 71]. The number of patients having sufficient control of heartburn was clearly higher compared with the stricter end points of complete relief of heartburn. This suggests that minor reflux symptoms are usually not a major problem for patients. Parallel with

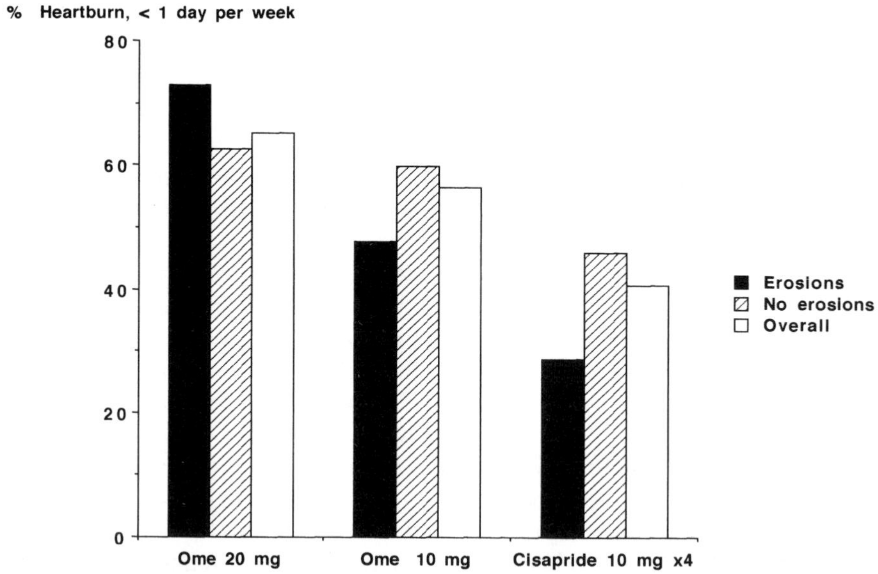

Figure 3. Absence of heartburn after 4 weeks of treatment with either omeprazole or cisapride [15].

these effects on control of reflux symptoms, measurements showed that patients had a normalisation of their quality of life. Of importance was the finding that control of heartburn occurred more frequently in endoscopy-negative patients with abnormal levels of oesophageal acid exposure then in those who had normal acid reflux variables [18]. It is also worth noting that a less effective treatment response was observed in patients who scored higher for other concomitant complaints such as irritable bowel symptoms and anxiety [13, 16].

PPIs in the long-term treatment

Reflux disease is usually a significant recurrent problem if the pretreatment symptoms are troublesome enough to cause significant disability and impaired quality of life. In patients with relatively severe oesophagitis, withdrawal of short-term therapy has been associated with symptomatic and endoscopic relapse in most patients. The response to short-term PPI treatment has proved to be a reliable predictor of efficacy during long-term treatment [40, 48, 70]. PPIs have been shown to be effective and safe when used as maintenance therapy [72–77]; omeprazole 20 mg daily is more effective than a daily dose of 10 mg in preventing symptom recurrence and in keeping the oesophageal mucosa completely healed when given over 6 months. Comparative trials have shown that both 20 and 10 mg of omeprazole are significantly more effective than placebo, H_2-receptor antagonists or cisapride (Fig. 4). As with omeprazole, trials of long-term therapy with lanzoprazole have shown that both 30 and 15 mg daily are superior to placebo and ranitidine [78–80]. In order to minimise drug exposure and cost, maintenance treatment may therefore be started with or stepped down to a lower dose of PPI given once daily. However, the physician should be prepared to return to full dosage if relapse of symptoms indicates this dose to be suboptimal. This strategy is based on the evidence that relief from heartburn is highly predictive of maintained healing of oesophagitis [70]. Even in patients with more severe grades of oesophagitis, omeprazole 20 mg daily is adequate in all but a minority of cases, and this effect can be maintained for years [81, 82].

Symptom relapse also occurs in most endoscopy-negative reflux disease patients after cessation of treatment. Therefore, long-term maintenance therapy needs to be developed also for this patient group [20]. Two therapeutic approaches with omeprazole have been evaluated, either continuous [83] or “on demand” treatment [84]. Continuous treatment maintains most patients in clinical remission, but a similar effect on patient satisfaction was obtained with omeprazole therapy on demand (Fig. 5). On an average, omeprazole 20 mg was taken every other day when the on-demand strategy was tested. It is important to identify patients who complain of frequent and severe reflux symptoms and who will sub-

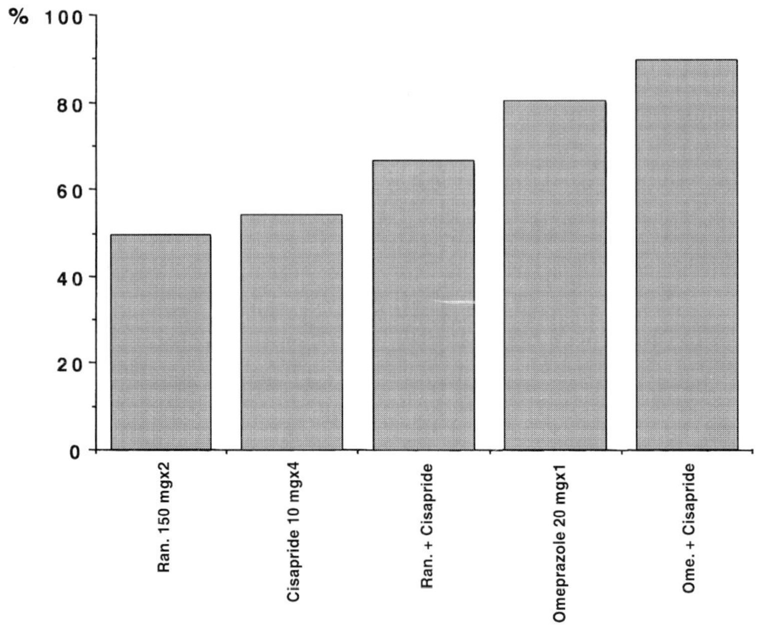

Figure 4. Remission rates (presented as percentage of healed oesophagitis reported at 12 months on therapy with different maintenance regimens). Adopted from ref. 77.

sequently require long-term therapy, either in the form of continuous or on-demand regimen.

Some reflux disease patients present with oesophageal stricture. They are often elderly and have no prior history of obvious and/or severe reflux symptoms. It is believed that stricture forms owing to deep ulcers and circumferential erosions which cause fibrous scarring. Identification of severe reflux oesophagitis at a young age and effective treatment with PPIs should decrease the risk of oesophageal stricture [80, 85, 86]. For those who have already developed a peptic oesophageal stricture, it is mandatory that any dilatation procedure be followed by effective antireflux therapy in the form of PPIs. These drugs have shown to be effective in preventing relapse of stricture and all of the associated risks and costs.

Resistance to healing of oesophagitis with PPIs is rare, but when it occurs is associated with persistently abnormal oesophageal acid exposure on treatment. This may relate to reduced responsiveness to acid inhibition, which may be associated with, or independent of, for instance, Zollinger-Ellison syndrome. Usually this problem can be overcome by dose escalation to high levels. Some patients on PPI therapy may continue to suffer from regurgitation (volume reflux) of nonacidic gastric contents [87], although most clinical trials with PPIs have shown beneficial effects on regurgitation in patients in whom it is not especially voluminous. The question whether PPI therapy is a suitable alternative to antireflux surgery

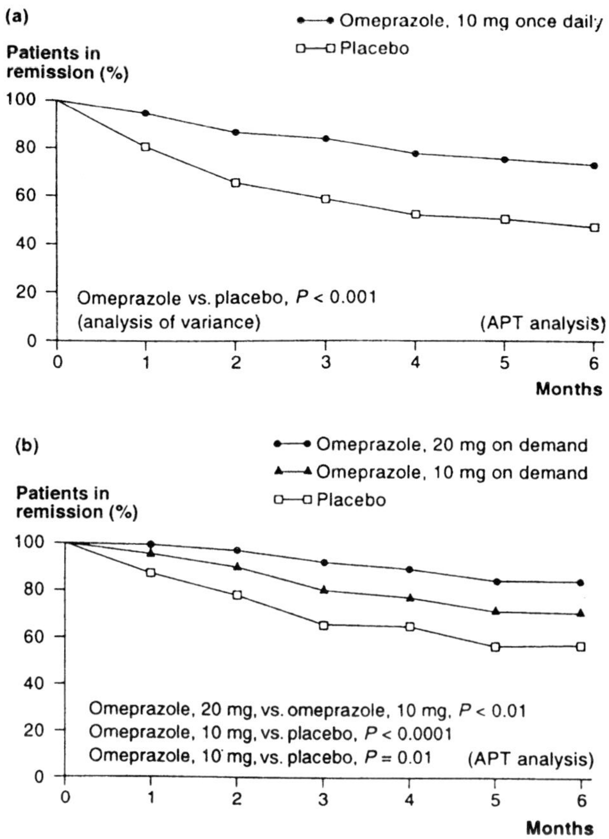

Figure 5. Sufficient control of heartburn during 6 months of maintenance therapy in endoscopy-negative reflux disease. Omeprazole was either given "on demand" (*b*) in doses of 10 or 20 mg or as continuous therapy (*a*) with 10 mg daily compared with placebo. Adopted from refs. 83 and 84.

in the long-term management of GORD is an important one that requires objective evaluation. Very recently, 3-year follow-up data from a randomised clinical trial comparing antireflux surgery with omeprazole showed that antireflux surgery and long-term PPI therapy have comparable benefits provided that there is an opportunity to increase omeprazole if the response to the standard dosage is suboptimal [88].

Conclusions

In contrast to previously available medical therapies, PPIs have proved to be effective in all clinical situations where pharmacological intervention in GORD is indicated. These drugs are very safe and well tolerated [89–91]. In the short term, they heal oesophageal mucosal breaks and relieve symptoms effectively. However, no medical therapy permanently corrects the various pathophysiological disturbances typical of GORD, and unless changeable lifestyle factors are responsible for the condition, relapse is very likely to occur when therapy is stopped. PPIs are very well suited for long-term therapy of reflux disease due to their high efficacy, convenience and reassuring safety profile.

References

1 Spechler SJ (1992) Epidemiology and natural history of gastro-oesophageal reflux disease. *Digestion* 51 (Suppl 1): 24–29
2 Nebel OT, Fornes MF, Castell DO (1976) Symptomatic gastroesophageal reflux: incidence and precipitating factors. *Dig Dis* 21: 953–956
3 Galmiche J-P, Bruley des Varannes S (1994) Symptoms and disease severity in gastro-oesophageal reflux disease. *Scand J Gastroenterol* 29 (Suppl 201): 62–68
4 Jones RH, Lydeard SE, Hobbs FDR et al (1990) Dyspepsia in England and Scotland. *Gut* 31: 401–405
5 Glise H, Hallerbäck B, Johansson B (1995) Quality of life assessments in the evaluation of gastroesophageal reflux and peptic ulcer disease before, during and after treatment. *Scand J Gastroenterol* 208: 133–135
6 Dimenäs E, Glise H, Hallerbäck B et al (1995) Well-being and gastrointestinal symptoms among patients referred to endoscopy owing to suspected duodenal ulcer. *Scand J Gastroenterol* 30: 1046–1052
7 Armstrong D, Emde C, Inauen W et al (1992) Diagnostic assessment of gastroesophageal reflux disease: what is possible vs what is practical. *Hepatogastroenterology* 39 (Suppl): 3–13
8 Robertson D, Aldersley M, Shepherd H et al (1987) Patterns of acid reflux in complicated oesophagitis. *Gut* 28: 1484–1488
9 Johnsson L, Adlouni W, Johnsson F et al (1992) Timing of reflux symptoms and esophageal acid exposure. *Gullet* 2: 58–62
10 Kister E, Ros E, Toledo-Pimental V et al (1994) Predictive factors of long-term outcome in gastro-oesophageal reflux disease; six years follow-up of 107 patients. *Gut* 35: 8–14
11 McDougall NI, Johnston BT, Kee F et al (1996) Natural history of reflux oesophagitis: a 10-year follow-up of its effect on patient symptomatology and quality of life. *Gut* 38: 481–486
12 Klauser AG, Schindlbeck NE, Müller-Lissner SA (1990) Symptoms in gastro-oesophageal reflux disease. *Lancet* 335: 205–208
13 Carlsson R, Dent J, Watts R et al (1998) Gastro-oesophageal reflux disease (GORD) in primary care – an international study of different treatment strategies with omeprazole. *Eur J Gastroenterol Heptatol* 10: 119–124
14 Green JRB (1993) Is there such an entity as mild oesophagitis? *Eur J Clin Res* 4: 29–34
15 Galmiche J-P, Barthelemy P, Hamelin B (1997) Treating the symptoms of gastroesophageal reflux disease. A double-blind comparison of omeprazole and cisapride. *Aliment Pharmacol Ther* 11: 765–773
16 Lind T, Havelund T, Glise H et al (1995) Omeprazole improves quality of life in patients with endoscopy negative reflux disease. *Gastroenterology* 108: A151
17 Shi G, Bruley des Varannes S, Scarpignato C et al (1995) Reflux-related symptoms in patients with normal oesophageal exposure to acid. *Gut* 37: 457–464
18 Lind T, Havelund T, Carlsson R et al (1997) Heartburn without oesophagitis: efficacy of omeprazole therapy and features determining therapeutic response. *Scand J Gastroenterol* 32: 974–979
19 Bate CM, Griffin SM, Keeling PWN et al (1996) Reflux symptom relief with omeprazole in patients without unequivocal oesophagitis. *Aliment Pharmacol Ther* 10: 547–555
20 Lundell L (1997) New information relevant to long-term management of endoscopy-negative reflux disease. *Aliment Pharmacol Ther* 11 (Suppl 2): 93–98
21 Sharma BK, Walt RP, Pounder RE et al (1984) Optimal dose of oral omeprazole for maximal 24-hour decrease of intragastric acidity. *Gut* 25: 957–964

22 Robinson M, Maton PN, Allen ML et al (1991) Effect of different doses of omeprazole on 24-hour oesophageal acid exposure in patients with gastro-oesophageal reflux. *Aliment Pharmacol Ther* 5: 645–661
23 Holloway RH, Dent J, Narielvala F et al (1996) Relation between oesophageal acid exposure and healing of oesophagitis with omeprazole in patients with severe reflux oesophagitis. *Gut* 38: 649–654
24 Chauhan A, Petch MC, Schofield PM (1996) Cardio-oesophageal reflux in humans as a mechanism for "linked angina". *Eur Heart J* 17: 407–413
25 Waring JP, Lacayo L, Hunter J et al (1995) Chronic cough and hoarseness in patients with severe gastroesophageal reflux disease. *Dig Dis Sci* 40: 1093–1097
26 Wiener GJ, Koufan JA, Wu WC et al (1989) Chronic hoarseness secondary to gastroesophageal reflux disease: documentation with 24-hr ambulatory pH monitoring. *Am J Gastroenterol* 84: 1503–1508
27 Wilson JA, White A, von Haacke NP et al (1989) Gastro-oesophageal reflux and posterior laryngitis. *Ann Otol Rhinol Laryngol* 98: 405–410
28 Mehta AJ, de Caestecker JS, Camm AJ et al (1996) Gastro-oesophageal reflux in patients with coronary artery disease: how common is it and does it matter? *Eur J Gastroenterol Hepatol* 8: 973–978
29 Heading RC (1989) Epidemiology of oesophageal reflux disease. *Scand J Gastroenterol* 24 (Suppl 168): 33–37
30 Schenk BE, Kuipers EJ, Klinkenberg-Knol EC, Festen HPM, Jansen EH, Tuynman HARE, Schrijver M, Dieleman KA, Meuwissen SGM (1997) Omeprazole as a diagnostic tool in gastroesophageal reflux disease. *Am J Gastroenterol* 92: 1997–2000
31 Jaup BH (1995) Effective acid inhibition as a diagnostic tool for gastroesophageal reflux disease. *Gut* 37 (Suppl 2): A36
32 Schindlbeck NE, Klauser AG, Voderholzer WA et al (1995) Empiric therapy for gastroesophageal reflux disease. *Arch Intern Med* 155: 1808–1812
33 Johnsson F, Weyvadt L, Solhaug JH et al (1998) One-week omeprazole treatment as a diagnostic test for gastro-oesophageal reflux disease. *Scand J Gastroenterol* 33: 15–20
34 Depla AC, Bartelsman JF, Roos CM et al (1988) Beneficial effect of omeprazole in a patient with severe bronchial asthma and gastro-oesophageal reflux. *Eur Respir J* 1: 966–968
35 Harding SM, Richter JE, Guzzo MR et al (1996) Asthma and gastroesophageal reflux: acid suppressive therapy improves asthma outcome. *Am J Med* 100: 395–405
36 DalNegro R, Pomari C, Turco P et al (1994) Gastroesophageal reflux and bronchial asthma: a cross-over omeprazole vs placebo comparison. *Respir Crit Care Med* 149: 4
37 Ford GA, Oliver PS, Prior JS et al (1994) Omeprazole in the treatment of asthmatics with nocturnal symptoms and gastro-oesophageal reflux: a placebo-controlled cross-over study. *Postgrad Med J* 70: 350–354
38 Meier JH, McNally PR, Punjy MM et al (1994) Does omeprazole improve respiratory function in asthmatics with gastroesophageal reflux? *Dig Dis Sci* 39: 2127–2133
39 Kamel PL, Hanson D, Kahrilas PJ (1994) Omeprazole for the treatment of posterior laryngitis. *Am J Med* 96: 321–326
40 McNally PR, Maydonovitch CL, Prosek RA et al (1989) Evaluation of gastroesophageal reflux as a cause of idiopathic hoarseness. *Dig Dis Sci* 34: 1900–1904
41 Hetzel DJ, Dent J, Reed WR et al (1988) Healing and relapse of severe peptic esophagitis after treatment with omeprazole. *Gastroenterology* 95: 903–912
42 Naesdal J, Bodemar G, Walan A (1984) Effect of omeprazole, a substituted benzimidazole, on 24-h intragastric acidity in patients with peptic ulcer disease. *Scand J Gastroenterol* 19: 916–922
43 Hemery P, Galmiche JP, Roze C (1987) Low-dose omeprazole effects on gastric acid secretion in normal man. *Gastroenterol Clin Biol* 11: 148–153
44 Hendell J, Hendel L, Aggestrup S (1995) Morning or evening dosage of omeprazole for gastro-oesophageal reflux disease. *Aliment Pharmacol Ther* 9: 693–697
45 Klinkenberg-Knol EC, Jansen JMBJ, Festen HPM et al (1987) Double-blind multicentre comparison of omeprazole and ranitidine in the treatment of reflux oesophagitis. *Lancet*: I: 349–351
46 Havelund T, Laursen LS, Skoubo-Kristensen E et al (1988) Omeprazole and ranitidine in treatment of reflux oesophagitis: double-blind comparative trial. *Br Med J* 296: 89–92

47 Vantrappen G, Rutgeerts L, Schurmans P et al (1988) Omeprazole (40 mg) is superior to ranitidine in short-term treatment of ulcerative reflux esophagitis. *Dig Dis Sci* 33: 523–529
48 Sandmark S, Carlsson R, Fausa O et al (1988) Omeprazole or ranitidine in the treatment of reflux esophagitis. *Scand J Gastroenterol* 23: 625–632
49 Zeitoun P, Barbier P, Cayphas JP et al (1989) Comparison of two dosage regimens of omeprazole – 10 mg once daily and 20 mg weekends – as prophylaxis against recurrence of reflux esophagitis. *Hepatogastroenterology* 36: 279–280
50. Dehn TCB, Shepherd HA, Colin-Jones D et al (1990) Double-blind comparison of omeprazole (40 mg od) vs cimetidine (400 mg qd) in the treatment of symptomatic erosive reflux oesophagitis, assessed endoscopically, histologically and by 24-h pH monitoring. *Gut* 31: 509–513
51 Bate CM, Keeling PWN, O'Morain C et al (1990) Comparison of omeprazole and cimetidine in reflux oesophagitis: symptomatic, endoscopic and histological evaluations. *Gut* 31: 968–972
52 Sontag SJ, Hirschowitz BI, Holt S et al (1992) Two doses of omeprazole vs placebo in symptomatic erosive esophagitis: the U.S. multicenter study. *Gastroenterology* 102: 109–118
53 Bate CM, Booth SN, Crowe JP et al (1993) Does 40 mg omeprazole daily offer additional benefit over 20 mg daily in patients requiring more than 4 weeks of treatment for symptomatic reflux oesophagitis? *Aliment Pharmacol Ther* 7: 501–507
54 Dammann HG, von Zur Mühlen A, Balks HJ et al (1993) The effects of lansoprazole, 30 or 60 mg daily, on intragastric pH and on endocrine function in healthy volunteers. *Aliment Pharmacol Ther* 7: 191–196
55 Londong W (1994) Effect of pantoprazole on 24-h intragastric pH and serum gastrin in humans. *Aliment Pharmacol Ther* 8 (Suppl 1): 39–46
56 Benhaim MC, Evreux M, Salducci J et al (1990) Lansoprazole and ranitidine in treatment of reflux oesophagitis: double-blind comparative trial. *Gastroenterology* 98: A20
57 Bardhan KD, Long R, Hawkey CJ et al (1991) Lansoprazole, a new proton-pump blocker, vs Ranitidine in the treatment of erosive reflux esophagitis. *Gastroenterology* 100: A30
58 Robinson M, Sahba B, Avner D et al (1995) A comparison of lansoprazole and ranitidine in the treatment of erosive oesophagitis. *Aliment Pharmacol Ther* 9: 25–31
59 Koop H, Schepp W, Dammann HG et al (1995) Comparative trial of pantoprazole and ranitidine in the treatment of reflux esophagitis. *J Clin Gastroenterol* 20: 192–195
60 Castell DO, Richter JE, Robinson M et al (1996) Efficacy and safety of lansoprazole in the treatment of erosive esophagitis. *Am J Gastroenterol* 91: 1749–1757
61 van Rensburg CJ, Honiball PJ, Grundling HK et al (1996) Efficacy and tolerability of pantoprazole 40 mg vs 80 mg in patients with reflux oesophagitis. *Aliment Pharmacol Ther* 10: 397–401
62 Tolman KG, Sanders SW, Buchi KN (1994) Gastric pH levels after 15 mg and 30 mg of lansoprazole and 20 mg omeprazole. *Gastroenterology* 106: A197
63 Florent C, Forestier S, Akrour O (1996) Comparison of the 24 hour intragastric pH profiles after 30 mg lansoprazole and 40 mg pantoprazole in healthy volunteers. *Gastroenterology* 110: A109
64 Mee AS, Rowley JL (1996) The Lanzoprazole Clinical Research Group. Rapid symptom relief in reflux oesophagitis: a comparison of lansoprazole and omeprazole. *Aliment Pharmacol Ther* 10: 757–763
65 Mulder CJ, Dekker W, Gerretsen M (1996) Lansoprazole 30 mg vs omeprazole 40 mg in the treatment of reflux oesophagitis grade II, III and IVa (a Dutch multicentre trial). *Eur J Gastroenterol Hepatol* 8: 1101–1106
66 Mössner J, Hölscher AH, Herz R et al (1995) A double-blind study of pantoprazole and omeprazole in the treatment of reflux oesophagitis: a multicentre trial. *Aliment Pharmacol Ther* 9: 321–326
67 Corinaldesi R, Valentini M, Belaïche J et al (1995) Pantoprazole and omeprazole in the treatment of reflux oesophagitis: a European multicentre study. *Aliment Pharmacol Ther* 9: 667–671
68 Hotz J, Gangl A, Heinzerling H (1996) Pantoprazole vs. Omeprazole in acute reflux esophagitis. *Gastroenterology* 110: A136
69 Hatlebakk JG, Berstad A, Carling L et al (1993) Lansoprazole vs omeprazole in short-term treatment of reflux oesophagitis. *Scand J Gastroenterol* 28: 224–228

70 Carlsson R, Galmiche JP, Dent J, Lundell L, Frison L (1997) Prognostic facors influencing relapse of oesophagitis during maintenance therapy with antisecretory drugs: a meta-analysis of long-term omeprazole trials. *Aliment Pharmacol Ther* 11: 472–482
71 Venables T, Newland R, Patel AC et al (1997) Omeprazole 10 mg once daily, omeprazole 20 mg once daily or ranitidine 150 mg twice daily, evaluated as initial therapy for the relief of gastro-oesophageal reflux disease in general practice. *Scand J Gastroenterol* 32: 965–973
72 Staerk-Laursen LS, Havelund T, Bondesen S et al (1995) Omeprazole in the long-term treatment of gastro-oesophageal reflux disease. A double-blind randomized dose-finding study. *Scand J Gastroenterol* 30: 839–846
73 Sontag S, Robinson M, Roufail W et al (1997) Daily omeprazole surpasses intermittent dosing in preventing relapse of esophagitis: a US multicenter double-blind study. *Aliment Pharmacol Ther* 11: 373–380
74 Hallerbäck B, Unge P, Carling L et al (1994) Omeprazole or ranitidine in long-term treatment of reflux esophagitis. *Gastroenterology* 107: 1305–1311
75 Dent J, Yeomans ND, Mackinnon M et al (1994) Omeprazole v ranitidine for prevention of relapse in reflux esophagitis. A controlled double-blind trial of their efficacy and safety. *Gut* 35: 590–598
76 Bate CM, Booth SN, Crowe JP et al (1995) Omeprazole 10 mg or 20 mg once daily in the prevention of recurrence of reflux oesophagitis. *Gut* 36: 492–498
77 Vigneri S, Termini R, Leandro G et al (1995) A comparison of maintenance therapies for reflux esophagitis. *N Engl J Med* 333: 1106–1110
78 Robinson M, Lanza F, Avner D et al (1996) Effective maintenance treatment of reflux esophagitis with low-dose lansoprazole. *Ann Intern Med* 124: 859–867
79 Gough AL, Long RG, Cooper BT et al (1996) Lansoprazole vs ranitidine in the maintenance treatment of reflux oesophagitis. *Aliment Pharmacol Ther* 10: 529–539
80 Swarbrick ET, Gough AL, Foster CS et al (1996) Prevention of recurrence of oesophageal stricture, a comparison of lansoprazole and high-dose ranitidine. *Eur J Gastroenterol Hepatol* 8: 431–438
81 Klinkenberg-Knol EC, Festen HMP, Jansen JBMJ et al (1994) Long-term treatment with omeprazole for refractory reflux esophagitis: efficacy and safety. *Ann Intern Med* 121: 161–167
82 Lundell L (1992) Acid suppression in the long-term treatment of peptic stricture and Barrett's oesophagus. *Digestion* 51 (Suppl 1): 49–58
83 Venables TL, Newland RD, Patel AC, Hole J, Copeman MB, Turbitt ML (1997) Maintenance treatment for gastro-oesophageal reflux disease. A placebo-controlled evaluation of 10 milligrams omeprazole once daily in general practice. *Scand J Gastroenterol* 32: 627–632
84 Lind T, Havelund T, Carlsson R et al (1996) The effect of omeprazole (ome) 20 mg and 10 mg daily on heartburn in patients with endoscopy-negative reflux disease (ENRD) treated on an on demand basis. *Gastroenterology* 110: A178
85 Marks RD, Richter JE, Rizzo J et al (1994) Omeprazole vs H_2-receptor antagonists in treating patients with peptic stricture and esophagitis. *Gastroenterology* 106: 907–915
86 Smith PM, Kerr GD, Cockel R et al (1994) A comparison of omeprazole and ranitidine in the prevention of recurrence of benign esophageal stricture. *Gastroenterology* 107: 1312–1318
87 Lundell L, Dalenbäck J, Hattlebakk J, et al (1998) Outcome of open antireflux surgery as assessed in a Nordic Multicentre, prospective clinical trial. *Eur J Surg* 164: 751–757
88 Lundell L, Dalenbäck J, Hattlebakk J, Janatuinen E et al (1998) Omeprazole or antireflux surgery in the long-term management of gastro-oesophageal reflux disease (GERD). Results of a multicentre, randomised clinical trial. AGA, New Orleans, May 1998
89 Fried M, Siegrist H, Frei R et al (1994) Duodenal bacterial overgrowth during treatment in outpatients with omeprazole. *Gut* 35: 23–26
90 Kuipers EJ, Lundell L, Klinkenberg-Knol EC et al (1996) Atrophic gastritis and *Helicobacter pylori* infection in patients with reflux esophagitis treated with omeprazole or fundoplication. *N Engl J Med* 334: 1018–1022
91 Lundell L, Havu N, Andersson A et al (1997) Gastritis development and acid suppression therapy revisited. Results of a randomised clinical study with long-term follow-up. *Gastroenterology* 112: A28

Socio-economic impact of acid-related diseases

Proton Pump Inhibitors
ed. by L. Olbe

Socio-economic impact of acid-related diseases

Hans Glise[1] and Bengt Hallerbäck[2]

[1] *ASTRA Hässle, Göteborg and Department of Surgery University Hospital, S-581 85 Linköping, Sweden*
[2] *Department of Surgery, NÄL S-461 85 Trollhättan, Sweden*

Introduction

Dyspeptic symptoms has been of interest to mankind since the beginning of history, and treatment regimens can be dated back thousands of years. Some early treatments have been found to have a buffering capacity in common with some of today's treatments, aiming to neutralise or inhibit acid production.

In recent years acid-related disorders have been recognised to be very common. Peptic ulcer was early known to be associated with acid: "No acid, no ulcer," Schwarz quipped. Several other upper gastrointestinal conditions were subsequently associated with acid, as the medical treatment improved and acid-reducing agents were shown to be effective in conditions like dyspepsia and nonesophagitis heartburn.

Socio-economic impact is a broad term, including aspects that concern both the individual and society. In this chapter we would like to provide some background for these concepts and to consider how they influence our view of the socio-economic impact of acid-related disorders.

Definition

Acid-related disorders include both organic disease, and functional disorders. Organic diseases are conditions for which anatomical, physiological or histological changes can be identified, taken as proof of the condition and treated. Examples of such diseases are peptic ulcer and gastroesophageal reflux disease (GERD). In functional disorders, like functional dyspepsia, no such changes are evident. The often-used definition of dyspepsia, "persistent or recurrent abdominal pain or abdominal discomfort centred in the upper abdomen" [1], describes symptom profiles in both organic and functional disease.

GERD relates to patients with heartburn and regurgitation indicating reflux disease, which can or cannot be verified at endoscopy. This means that patients without any endoscopic signs of esophagitis as well as patients with normal endoscopic findings are included. It is well known that there is also an overlap between symptoms due to GERD and functional dyspepsia [1].

Prevalence and incidence of acid-related disorders

Peptic ulcer disease is claimed to affect about 10% of the population over a lifetime and 3% annually [2]. Peptic ulcer prevalence seems to be a cohort phenomenon closely connected to *Helicobacter pylori* (*Hp*) infection [3], which is decreasing in the industrialized world due to the lower infection rate among younger people [2, 4]. Diagnosis of peptic ulcer is based on endoscopy or X-ray. In patients with earlier confirmed ulcer and repeated symptoms, diagnosis can be made on this ground.

Heartburn, the principal symptom of GERD, has been reported to affect 40% of the adult population monthly and 7% daily. Heartburn is not always reported as the main symptom in patients with reflux disease, which makes the condition possibly even more common than reported. These problems have led to the construction of specific questionnaires to better identify heartburn patients [5]. Among patients with heartburn, 20–25% have been reported to consult a doctor and 30% of those investigated have signs of reflux esophagitis. On the other hand, severe reflux esophagitis may give rise to very few subjective symptoms. The prevalence of reflux esophagitis has been estimated to 2% in the western world. With the increased interest in reflux disease and access to endoscopy, the diagnosis of reflux esophagitis in British endoscopy units rose from 3 to 19% from 1977 to 1986. The annual incidence of esophagitis has also increased during the last decades. In recent reports the incidence of reflux esophagitis is estimated at 120 per 100,000. Heartburn is more common, with an annual incidence of 0.75–2% [4].

Functional dyspepsia is the most common gastrointestinal disorder. The prevalence of functional dyspepsia is between 14 and 40% [6], and the annual incidence 1% and higher [4]. Patients with functional disorders are generally younger, and females are represented in higher numbers than in the organic diseases. It must be emphasized that not all of the symptoms in this group are acid-related. Acid-inhibitory treatment is effective in less than 50%.

Quality of life in acid related diseases

Instruments used

Patients with acid-related gastrointestinal diseases have been extensively studied with regard to the effect of these disorders on quality of life (QoL).

Interviews have been conducted before diagnosis and during treatment and follow-up after treatment, using diverse instruments, both generic and specific. Generic instruments address the general impact of the disease on patients, daily living and well-being [7]. These instruments can be used for a broad range of medical as well as other conditions of life. The specific instruments focus on symptoms of a specific condition and may be used to follow changes during treatment [7]. Besides these instruments, a variety of psychological instruments have been applied to these groups of patients to assess how acidic related conditions affect individuals [8].

Result of investigations

In patients investigated for abdominal complaints, QoL has been found to be low in patients with duodenal ulcer, gastric ulcer, reflux esophagitis and also with no findings at endoscopy [7, 9]. In fact, QoL is lower in these conditions than in angina pectoris due to surgery and congestive heart failure [7].

In functional and organic conditions, such as nonesophagitis heartburn and reflux esophagitis, QoL outcomes are very similar, indicating that the subjective severity of symptoms, and not objective manifestations of the disease, is the main determinant of impact on well-being [5, 7, 9].

Rates of anxiety are higher with functional conditions, such as dyspepsia, compared with peptic ulcer disease [8], which may influence QoL as well as the consequences of the symptoms [10].

Costs associated with acid-related disorders

The expenditures for a condition/disease can be divided into direct and indirect costs. Individual aspects, such as QoL, can be included among indirect costs. Any comprehensive evaluation must include the view of all parties, that is individuals, employers, the social system, health care providers and other payers such as insurance companies (Tab. 1).

Table 1. Factors for consideration in the socio-economic impact of disease

Direkt costs	Indirect costs
Cost of therapy	Loss of productivity
Consultations	Consultations
Investigations	Sick leave
Travel	Lower working capacity
	Social aspects
	– Impact of disease on the individual
	– QoL

Few studies have been performed to evaluate the total cost associated with specific diseases, and acid-related disorders are no exception. Much early work is inapplicable to the increasing numbers of patients with acid-related diseases. More recent work often focuses on specific aspects of acid-related diseases, seen from a single vantage such as that of a health maintenance organisations (HMO) [11, 12, 13].

Direct costs

The pattern of expenditures for acid-related disorders has changed dramatically since the mid-1970s. New investigational tools such as endoscopy, esophageal 24-h pH metry and *Hp* diagnostics have made diagnoses more reliable. The introduction of new medical treatment regimens, such as H_2-receptor antagonists, proton pump inhibitors and *Hp* eradication treatments, have changed the mode of treatment, resulting in shorter treatment periods, better treatment results and also a decrease in surgical procedures. In California the rate of hospitalisations and surgical procedures for acid-related disorders decreased steadily from 1976 to 1985 [13]. In a calculation of the California Medicaid program, 1976–1985, the total cost for acid-related disorders was reduced by 13%. In the same period the expenditure for drugs was doubled, and costs for hospitalisation/surgery were halved (Fig. 1).

In the United States as a whole, the decrease in hospitalisations for peptic ulcer disease during the late 1970s was found primarily among younger patients. A decline of 24% between 1970 and 1977 and a further 42% from 1978 to 1986 was found for the <65-year group. Among elderly patients,

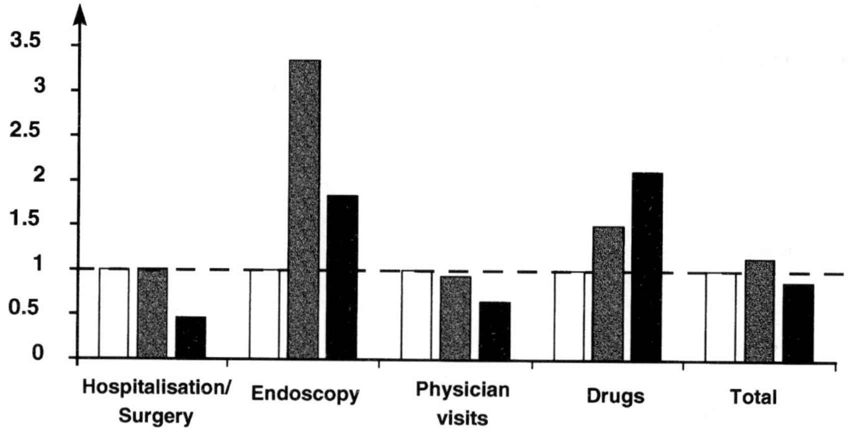

Figure 1. Total relative expenditure for acid-related diseases from 1976 to 1985 in the California Medicaid program divided on the major cost groups. 1976 has been set as 1.0, and 1980 and 1985 show the relative changes from 1976. □ 1976, ▩ 1980, ■ 1985. From ref. 17.

>65 years, there has been no decrease in hospitalisations for peptic ulcer disease, and the death rate has even been reported to have increased, possibly due to the non-steroidal anti-inflammatory drug (NSAID) use.

In another HMO survey, 5.8% of all members were estimated to have an acid-related disorder requiring medical attention, and this prevalence is advancing with age [11]. In the same survey hospital costs were found to be higher for peptic ulcer patients than for GERD or dyspepsia patients. Outpatient costs, on the other hand, were higher among GERD patients, mostly due to the higher prevalence of this condition. Of the total health plan costs of acid-related disorders, GERD (including erosive and non-erosive reflux patients) accounted for 40.6%, peptic ulcer for 36.8% and gastritis/dyspepsia for 22.6% [11]. These cost estimates only consider direct costs measurable in the HMO follow-up systems.

Use of consultations and medication would appear to be hard to evaluate. In dyspepsia, only 1 out of 4 or 5 patients is estimated to make use of health-care resources, but dyspepsia is still one of the most common conditions in ambulatory practice, where 3–7% of physician consultations are believed to be due to dyspepsia [6]. In connection with consultations, over 80% of patients will receive a drug prescription [11, 14], and 25–30% of individuals with dyspepsia or reflux problems will have used drugs to relieve their symptoms during a 3-month period.

Indirect costs

The indirect costs associated with acid-related disorders may well be considerably higher than the direct costs. Indirect costs include sick leave, lower working capacity and social effects of disease. Sick leave has reportedly increased among patients with peptic ulcer and dyspepsia compared with the general population (Fig. 2). In functional dyspepsia, sick leave is also increased due to nonabdominal complaints, mostly musculoskeletal [14], which may be difficult to pinpoint in some statistics. The increase in sick leave among dyspeptic patients may be related to psychological factors, indicated by symptom profiles similar to those of peptic ulcer patients, but higher anxiety and other psychopathology levels in the dyspepsia group [8, 14]. In one study 34% of dyspeptic patients were classified as having a psychiatric condition, mostly anxiety, compared with 15% of peptic ulcer patients and 1% of controls [8]. The rates of psychopathology and anxiety found may explain the increase in consultations for patients with reflux or dyspeptic symptoms [10].

In a recent epidemiological study in a random Swedish population, sick-listing was increased in patients with reflux symptoms or dyspepsia (Fig. 3). For dyspepsia, Nyrén estimated that in 1985, 90% of total costs were related to short-term sick leave, 7% to outpatient care and 2% to drug costs [15].

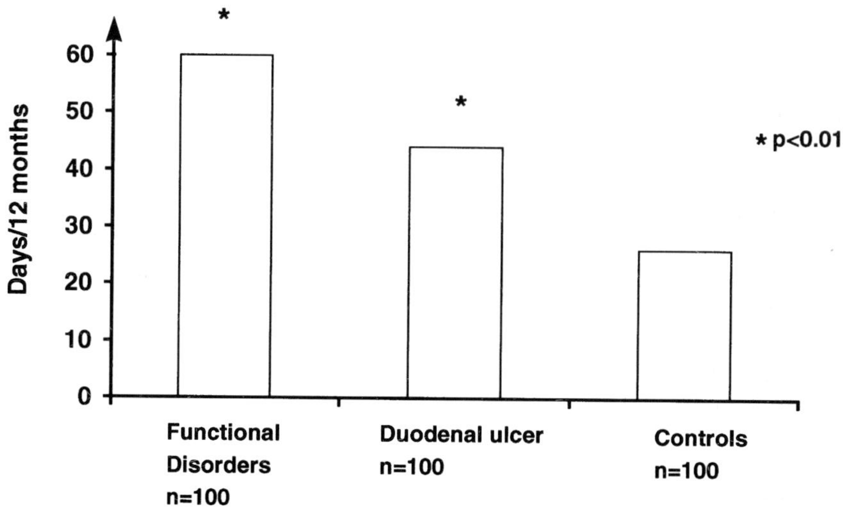

Figure 2. Sick leave during 12 months among controls, duodenal ulcer and functional dyspepsia patients. From ref. 8.

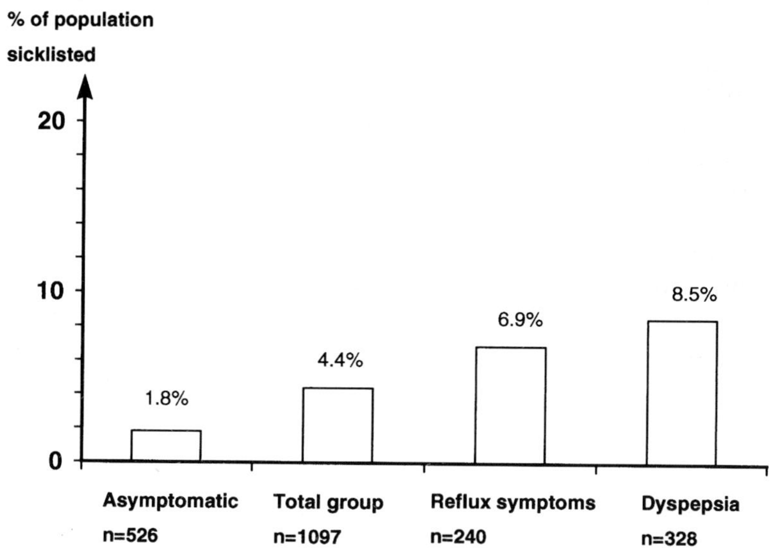

Figure 3. Sick listing at any stage during a 3-month period in a Swedish random study. Individuals have been grouped based on no symptoms or symptoms or reflux and dyspepsia. From ref. 4.

Effect of therapy

Costs for acid-related diseases are also affected by the treatment history and the health-care system. Several studies have shown that different types of medication affect global costs considerably. Treatment effect is significant in terms of both total cost and patients, social situation and QoL. A comparison of different regimens should preferably include both the cost of medication and the outcome of sick leave, hospital use, surgery and QoL. Studies in *Hp* eradication and acid-related disorders have shown that the most effective medication generally seems to be the most cost-effective, due to the relatively small impact of drug cost [16].

There has been a marked change in how patients with acid-related diseases are treated. Today medical treatment is the dominant option. This option started with the introduction of the H_2-receptor antagonists and has been further reinforced with the advent of proton pump inhibitors. Omeprazole, the first proton pump inhibitor, has been proven effective in all acid-related disorders. But the effect of these inhibitors in the functional disorders dyspepsia and nonesophagitis heartburn is generally not as good as in peptic ulcer and reflux esophagitis [5]. This may be explained in part by patient complaints not being acid-related, and in part by the psychological burden of higher levels of anxiety [5, 8, 11, 14], which seems to be a negative factor for treatment success [5]. In GERD, the effect of treatment in endoscopy-negative and -positive patients is clearly related to the medication used. When omeprazole is compared with cisapride or ranitidine, the effect of treatment is far better with omeprazole in both endoscopy-positive patients and endoscopy-negative patients.

Pretreatment anxiety levels, as determined by QoL instruments, predicted treatment outcome. Patients with high levels of anxiety had a lower symptom relief rate than those with low levels of anxiety [5]. Another aspect of medication is the impact on QoL and anxiety. In several studies effective acid inhibition has been shown to normalise QoL in acid-related conditions. Anxiety is the dimension most affected by effective symptomatic treatment in GERD patients.

Total socio-economic impact

The total socio-economic impact of acid-related diseases is difficult, and perhaps impossible, to evaluate. To judge from dyspepsia, the overwhelming cost factor is indirect, which probably is also true for other acid-related conditions.

Effective medical treatment is the ultimate predictor of lower direct costs. Its importance is further emphasised by its effect on symptoms, QoL and general well-being (Fig. 4). In all probability symptoms are the main determinant for short-term sick leave and reduced working capacity, due to

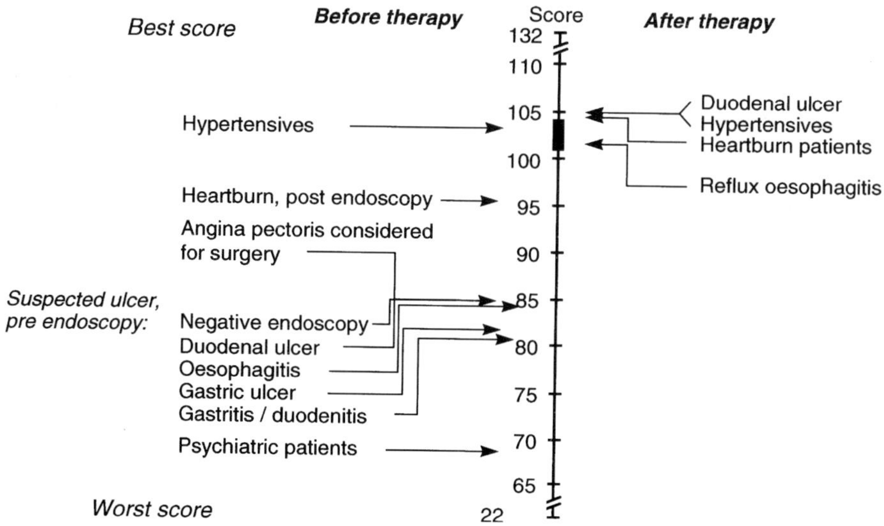

Figure 4. Effect of QoL – the Psychological General Well-Being Index (PGWB) among in patients with acid-related disorders, before and after treatment [7].

the link that seems to exist between symptoms, anxiety and psychopathology. The importance of treatment on these aspects in evaluating the socio-economic impact of acid-related diseases cannot be overstated.

References

1 Talley NJ, Colin-Jones D, Koch KL, Koch M, Nyrén O and Stanghellini V (1991) Functional dyspepsia: a classification with guidelines for diagnosis and management. *Gastroenterol Int* 4: 145–160
2 Sonnenberg A, Everhart JE (1996) The prevalence of self-reported peptic ulcer in the United States. *Am J Public Health* 86: 200–205
3 Van der Hulst RWM, Tytgat GNJ (1996) *Helicobacter pylori* and peptic ulcer disease. *Scand J Gastroenterol* 31: (Suppl 220) 10–18
4 Agreus L (1993) The abdominal symptom study, an epidemiological survey of gastro-intestinal and other abdominal symptoms in the adult population of Östhammar, Sweden. Thesis, Uppsala University, Sweden
5 Carlsson R (1998) Gastroesophageal reflux disease – a study of pathophysiology, clinical diagnosis and management. Thesis, Department of Surgery, University of Göteborg, Sweden
6 Chiba N (1998) Definitions of dyspepsia: time for a reappraisal. *Eur J Surg* (Suppl) 583; *in press*
7 Glise H, Hallerbäck B, Wiklund I (1996) Quality of life: a reflection of symptoms and concerns. *Scand J Gastroent* 31 (Suppl 221): 14–17
8 Haug TT, Svebak S, Wilhelmsen I, Berstad A, Ursin H (1994) Psychological factors and somatic symptoms in functional dyspepsia. A comparison with duodenal ulcer and healthy controls. *J Psycosomatic Res* 38: 281–291
9 Dimenäs E, Glise H, Hallerbäck B, Hernqvist H, Svedlund J, Wiklund I (1995) Well-being and gastrointestinal symptoms among patients referred to endoscopy owing to suspected duodenal ulcer. *Scand J Gastroenterol* 30: 1046–1052
10 Lydeard S, Jones R (1989) Factors affecting the desicion to consult with dyspepsia: comparison of consulters and non-consulters. *J Royal Coll General Practitioners* 39: 495–498

11 Levin TR, Kunz K, Henke CJ, Selby JV (1997) Costs of acid-related disorders to a helth maintenance organization. *Am J Med* 103: 520–528

12 Selby JV, Ray GT, Zhang D, Colby CJ (1997) Excess costs of medical care for patients with diabetes in a managed care population. *Diabetes Care* 20: 1396–1402

13 Bloom BS, Fox NA, Jacobs J (1989) Patterns of care and expenditures by California medicaid for peptic ulcer and other acid related diseases. *J Clin Gastroenterol* 11: 615–620

14 Nyrén O (1985) Non-ulcer dyspepsia. Studies on epidemiology, pathophysiology and therapy. Thesis, Department of Surgery, Uppsala University, Sweden

15 Nyrén O, Lindberg G, Lindström E, Marké L-Å, Seensalu R (1992) Economic costs of functional dyspepsia. *PharmacoEconomics* 1 (5): 312–324

16 Segal R, Russel WL, Ben-Joseph R, Mansheim B (1996) Cost of acid peptic disorders in a managed-care organization. *Clin Ther* 18 (2): 319–333

17 Bloom BS, Fox NA, Jacobs J (1989) Patterns of Care and Expenditures by California Medicaid for Peptic Ulcer and Other Acid-Related Diseases. *J Clin Gastroenterol* 11(6): 615–620

Subject index

absorption 143, 165
absorption of protein-bound vitamin B_{12} 215
achlorhydria 91, 101
achlorhydria, in Zollinger-Ellison syndrome (ZES) 214
acid hyposecretion 87, 215
acid peptic attack 193
acid secretion, inhibition of 132
acid stability 146
acid suppression 194
acid tolerance 117
acidophile 117
activation, acid 146
activation, extragastric 146
activation, rates of 148
alkalophile 117
allergic reaction 167
anticholinergic agent probanthine 209
antrectomy 84
anxiety 241, 243, 245
apoptosis 129
aspirin 193
α, β association 39
autocrine growth factor 107
ATPase, P-type 24
atrophic corpus 95
atrophic gastritis 92, 93, 105

bacterial genome of *H. pylori* 120
bacterial overgrowth 99–101, 108
bioavailability 143, 166
bioavailability, interfering factors 145
bioenergetics 118

calcitonine gene-related peptide (CGRP) 82
carcinoid 93, 106
carcinoid tumour, of the stomach 214
catalytic subunit 31
chief cell 83
cimetidine 205
colorectal cancer 108
colorectal tumour 107
comparative study 200
confocal 128
conscious dog 5
cyclic adenosine monophosphate (cAMP) 65
cyclic adenosine monophosphate (cAMP)-stimulated acid secretion 8
cytoprotective effect 194

dispersion, in liquids 166
distribution 145
dog 80
drug interaction, induction of CYP 1A 152
drug interaction, lansoprazole 152
drug interaction, omeprazole 150
drug interaction, pantoprazole 152
drug interaction, rabeprazole 153
duration of action 209

effect of long-term omeprazole treatment on body iron stores 215
elimination, proton pump inhibitors 149
elimination half-life 218
end-of-life tumour 86
endoscopic study 196
endoscopy-negative reflux 224–226, 228, 229, 231
enteric-coated dosage form 164
enterochromaffin-like (ECL) cell 65, 83
enterochromaffin-like (ECL) cell carcinoid 84
enterochromaffin-like (ECL) cell hyperplasia 92, 93
extemporaneous reconstitution 167

famotidine 205
food consumption 81
functional dyspepsia 243, 245
fundectomy 214

gastric acid 64
gastric acid, inhibition of 66
gastric acid hypersecretion 205
gastric acid pump 24
gastric acid secretion 4, 47
gastric adenocarcinoma 106
gastric carcinoid 92, 106
gastric carcinoma 101
gastric endocrine cells 93
gastric emptying 164
gastric enterochromaffin-like (ECL) cell 213
gastric gland, isolated 11
gastric hypersecretory state 205
gastric mucosa, human 10
gastric mucosa, isolated 8
gastric resection 108
gastric vesicle, isolated 11
gastrin 81, 107
gastrin-17, long-term infusion 214

gastrin level 81
gastrin level, elevated 92, 107
gastro-oesophageal reflux disease (GORD) 223–232
GI hormone 81
growth rate 81

H,K ATPase 10, 24
H,K ATPase, gastric 47
H,K ATPase, gastric, activation of 28
H,K ATPase, gastric, 2D structure of 31
H,K ATPase, reversible K-site antagonists of 48
H,K ATPase, structure function model of 39
H,K ATPase, synthesis and turnover 30
H_2-receptor antagonist 65, 226, 229
H_2-receptor blocker 83
heartburn 224, 226, 229, 231, 240, 241, 245
Heliobacter pylori 98, 117, 131–137, 201
Heliobacter pylori, acid adaptation 124
Heliobacter pylori, bioenergetic profile 123
Heliobacter pylori, metabolism 122
Heliobacter pylori, survival 121
Heliobacter pylori status 94
histamine H_2-receptor antagonist 49
histamine H_2-receptor antagonist, high doses, side effects 207
24-hour pH monitoring 224, 225
hypergastrinaemia 91, 92, 101, 106, 107, 214
hyperplastic/hypertrophic response 84

indirect costs 241, 243
influence of antacid 166
influence of food 165
inhibition of stimulated acid secretion 80
instability 162
intravenous omeprazole in Zollinger-Ellison syndrome (ZES) 216

kinetics 26

lactation 145
lansoprazole 48, 66, 69, 79, 161, 205, 227
lansoprazole, in Zollinger-Ellison syndrome (ZES) 213
long-term study ($\geq$1 year) 80
long-term omeprazole treatment in Zollinger-Ellison syndrome (ZES), safety 213
long-term omeprazole treatment in Zollinger-Ellison syndrome (ZES), side-effects 213
long-term proton pump inhibitor (PPI) therapy 229–231
long-term tachyphylaxis 211
loss of heterozygosity 214
low water solubility 162
loxtidine 86
lyophilised substance 167

M5/M6 domain in cation transport 36
macroscopic finding 83
maintenance 198
malabsorption 99
metabolism, enzymes involved in 149
metabolism, slow metabolizers 149
metiamide 205
microscopic finding 83
mouse 80
multiple endrocine neoplasia-type 1 (MEN-I) 214

neuropeptide Y (NPY) 82
neutralophile 117
nitrosation 100
N-nitroso compound 100
non-steroidal anti-inflammatory drug (NSAID) 193

oesophagitis 227–230
omeprazole 17, 48, 66, 67, 79, 161, 209, 211, 225–229
oral dosage form 163
oxyntic mucosa 83

pantoprazole 48, 66, 71, 79, 161, 205, 227
pantoprazole, in Zollinger-Ellison syndrome (ZES) 213
parenteral dosage form 167
parenteral histamin H_2-receptor antagonist 216
parietal cell 10
partial corpectomy 214
pepsin 67
pepsinogen concentration 83
peptic ulcer disease 240, 241
peptide histidine isoleucine (PHI) 82
perforation 193
pernicious anaemia 91, 101, 214
pharmacodynamics of intravenous (i.v.) and oral omeprazole in Zollinger-Ellison syndrome (ZES) 218
pharmacokinetics of intravenous (i.v.) and oral omeprazole in Zollinger-Ellison syndrome (ZES) 218
pharmacokinetics 144
pharmacological study 10
pK_a value 162
plasma gastrin level, elevated 101
pregnancy 145
prophylaxis 200
prostaglandin synthesis 193

proton pump 132
proton pump inhibitor (PPI) 3, 131, 133–137, 161
proton pump inhibitor (PPI), safety 231
pyridyl methylsulfinyl benzimidazole 24

quality of life 229, 240, 241, 245

rabeprazole 48, 66, 72, 161
ranitidine 205
ranitidine, high-dose 214
rat 80

SCH 28080 42
serum ferritin level 215
serum vitamin B_{12} level, in achlorhydria 216
short-term proton pump inhibitor (PPI) therapy 226–229
sick leave 243, 244
SK&F93479 86
socio-economic impact 241, 245
stability, dependent on pH 162
steatorrhea 100
stomach weight 83
storage stability 166
substituted benzimidazole 12, 161
subunit α and β, association of 35
subunit β 35

tachyphylaxis 80
target for drugs 40
testing, *in vitro* 164
tolerability 153
transmembrane domain 33
transport reaction 25
transporter 120
twice-a-day dose 211

ulcer bleeding 193
ulcer disease 193
ulcer healing 198
urea transporter 126
urease activity 117

vagotomy 92, 93, 101, 108
vasoactive intestinal peptide (VIP) 82
vitamin B_{12} absorption 215

water intake 81
weight gain 81

Zollinger-Ellison syndrome (ZES) 205, 214
Zollinger-Ellison syndrome (ZES), long-term treatment with omeprazole 211

Detailed information about all our titles also available on the internet:
http://www.birkhauser.ch
Check our Highlights for new and notable titles selected monthly in each field

PIR
Progress in Inflammation Research

Medicinal Fatty Acids in Inflammation

Kremer, J.M.,
Albany Medical College, Albany, USA
(Ed.)

This volume is a unique assembly of contributions focusing on the biochemical, immunological and clinical benefits of n-3 fatty acids in inflammation.

Leading clinical investigators from fields as diverse as rheumatology, dermatology, nephrology, gastroenterology and neurology have authored chapters. The basic scientific underpinnings of their findings are elucidated as well.

The work is a highly accessible, one-of-a-kind source which will well serve lipid researchers, graduate students, dieticians and members of the food industry.

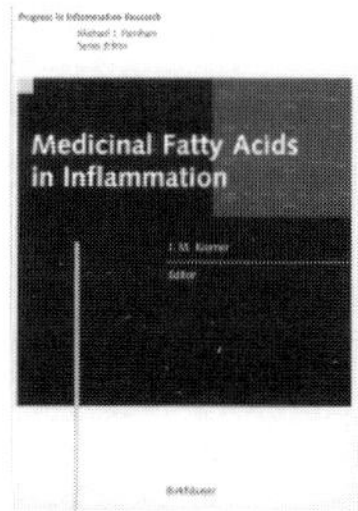

Contents

List of contributors

Preface

Calder, P. C.:
n-3 Polyunsaturated fatty acids and mononuclear phagocyte function

Zurier, R. B.:
Gammalinolenic acid treatment of rheumatoid arthritis

Ziboh, V. A.:
The role of n-3 fatty acids in psoriasis

Horrobin, D. F.:
n-6 Fatty acids and nervous system diorders

Fernandes, G.:
n-3 Fatty acids on autoimmune disease and apoptosis

Belluzzi, A. and Miglio, F.:
n-3 Fatty acids in the treatment of Crohn's disease

Rodgers, J. B.:
n-3 Fatty acids in the treatment of ulcerative colitis

Geusens, P. P.:
n-3 Fatty acids in the treatment of rheumatoid arthritis

Grande, J. P. and Donadio, J. V.:
n-3 Polyunsaturated fatty acids in the treatment of patients with IgA nephropathy

Subject index

PIR – Progress in Inflammation Research
Kremer, J.M., (Ed.)
Medicinal Fatty Acids in Inflammation
1998. 162 pages. Hardcover
ISBN 3-7643-5854-8

BioSciences with Birkhäuser

(Prices are subject to change without notice. 01/99)

For orders originating from all over the world except USA and Canada:

Birkhäuser Verlag AG
P.O. Box 133
CH-4010 Basel / Switzerland
Fax: +41 / 61 / 205 07 92
e-mail: orders@birkhauser.ch

For orders originating in the USA and Canada:

Birkhäuser Boston, Inc.
333 Meadowland Parkway
USA-Secaucus, NJ 07094-2491
Fax: +1 / 201 348 4033
e-mail: orders@birkhauser.com

Birkhäuser

Detailed information about all our titles also available on the internet:
http://www.birkhauser.ch
Check our Highlights for new and notable titles selected monthly in each field

PIR
Progress in Inflammation Research

Cytokines in Severe Sepsis and Septic Shock

Redl, H. / Schlag, G. †,
Ludwig Boltzmann Institute for Experimental and Clinical Traumatology, Vienna, Austria (Ed.)

[Infotext]This book deals with the central role of cytokines in the generalized inflammatory response of the host as the consequence of severe infection/endotoxin action. International specialists cover several aspects in 20 chapters starting with the agents responsible (endotoxin, superantigens) and recognition during cytokine induction. Further chapters deal with the signal transduction cascade, its modulation due to sex or genetic polymorphism, and the possibilities and problems in detection (including surrogate markers). Major targets of actions are covered in the chapters on coagulation/fibrinolysis, adherence molecules, vasoactive factors, apoptosis and metabolism. As not all actions of cytokines are beneficial, several chapters deal with the prevention of induction, modulation of the cytokine generation or scavenging cytokines including gene therapy approaches. Models are necessary for obtaining pathophysiological information and for testing therapeutic approaches, and thus all chapters deal with experimental models as well as clinical trials. The reasons why these have failed so far are the subject of the final chapter.

Researchers and students of Critical Care Medicine and Biomedicine will find up-to-date reviews and data in this book.

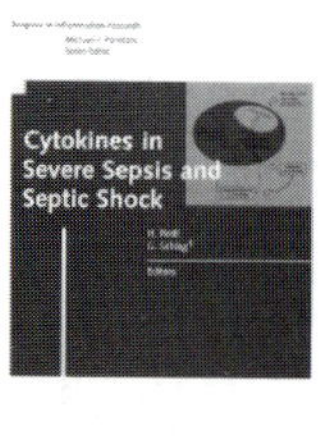

PIR – Progress in Inflammation Research
Redl, H. / Schlag, G. † (Ed.)
Cytokines in Severe Sepsis and Septic Shock
1998. 384 pages. Hardcover
ISBN 3-7643-5877-7

BioSciences with Birkhäuser

(Prices are subject to change without notice. 01/99)

For orders originating from all over the world except USA and Canada:

Birkhäuser Verlag AG
P.O. Box 133
CH-4010 Basel / Switzerland
Fax: +41 / 61 / 205 07 92
e-mail: orders@birkhauser.ch

For orders originating in the USA and Canada:

Birkhäuser Boston, Inc.
333 Meadowland Parkway
USA-Secaucus, NJ 07094-2491
Fax: +1 / 201 348 4033
e-mail: orders@birkhauser.com

Birkhäuser